This book project was supported by

D1609770

KARL STORZ GmbH & Co. KG
Mittelstraße 8
78532 Tuttlingen
Telefon +49 (0) 74 61/708-0
Telefax +49 (0) 74 61/708-105
info@karlstorz.de
www.karlstorz.com

MAQUET

MAQUET Vertrieb und Service
Deutschland GmbH
Kehler Straße 31
76437 Rastatt
Telefon +49 (0) 1803 212133
Telefax +49 (0) 1803 212177
info.vertrieb@maquet.de
www.maquet.com

ERBE

ERBE Elektromedizin GmbH
Waldhörnlestraße 17
72072 Tübingen
Telefon +49 (0) 70 71/755-0
Telefax +49 (0) 70 71/755-179
sales@erbe-med.de
www.erbe-med.com

Edmund A. M. Neugebauer, Stefan Sauerland,
Abe Fingerhut, Bertrand Millat, Gerhard Buess
Editors

EAES Guidelines for Endoscopic Surgery

Twelve Years Evidence-Based Surgery in Europe

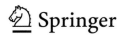 Springer

Edmund A.M. Neugebauer, Professor, PhD
University Witten-Herdecke
Institute for Research in Operative Medicine
Director and Chair for Surgical Research
Ostmerheimer Str. 200
51109 Cologne, Germany

Stefan Sauerland, MD, MPH
University Witten-Herdecke
Institute for Research in Operative Medicine
Ostmerheimer Str. 200
51109 Cologne, Germany

Abe Fingerhut, Professor, MD
Centre Hopitalier Intercommunale
Service de Chirurgie Viscérale Digestive
Rue de Champ Gaillard 10
78300 Poissy, France

Bertrand Millat, Professor, MD
Hôpital Saint Eloi
Service de Chirurgie Viscérale Digestive
34295 Montpellier, France

Gerhard Buess, Professor, MD
University Tübingen
Section for Minimally Invasive Surgery,
Hoppe-Seyler-Straße 3
72072 Tübingen, Germany

ISBN-10   3-540-32783-5 Springer Berlin Heidelberg New York
ISBN-13   978-3-540-32783-7 Springer Berlin Heidelberg New York

Library of Congress Control Number 2006923763

Cataloging-in-Publication Data applied for
A catalog record for this book is available from the Library of Congress.

Springer is a part of Springer Science+Business Media

springer.com

© Springer Berlin Heidelberg 2006
Printed in Germany

Editor: Gabriele M. Schröder, Heidelberg, Germany
Desk Editor: Stephanie Benko, Heidelberg, Germany
Production: LE-TeX Jelonek, Schmidt & Vöckler GbR, Leipzig
Cover design: Frido Steinen-Broo, eStudio Calamar, Spain
Typesetting: K + V Fotosatz, Beerfelden, Germany

Printed on acid-free paper   24/3100Di – 5 4 3 2 1 0

Preface

Every new idea needs enthusiasts convinced that the idea is solid and prosperous. The concept of minimally invasive surgery was introduced to the field of visceral surgery first by Gerhard Bueß, who performed the first clinical operations in transanal endoscopic microscopy in 1983. Cholecystectomy was performed by a special approach used by Erich Mühe in 1985. In 1987 the first laparoscopic cholecystectomy with the technique we are using today was performed by Mouret from France.

This laparoscopic approach was the idea which infected surgeons around the globe. Without doubt, the idea of minimally invasive surgery, and in particular laparoscopic or endoscopic surgery, can nowadays be considered as a major breakthrough in surgical technique which, with appropriate associated technology, has translated into tremendous improvements in clinical diagnostics, clinical outcomes, as well as surgical education.

At the very beginning of the laparoscopic revolution, clinical intuition and personal experience of pioneers were the only "evidence" base as concerned performance and teaching of this new approach to surgery. Heavily supported by the medical device industry, laparoscopic surgery started a legendary career, without any prior solid scientific testing and often outside centers of excellence. As a result, serious complications of laparoscopic surgical procedures were reported. Moreover, the advent of laparoscopic surgery was accused of contributing significantly to the rising healthcare expenditure in times of money shortages. Therefore, the executive office of the European Association of Endoscopic Surgery (EAES) under the presidency of Hans Troidl (Cologne) decided in 1993 to appoint an ad hoc working group to critically review and systematically assess the progress of laparoscopic surgery in the different developing fields of surgery. The scientific mandate was given to Edmund Neugebauer.

At that time consensus development conferences (CDCs), according to the policy of the National Institute of Health (NIH), was the accepted method of choice. However, the NIH format was time-consuming, expensive, and did not adequately reflect the needs for rapid assessment in the evolving field of laparoscopic surgery. The EAES executive office felt that there was dire need for a more practical approach in order to provide specific guidelines as soon as possible, early in the development of new indications when evidence was still sparse, to prevent harm and to critically appraise the potential benefits of this new technology. A novel type of CDC was developed including essential elements of the NIH process such as panel selection by specific transparent criteria, a formal consensus procedure, and specific statements formulated as guidelines. Up until 1999, six CDCs took place including topics such as laparoscopic cholecystectomy, appendectomy, hernia repair, surgery for gastroesophageal reflux disease, treatment of common bile duct stones, and colonic diverticular disease.

Owing to the evolving field of evidence-based medicine with rigorous evaluation of the scientific evidence and the necessity to keep CDC statements in synchronous pace with medical knowledge, the EAES ad hoc committee, under the guidance of Neugebauer and within the Scientific Committee of the EAES, started a critical revision of the consensus methodology at the EAES conference in 1999 in Linz, Austria. Moreover, it was felt that there was a need for improved methods of dissemination and implementation of these EAES guidelines. One of the key factors for acceptance and impact of clinical practice guidelines is the strength and validity of the development process itself. The critical appraisal and analysis showed that further improvement was needed in identification, evaluation, synthesis of scientific evidence, as well as for the transparency of the recommendations. This was achieved by connecting the levels of scientific evidence with the grades of recommendation, through participation of all relevant stakeholders in the guideline panel, and application of formal consensus development methods. With use of this updated methodology, starting in Maastricht in 2001, evidence-based guidelines have been developed for the creation of pneumoperitoneum, laparoscopic surgery in colonic cancer, quality of life after laparoscopic surgery, obesity surgery, and laparoscopy for abdominal emergencies. After open discussion between the panel and all members of the EAES at the annual congresses of the EAES in 2-h plenary sessions, and diligent work of the ad hoc committee, all evidence-based guidelines have been expediently published over the years in *Surgical Endoscopy*, the official organ of the EAES, for quick and wide dissemination.

Endoscopic surgery is still an area of rapid development. Nearly not one month goes by without new studies being published that need to be examined to link and relate the new information to the impact on existing guidelines. Regular updates are therefore necessary. The first update, concerning the guidelines developed from the start until 1999, was published in the Springer booklet released at the EAES Congress in Nice (2000) [1]. It was only natural that a new book be undertaken. The Berlin EAES and World Congress was the ideal occasion to publish a further and ever so necessary update. It summarizes all the original recommendations, followed by updates in 2006 originating from leading laparoscopic surgeons in Europe. All statements are based not only on the expert's opinion, but also on formal assessment of the scientific evidence as it has appeared in the literature since the publication of the guidelines in *Surgical Endoscopy*. Therefore, this book allows the readers to gain an overview of the cutting edge of laparoscopic surgical research. All recommendations described herein are those surgical procedures and techniques for which a benefit has been proven. Most guidelines contain key statements and all chapters follow a structured format to enhance easy and quick identification of all useful information.

Guidelines can only be as good as the evidence available. During the process of guideline development it became apparent that we still have weak evidence in several fields of endoscopic surgery. This should be taken as a request to our readers to perform more randomized controlled studies in "their institution" and to provide patients for multicenter trials.

Several and sometimes wide variations may appear according to differences in surgeons' fields of competence, accreditation for practice, and social health care and reimbursement systems in Europe and other places of the world. Local adaptations of the guidelines are therefore needed and mandatory.

The editors think that this book gives a perfect overview of what laparoscopic surgery has achieved within a little more than one decade of performance as expressed in our subtitle: *Twelve Years Evidence-Based Surgery in Europe*. It is our intention to follow up with this same book format in regular time frames under the auspices of the EAES while developing new evidence-based guidelines in parallel. All our efforts, however, will be useless if these guidelines are not translated into practice. It is therefore our hope that they will be introduced in teaching courses and clinical algorithms in our hospitals, throughout Europe, and the rest of the world.

The editors of this book would finally like to thank all contributors for the excellent work without which this book would not have been possible, the EAES for its support and generous sponsorship, as well as Springer, and especially Stephanie Benko, Desk Editor Clinical Medicine, for her professional service.

Cologne, August 2006   Edmund A. M. Neugebauer
                                                (for the Editors)

References

1. Neugebauer E, Sauerland S (eds) (2000) Recommendations for evidence based endoscopic surgery – the updated EAES Consensus Development Conference. Springer, Berlin Heidelberg New York

Contents

G. Scozzari
Chirurgia Generale II e Centro di Chirurgia Mini-Invasiva, Department of Surgery, University of Turin, 10126 Turin, Italy

A. Shamiyeh
Ludwig Boltzmann Institute for Operative Laparoscopy, II Surgical Department, Academic Teaching Hospital Linz, AKH Linz, Krankenhausstr. 9, 4020 Linz, Austria

P. Spinelli
Divisione di Diagnostica e Chirurgia Endoscopica, Istituto Nazionale per lo Studio e la Cura dei Tumori, 20133 Milano, Italy

A. Szold
Department of Surgery B, Sourasky Medical Center, Weizmann Street 6, 64239 Tel Aviv, Israel

R. Tacchino
Department of Surgery, Catholic University of Rome, Viale della Tecnica 205, 00144 Roma, Italy

E. Targarona
Department of General and Digestive Surgery, Hospital de Sant Pau C/Padre Claret 167, 08025 Barcelona, Spain

Y. Tekant
Hepatopancreatobiliary Surgery Unit, University of Istanbul, Istanbul 55004, Turkey

I. Tomasi
1^a Chirurgia Clinicizzata, Ospedale di Borgo Trento, Piazzale A. Stefani 1, 37126 Verona, Italy

J. Treckmann
Clinic for General Surgery and Transplantation, University Hospital Essen, Hufelandstr. 55, 45122 Essen, Germany

H. Troidl
Surgical Clinic Merheim, II Department of Surgery, University of Cologne, Ostmerheimer Str. 200, 51109 Cologne, Germany

S. Uranues
Departments of General Surgery and Surgical Research, University Surgical
Clinic, Auenbruggerplatz 29, 8036 Graz, Austria

B. Ure
Department of Paediatric Surgery, Medical University of Hannover,
Carl-Neuberg Str. 1, 30623 Hannover, Germany

R. Veldkamp
Department of Surgery, Medisch Centrum Rijnmond-Zuid, Locatie Zuider,
Groene Hillerdijk 315, 3075 Rotterdam, The Netherlands

N. Veyrie
Hôpital Hôtel Dieu, AP-HP, 75004 Paris, France

W. Wayand
Ludwig Boltzmann Institute for Operative Laparoscopy, II Surgical
Department, Academic Teaching Hospital Linz, AKH Linz, Krankenhausstr. 9,
4020 Linz, Austria

R. Weiner
Department of Surgery, Krankenhaus Sachsenhausen, Schulstr. 31,
60594 Frankfurt, Germany

S. D. Wexner
Department of Colorectal Surgery, Cleveland Clinic Florida, 33331 Weston,
FL, USA

R. L. Whelan
Section of Colon and Rectal Surgery, Columbia University College
of Physicians & Surgeons, New York, NY 10025, USA

S. Wood-Dauphinée
Department of Epidemiology and Biostatistics, School of Physical
and Occupational Therapy, McGill University, 3630 Promenade
Sir-William-Osler, Montreal, Quebec H3G 1Y5, Canada

J. Zehetner
Ludwig Boltzmann Institute for Operative Laparoscopy, II Surgical
Department, Academic Teaching Hospital Linz, AKH Linz, Krankenhausstr. 9,
4020 Linz, Austria

The EAES Clinical Practice Guidelines on the Evaluation of Quality of Life After Laparoscopic Surgery (2004)

Dragan Korolija, Stefan Sauerland, Sharon Wood-Dauphinée, Claude C. Abbou, Ernst Eypasch, Manuel García Caballero, Mary A. Lumsden, Bertrand Millat, John R. T. Monson, Gunilla Nilsson, Rudolf Pointner, Wolfgang Schwenk, Andreas Shamiyeh, Amir Szold, Emilio Targarona, Benno Ure, Edmund A. M. Neugebauer

Introduction

When a new procedure or technology is introduced, it is expected to achieve "better" or at least equal results than the more traditional approaches. Classical outcomes for the evaluation of surgical procedures are usually perioperative case fatality, morbidity, recurrence rate, and long-term survival. However, from the patient's point of view, the so-called heuristic end points, such as symptom resolution, duration of convalescence, patient satisfaction and well-being, and quality of life (QoL), are at least as important as the "classical" outcomes. Furthermore, although of particular interest to caregivers and payers, they are rarely considered in studies testing the efficacy and effectiveness of new surgical approaches [12].

Minimally invasive (laparoscopic) surgery promised to improve health-related outcomes. The classical outcomes of laparoscopic and open surgery have been extensively compared according to the literature and discussed in the previous consensus development conferences organized by the European Association for Endoscopic Surgery (EAES) [87]. Approximately 15 years after the first laparoscopic cholecystectomy, it is essential to answer the question of whether laparoscopic surgery, compared to open surgery, improves the patient's QoL.

An evidence-based approach was therefore undertaken to evaluate existing information about different areas of laparoscopic surgery and to assess for which diseases laparoscopic surgery results in better postoperative QoL compared to open surgery. QoL is a multidimensional construct comprising physical, psychological, social, and functional domains [88]. Our second aim was to appraise QoL instruments used in the literature and to give recommendations for their future use in laparoscopic surgery. These recommendations are based on a systematic review combined with a formal consensus development conference (CDC).

Methods

Selection of Topics

At the meeting of the scientific committee and the executive board of the EAES in Lisbon in June 2002, there was a unanimous vote to implement a mechanism to evaluate QoL after laparoscopic surgery. Topics of interest were selected according to their overall prevalence and the use of laparoscopic surgery as an operative approach: gastroesophageal reflux disease (GERD), achalasia, paraesophageal hernia, obesity, cholecystolithiasis, inguinal hernia, and colorectal spleen, kidney, ovarian, and uterine diseases. In addition, the pediatric aspects of some of these diseases were addressed. The Cologne Group was asked to organize a CDC, according to previously established methodology [86]. For this purpose, the methods of a systematic review and a CDC were combined.

Literature Searches

Under the guidance of a clinical epidemiologist (S.S.), a surgeon with education and experience in evidence-based medicine and systematic reviews (D.K.) performed comprehensive literature searches in Medline, Embase, the Cochrane Library, and other sources. The medical subject headings "Laparoscopy" and "Quality of life" were used. Additionally, Medline was searched using the words "laparosc*," "gynecol*," "urolog*," and "quality of life." The reference lists of obtained articles were also checked. There were no language restrictions. The search was limited to the years 1990–2002. Additionally, abstracts presented at the EAES congresses in 2001 and 2002 were searched by hand. If related abstracts were identified, contacts were made with the authors to obtain complete results.

Our primary intention was to identify existing systematic reviews or meta-analyses and relevant randomized controlled trials (RCTs). In the absence of such evidence, we searched for concurrent cohorts (CCHs), externally or historically controlled cohorts population-based outcome studies, and case series. All articles were graded according the hierarchy of evidence defined by Sackett et al. [110], as shown in Table 1.1. Critical appraisal of papers was carried out as recommended by Muir Gray [84]. Articles were considered relevant if they reported QoL outcomes using standardized or self-developed questionnaires. Multiple publications of the same study were included only once in the review. For each study, the first author, publication year, number of patients analyzed, type of questionnaire, type of procedure, length of follow-up, level of improvement, and characteristics of the control group were extracted.

As the surgical articles were being reviewed, QoL measures that had been employed as outcomes were noted. The focus was on known and standard-

Table 1.4. Ad hoc questionnaires and domains covered

	No. of studies	Physical	Psychological	Social relations	Functional capacity
GERD	5	[5, 20, 66, 103, 106]	[20, 66, 103, 106]	[103, 106]	
GERD in childhood	1	[75]		[75]	[75]
Obesity	1	[144]	[144]	[144]	[144]
Splenectomy	–				
Achalasia	1	[24]	[24]	[24]	[24]
Paraesophageal hernia	–				
Cholecystolithlosis	2	[56, 111]	[56, 111]	[56, 111]	[56, 111]
Colorectal	2	[71, 97]	[97]	[13, 71, 97]	[13, 71, 97]
Groin hernia	6	[18, 21, 77, 112, 113, 125]	[113, 125]	[18, 21, 77, 112, 113, 125]	[18, 21, 77, 112, 113, 125]
Nephrectomy	3	[3, 43, 78]	[43, 78]	[43, 78]	
Hysterectomy	7	[31, 39, 59, 89, 101, 114, 118]	[31, 39, 89, 101, 114]	[31, 39, 59, 89, 101, 114, 118]	[31, 39, 59, 89, 101, 114, 118]
Prostatectomy	–				

The numbers in *brackets* represent the references that report on particular domains

that measures be reexamined for their measurement properties, particularly validity, prior to applying them to a new patient population. Measurement studies revalidating the generic measures using appropriate diagnostic patient samples for this CDC were not found. Rather, investigators relied on information from patients with other diagnoses and used the measures. This leap of faith is often made in clinical research. It is probably reasonable since all the generic instruments have been extensively tested for reliability, validity, and responsiveness to change on a variety of patient samples. This statement pertains to the Short Form (SF) 36 [138], Quality of Life Index [119], Sickness Impact Profile [8], Nottingham Health Profile [50], EuroQol [34], Psychological General Well-Being Index [29], Hospital Anxiety and Depression Scale (HADS) [147], Linear Analogue Self-Assessment (LASA) [22] scales, and, to a lesser extent, the Health and Activity Limitation Index, which is relatively new [32].

Information about the content, mode of administration, scoring, and psychometric properties of the specific instruments is presented in Table 1.5. In addition, one investigator used a battery of standardized measures to capture QoL of people with inguinal hernia repair [41], and other investigators used the Visick Classification [94, 96, 102], which is very old and not well validated but traditionally accepted by the surgical community.

Table 1.5. Condition-specific measures of quality of life in related literature

Appraisal properties	Gastrointestinal					Colorectal				Obesity			Groin hernia	Nephrectomy
	GIQLI	GSRS	QOL-RAD	GERD-HRQL	Achalasia QOL index	FACT-C	FIQL	BIQ	SDS	EORTC-QLQ-C30	IWQOL-Lite	BAROS	Pain-O-Meter (tool)	PRS
Dimensions														
Physical	+		+		+	+	+	+	+	+	+	+		+
Emotional	+		+		+	+	+	+		+	+	+		
Cognitive									+	+				
Social	+		+		+	+	+		+	+	+	+		+
Symptoms	+	+	+	+	+	+			+	+	+	+	+	+
Response format														
Categorical	+	+	+	+	+	+	+	+	+	+	+	+	+	+
Mixed														+
VAS													+	+
Administrative mode														
Self-report	+	+	+	+	+	+	+	+	+	+	+	+		+
Interview		+								+			+	
Caregiver												+		
Scoring														
Subscale scores	+	+	+		+	+	+	+		+	+			
Total score	+	+	+	+		+			+	+	+		+	+
Classification												+		

	GIQLI	GSRS	QOLRAD	GERD-HRQL	Achalasia QOL	FIQL	FACT-C	SDS	BIQ	EORTC QLQ-C30	IWQOL-Lite	BAROS	Pain-O-Meter	PRS
Reliability														
Internal consistency	+	+	+	+	+	+	+	+	+	+	+	+		+
Test-retest	+					+		+				+		+
Validity														
Content	+	+	+	+		+	+	+	+	+	+	+		+
Criterion	+								+					
Construct-convergent	+	+	+	+		+	+	+	+	+	+	+		+
Construct-divergent	+	+	+	+		+	+		+	+	+	+		+
Factorial			+	+		+					+			
Responsiveness	+	+	+	+		+	+	+		+	+	+	+	+
Estimated time to administer														
<2 min	+		+				+							
3–10 min	+	+				+		+		+	+			+
>10 min	+					+		+				+		+

Gastrointestinal Quality of life Index (*GIQLI*) [37]; Gastrointestinal Symptom Rating Scale (*GSRS*) [122]; Quality of Life in Reflux and Dyspepsia Patients (*QOLRAD*) [146]; Gastroesophageal Reflux Disease – Health-Related Quality of Life (*GERD-HRQL*) [133]; Achalasia QOL Index [83]; Functional Assessment of Cancer Therapy – Colorectal (*FACT-C*) [135]; Fecal Incontinence Quality of Life (*FIQL*) [108]; Body Image Questionnaire (*BIQ*) [28]; Symptoms Distress Scale (*SDS*) [76]; European Organization for Research and Treatment of Cancer (*EORTC QLQ-C30*) [2]; Impact of Weight on Quality of Life–Lite questionnaire (*IWQOL-Lite*) [60]; Bariatric Analysis and Reporting Outcome System (*BAROS*) [92]; Pain-O-Meter [40]; Postoperative Recovery Scale (*PRS*) [136]

A number of investigators in each surgical area used ad hoc questionnaires or individual questions related to symptoms or QoL variables. Items in the ad hoc questionnaires were of interest to surgeons and often reflected the recovery of the patients postoperatively as well as their satisfaction with the surgery. Each item in the questionnaire was treated statistically as a unique piece of information; item scores (if present) were not summed. Items were compared by surgical group (i.e., open versus laparoscopic surgery).

Other investigators asked individual questions. Sometimes, questions were scaled in terms of response categories (i.e., no, mild, moderate, or severe pain), but most often the patient was asked to report time from operation (in days or weeks) to recovery of full physical activities or to return to usual social activities, to a "normal" lifestyle, to work, or to a pain-free state. Occasionally, patients were asked to provide information on medication use. As with the ad hoc questionnaires, responses between surgical groups were compared.

The answers of the experts were used at the CDC in Cologne when specific time points for QoL instrument application had been suggested. For example, if there were two QoL measures that addressed different domains, we selected the measure that included the clinically more relevant domain.

Gastroesophageal Reflux Disease

Key Points and Suggestion for QoL Assessment

Laparoscopic fundoplication provides faster improvement of QoL when compared with open fundoplication (EL 1b). Long-term improvement of QoL is not different when compared to open surgery (EL 1b).

For GERD we suggest the use of the SF-36 or the PGWB (generic measures) in addition to the GIQLI and the QOLRAD (disease-specific measures). If the interest is primarily in symptom resolution the GSRS or the GERD-HRQL (symptom scales) are alternatives. Preoperative QoL assessment may be a useful adjunct in clinical decision-making. The suggestion is that the first postoperative evaluation of QoL should be done between 1 and 3 months after surgery and repeated at least at 1 year.

Background and Evidence

Seven randomized trials and seven nonrandomized trials compared laparoscopic and open antireflux procedures. When assessing the trials, we did not differentiate between Nissen and Toupet fundoplication. In GERD, more than in other diseases, QoL assessment is very important for patient selection in routine practice. Kamolz et al. [55] have shown that some patient populations, such as those with major depression, showed less QoL improvement than other groups of patients, despite normal physiologic postoperative data.

In one of the seven RCTs, Heikkinen et al. [48, 49] compared laparoscopic and open Nissen fundoplication 1, 3, and 24 months after surgery (1b). They used the GIQLI [37] and a Visual Analogue Scale (VAS) [104] for pain as well as an ad hoc questionnaire on patient satisfaction. The laparoscopic group experienced less postoperative pain and returned earlier to work and normal life. Two years after the surgery, GIQLI scores were significantly improved, compared to preoperative data, but did not differ between the laparoscopic and open groups. In a similar study by Chrysos et al. [20], patients were given an ad hoc questionnaire after laparoscopic and open Nissen fundoplication (1b). Follow-up at 12 months included 106 patients. One year after surgery, the laparoscopic group reported significantly greater postoperative satisfaction when compared with the open group. Laine et al. [66] studied a total of 110 patients over a period of 12 months (1b). They used an ad hoc questionnaire. One year after surgery, all patients in the laparoscopic group and 86% of patients in the open group were satisfied with the operation. The fourth RCT by Bais et al. [5] also compared laparoscopic and open Nissen fundoplication (1b). They analyzed data on 103 patients from an ad hoc questionnaire. The follow-up was 2 years. The primary end points were dysphagia, recurrent GERD, and intrathoracic hernia. The laparoscopic group had significantly more patients with dysphagia 3 months after surgery. A further study by Nilsson et al. [91] compared laparoscopic Nissen with open Nissen fundoplication (1b). They used the standardized PGWB [29], together with an ad hoc questionnaire developed by the authors. The follow-up was for 6 months and included 60 patients. One and 6 months after surgery, there were no significant differences between the groups with regard to PGWB scores. Six months after surgery, the laparoscopic group reported significantly more sleep disturbances on the ad hoc questionnaire. In another publication from the same study, the authors used the GSRS [122] to analyze the differences in QoL between the two surgical approaches [143]. The GSRS scores did not differ between the two groups 1 and 6 months after surgery. Velanovich [130] compared laparoscopic and open Nissen and Toupet fundoplication (2b). The follow-up at 6 weeks used the GERD-HRQL [133] questionnaire and the SF-36, the generic QoL instrument developed for the Medical Outcomes Study [138]. There were 80 patients included in the study. The laparoscopic group had better results in the physical functioning scale of the SF-36. The results on the GERD-HRQL (symptoms) scale were not different between the groups.

Among the nonrandomized studies, Peters et al. [96] used the Visick score [134] and an ad hoc questionnaire to compare laparoscopic and open Nissen (2b). The follow-up was 54 months and incorporated 70 patients. There were no significant differences between the two groups. Blomqvist et al. [9] used three standardized scales to compare laparoscopic and open Nissen and Toupet patients (2b). Specifically, they applied the PGWB questionnaire [29], the GSRS [122] and a visual analog scale depicting specific reflux-related symptoms (RVAS) [4]. The follow-up was 12 months for the 50 patients enrolled in the study. There were no significant differences in PGWB scales. In the GSRS scale, differences were shown between the two procedures, with more dyspeptic and indigestion symptoms in patients having undergone a laparoscopic Nissen procedure. Rantanen et al. [102] compared laparoscopic and open Nissen groups (2b). Using the Visick scale [134] and VAS [4] for dysphagia, flatus, and bloating, they studied a total of 57 patients. Three years after the operation, there were no differences between the two groups except for belching ability and temporary dysphagia. Richards et al. [106] compared laparoscopic and open Nissen groups with an ad hoc questionnaire (2b) given to 232 patients over a 3-month period. The laparoscopic group returned to work and reported better general health earlier than the open group. In the study by Rattner and Brocks [103], 86 patients were evaluated over 12 months after laparoscopic and open Nissen fundoplication approaches (2b). The laparoscopic group returned to work earlier than the open group. Overall satisfaction scores as measured with an ad hoc questionnaire were similar, irrespective of the operative technique. Finally, a nonrandomized study reported by Pelgrims et al. [94] compared 210 patients after laparoscopic and open Nissen procedures (2b). One year after surgery, there were no significant differences in Visick scores between the groups.

GERD in Childhood

Key Points and Suggestion for QoL Assessment

In children, there is no evidence that laparoscopic antireflux surgery provides different QoL when compared to open antireflux surgery (EL 2b).

For children with GERD we suggest that the use of the Child Health Questionnaire (CHQ) [68] or the Pediatric Quality of Life Inventory (PedsQL) [128] be tried. Both questionnaires are generic and need to be evaluated for this condition. Disease-specific instruments are not available. QoL assessment is suggested 3, 6, and 12 months after surgery.

Background and Evidence

In children, many diseases are treated laparoscopically, but only GERD has been evaluated on QoL outcomes. Mattioli et al. [75] compared laparoscopic and open Nissen fundoplication in children aged 1–14 years (2b). Data on 66 children from an ad hoc questionnaire were analyzed. Six months after surgery, there were no differences between the groups in terms of pain relief and ability to play without symptoms. As in adults, the preoperative assessment of QoL is very important for patient selection, and further studies on QoL improvement after laparoscopic pediatric surgery are needed.

Obesity

Key Points and Suggestion for QoL Assessment

Randomized studies comparing open and laparoscopic vertical gastroplasty or gastric banding have not examined QoL. Laparoscopic gastric bypass provides QoL faster improvement of QoL when compared to open gastric bypass (EL 1b), but long-term results are similar (EL 1b).

For obesity surgery, we suggest the use of the SF-36 (generic measure) and the Impact of Weight on Quality of Life (IWQOL-Lite) (disease-specific measure). We recommend QoL evaluations for at least 2 years, but ideally they should be continued lifelong.

Background and Evidence

Two randomized trials compared laparoscopic and open gastric bypass for morbid obesity. On a sample of 155 patients, Nguyen et al. [90] used two standardized questionnaires to assess QoL (1b): the SF-36 [138] and the Moorhead–Ardelt quality-of-life questionnaire (BAROS) [92]. One month after surgery, SF-36 scores in four of the eight domains (physical functioning, social functioning, general health, and bodily pain) were significantly better in the laparoscopic group than in the open group. At 3 months after surgery, SF-36 scores in all eight domains had improved in the laparoscopic group and were equal to US norms, although physical functioning was still significantly impaired in the open group. Six months after surgery, SF-36 scores on all eight domains for both the laparoscopic and the open group were comparable with U.S. norms and were not significantly different between the groups. The Moorhead–Ardelt scores (BAROS) for sexual interest/activity at 3 months after surgery were significantly higher after laparoscopic surgery. At 6 months, there were no significant differences in any of the five QoL domains. Weight loss outcomes were comparable between the two groups at 1-year follow-up, but the laparoscopic group had significantly greater weight loss at 3 and 6 months. Westling and Gustavsson [144] administered an ad hoc questionnaire to 51 patients (1b). The laparoscopic group experienced less postoperative pain and shorter sick leave compared to the open group. One year after surgery there were no significant differences between the laparoscopic and open groups in weight loss and patient satisfaction, which was high in both groups.

QoL measurements in morbidly obese patients require long-term observations since weight loss takes time to complete and the incidence of complications, such as incisional hernia or band slippage, does not decrease considerably after the first postoperative year.

Splenectomy for Benign Diseases

Key Points and Suggestion for QoL Assessment

Laparoscopic splenectomy produces less pain in the early postoperative period compared to open splenectomy (EL 2b).

When splenectomy is undertaken for benign diseases, further information is required to make a recommendation for using the SF-36 (generic) or another instrument. QoL should be evaluated in the early postoperative period.

Background and Evidence

Only one nonrandomized study of 44 patients compared QoL results between laparoscopic and open splenectomy. In the study by Velanovich and Shurafa [132], the SF-36 was administered 6 weeks after the operation (2b). The laparoscopic group had significantly better scores in only one of eight domains (bodily pain).

Achalasia

Key Points and Suggestion for QoL Assessment

Laparoscopic Heller myotomy provides faster improvement of QoL when compared with open Heller myotomy (EL 2b).

For achalasia, we suggest the use of the SF-36 or the PGWB (generic measures) in addition to the GIQLI or the QOLRAD (disease-specific measures). If the interest is primarily in symptom resolution, the GSRS or the GERD-HRQL (symptom scales) are alternatives. The suggestion is that the first postoperative evaluation of QoL should be done between 1 and 3 months after surgery and repeated at least at 1 year.

Background and Evidence

In achalasia, short-term data are important in comparing results between laparoscopic and open surgery. However, achalasia is a disease that attacks the whole esophagus; therefore, long-term follow-up is more relevant for the patient's outcome. When examining GIQLI scores between 1 and 3 years after surgery, Decker et al. [23] noted a significant deterioration, but in their 40 patients postoperative results were still better than preoperative ones.

Two small nonrandomized studies compared laparoscopic and open Heller myotomy. Katilius and Velanovich [57] used a validated generic questionnaire (SF-36) [138] to evaluate QoL (2b). Although the study included only 26 patients, they were able to detect significant differences: six weeks after the operation, the laparoscopic group scored better on the subscales reflecting physical functioning, role-physical, and vitality. Dempsey et al. [24] used an ad hoc questionnaire that covered all domains of QoL (2b). The study examined the postoperative course of 22 patients over a 16 month follow-up. The laparoscopic group experienced less postoperative pain and returned to work earlier than the open surgery group. Notably, follow-up length differed between the groups.

Paraesophageal Hernia

Key Points and Suggestion for QoL Assessment

Laparoscopic paraesophageal hernia repair provides better QoL when compared to open surgery (EL 2b). Until further data are available, we suggest the same instruments and time shedule for paraesophageal hernia as for GERD.

Background and Evidence

Only one study compared laparoscopic and open paraesophageal hernia repair. Velanovich and Karmy-Jones [13] used the SF-36 [138] to evaluate QoL 6 weeks after the procedure (2b). The study included 38 patients. Patients in the laparoscopic group reported better scores in the physical functioning, role-physical, role-emotional, vitality, and social functioning scales. The authors did not report on the long-term QoL scores.

Cholecystolithiasis

Key Points and Suggestion for QoL Assessment

Laparoscopic cholecystectomy improves QoL faster than open surgery (EL 1b). Long-term results after laparoscopic cholecystectomy are slightly better or not different compared to those of open surgery (EL 1b). The suggestion is to use the SF-36 or the PGWB (generic instrument) in conjunction with the GIQLI (disease-specific instrument). If time and resources are limited, the GIQLI may be used alone because it incorporates all domains of a QoL assessment. Postoperatively, a QoL assessment is suggested at 1 and 6 months.

Background and Evidence

Two randomized and eight nonrandomized trials reported on QoL after laparoscopic or open cholecystectomy. Whereas the results on short-term outcomes are homogeneous, long-term data are conflicting.

In a randomized trial of laparoscopic versus open cholecystectomy, Barkun et al. [6] used the NHP, the GIQLI, and the VAS for QoL assessment (1b). Using paired analysis, significant improvement in the laparoscopic group was detected as early as 10 days after surgery with the VAS ($p = 0.047$) and at 1 month with the NHP and the GIQLI ($p = 0.0001$). The open group did not show significant improvement until 1 month after surgery with the GIQLI ($p = 0.002$) and until 3 months with the NHP ($p = 0.03$). The extent of improvement in all QoL scores after surgery was similar in both groups. The second randomized trial was performed by McMahon et al. [81] (1b). QoL results in terms of a modified SF-36 score and the Hospital Anxiety and Depression Scale (HADS) [147] were reported at the 1-, 4-, and 12-week follow-ups. The only significant long-term advantage for laparoscopic surgery was a higher satisfaction rate with the appearance of the scar. As early as 1993, Sanabria et al. [111] (2b) studied 120 patients over an 8-week period after laparoscopic or open cholecystectomy. A significantly faster recovery was found, but at the final evaluation, the patients' answers did not differ when asked to subjectively rate the change in the quality of their lives. In the second nonrandomized trial, Eypasch et al. [36] in 1993 compared QoL after open ($n = 21$) and laparoscopic ($n = 158$) cholecystectomy (2b). The GIQLI, the QOL-Index (QLI) [119], and a VAS were used to assess QoL 2 and 6 weeks after surgery. At both time points, there was a trend toward better QoL in the laparoscopic group. Similar data were reported by Ludwig et al. [113] in a comparative study of 103 patients (2b). The authors modified the GIQLI and found a slightly quicker convalescence after laparoscopic cholecystectomy. However, in the final evaluation 5 weeks after surgery, both groups experienced a similar QoL. In a prospective controlled study of 31 patients, Plaisier [98] reported NHP data for the 3-, 6-, and 12-month intervals after surgery (2b). A significant difference in favor of laparoscopic surgery was found 6 months after cholecystectomy, but this difference vanished after 1 year with the exception of questions related to nausea, stomach swelling, and fatty food avoidance. A study from China also confirmed that GIQLI scores were initially better after laparoscopic cholecystectomy, but Chen et al. [19] did not find any long-term benefit of laparoscopic surgery in their series of 51 patients over 16 weeks (2b). In a large study by Kane et al. [56] (2b), 2481 patients were mailed a questionnaire 6 months after cholecystectomy. After adjusting for baseline differences, it was found that patients were more likely to perform their usual activities after laparoscopic surgery. There were no differences in pain, symptoms, or general health as measured with an ad hoc questionnaire.

Topcu et al. [124] (2b) performed a retrospective comparative study on 200 patients. Prior to surgery, both groups were comparable, but 4 years after surgery laparoscopically treated patients reported significantly better QoL in all eight domains of the SF-36. In another study, Quintana et al. [99] used the SF-36 and GIQLI to compare laparoscopic and open cholecystectomy (2b). There were 887 patients followed during the first three postoperative months. Additionally, the authors used ad hoc questions that focused on satisfaction with the intervention and the number of days before returning to work and daily activities. No significant differences between the open and laparoscopic groups either in the SF-36 scores or in the GIQLI scores were detected.

The occurrence of a bile duct injury has a significant impact on QoL in the long term. Moreover, the incidence of bile duct injury remains as high as 1.4%. Boerma et al. [10] used the SF-36 to examine QoL 5 years after bile duct injury during laparoscopic cholecystectomy. Despite the excellent objective outcome, QoL was both physically and mentally reduced when compared with controls ($p < 0.05$). In a similar observational study by Melton et al. [82], 89 patients were asked about their QoL after successful surgical repair of a major bile duct injury. However, the QoL instrument used in that study was developed for and validated in cancer patients only. QoL scores of bile duct injured patients were comparable to those of patients undergoing uncomplicated laparoscopic cholecystectomy and healthy controls in the physical and social domains but were significantly worse in the psychological domain.

Colorectal Diseases

Colorectal Cancer

Key Points and Suggestion for QoL Assessment
Laparoscopic colectomy produces less postoperative pain compared to open colectomy (EL 1b). In the early postoperative period, a higher QoL is reported earlier after laparoscopic than after open colectomy (EL 1b).

For patients with colorectal carcinoma, either the FACT-C or the EORTC QLQ-C30/CR38 will provide comprehensive information about all QoL domains, including symptoms. If fecal incontinence is an issue, the FIQL could be added. Because significant differences have been shown as long as 1 month after surgery but not at 2 months, QoL should be measured at least during the short-term follow-up. Long-term studies are needed.

Background and Evidence
Four randomized controlled trials and two nonrandomized trials reported on QoL outcomes in laparoscopic versus open colorectal procedures. Weeks et al. [141] used the Symptoms Distress Scale (SDS) [76], the QLI [119], and

the Global Rating Scale (GRS) [126] to study 428 patients over 2 months (1b). The laparoscopic group had significantly better GRS scores 2 weeks after surgery. This group also needed less postoperative analgesics. Two months after surgery there were no significant differences between the laparoscopic and open groups. The second randomized study, by Schwenk et al. [115], used the EORTC QLQ-C30 to compare QoL after laparoscopic or open colorectal resection (1b). One week after surgery, physical and emotional functions were more impaired in the open group ($p < 0.05$). Four weeks after surgery, only physical function differed between the two groups, and after 3 months the differences were no longer detectable. In addition to the QLQ-C30, a disease-specific add-on module, the QLQ-CR38, has been developed and validated by the EORTC [120].

Braga et al. [13] measured early postoperative morbidity in a randomized trial that included 269 patients. They used the time until return to full physical and social activities as a surrogate for QoL. The laparoscopic group recovered after 32 days, compared to 65 days for the open group. Finally, Liang et al. [71] reported on pain and return to partial activity, full activity, and work after laparoscopic or open sigmoid resection for large sigmoid polyps. Despite the small sample size, the authors found that patients in the laparoscopic group had a significantly lower incidence of pain. Return to full functional recovery was measured blindly and was 2 weeks earlier in the laparoscopic group ($p < 0.05$).

Dunker et al. [27] followed 35 patients over a period of 15 months (2b). They used the SF-36, the GIQLI, and the Body Image Questionnaire (BIQ) [28]. The laparoscopic group was significantly more often satisfied with the cosmetic result of the operation. There were no significant differences in other QoL scores. Pfeifer et al. [97] used an ad hoc questionnaire to assess QoL in 69 patients undergoing colorectal resection for a variety of diseases, including cancer (2b). There were no significant differences 2 months after surgery. In addition to the previous comments, some experts noted that there are no data on QoL outcomes from randomized controlled trials with total mesorectal excision.

Diverticular Disease

Key Points and Suggestion for QoL Assessment
For diverticular disease, laparoscopic and open approaches have similar long-term results in QoL improvement (EL 2b).

For patients with diverticular disease, the SF-36 will provide comprehensive information about QoL. If fecal incontinence is an issue, the FIQL could be added. QoL should be measured 1 month after surgery and repeated after 12 months. Further studies comparing QoL outcomes after laparoscopic and open surgery are needed.

Background and Evidence

There is only one retrospective comparative study on QoL after laparoscopic and open surgery for diverticular disease. Five years after surgery, Roblick et al. [107] asked 45 matched patient pairs to assess their QoL using the SF-36 (2b). No significant differences were found at this late point in time after the surgery. Short or intermediate-term results were not available.

Groin Hernia

Key Points and Suggestion for QoL Assessment

Compared to open hernia repair, laparoscopic surgery (TAPP and TEP) improves QoL more quickly (EL 1a). This is also true for bilateral hernia repair (EL 1b). Long-term restoration of QoL is not different (EL 1a).

The SF-36 (generic measure) is suggested as the primary HRQL measure of outcome. In addition, the VAS or a single-item rating of pain is recommended. The status of QoL should be measured after 1 and, at least, 6 and 12 months postoperatively.

Background and Evidence

Three meta-analyses, one systematic review, ten randomized trials, and nonrandomized trial compared QoL outcomes using standardized or ad hoc questionnaires.

The Cochrane review by the European Hernia Trialists was first published in 2000 and updated in 2003 (1a) [77]. The reviewers compared TAPP and TEP with open mesh and nonmesh procedures. As can be expected from the large number of primary trials, the duration and completeness of follow-up varied considerably among the studies. In the meta-analysis, a significant reduction in persisting postoperative pain (overall 290/2101 versus 459/2399; Peto OR = 0.54; 95% CI, 0.46–0.64; $p < 0.0001$) and in sick leave (HR 0.56; 95% CI, 0.51–0.61; $p < 0.0001$; equivalent to 7 days) was found. The other systematic reviews by Chung and Rowland [21] (1a), Cheek et al. [18] (1a), and Schmedt et al. [113] (1a) gave very similar results since they mainly included the same primary studies.

Among these primary RCTs, the study by Lawrence et al. [69] was one of the first that examined QoL (1b). A linear analogue scale for pain, the SF-36, and the Euroqol (linear analogue section) [34] were used to compare TAPP with Lichtenstein repair in 124 patients. The laparoscopic group had less pain and significantly higher scores in social function and energy by 10 days and at 6 weeks after the operation. When describing later results, 3 and 6 months postoperatively (1b) [70], the SF-36 demonstrated no differences in scores. In a second RCT including 258 patients, Liem et al. [72] used the SF-36 to compare laparoscopic extraperitoneal hernia repair with the Lichtenstein procedure (1b). QoL was better in the laparoscopic group both 1 and 6 weeks after surgery. The differences were significant for physical functioning, role-physical, bodily pain, social functioning. In a smaller third trial of only 53 patients, the Sickness Impact Profile (SIP) [8] and the Pain-O-Meter [40] were applied to compare the 6-week results after TAPP or Lichtenstein repair (1b) [40]. The laparoscopic group had less pain postoperatively and returned to work earlier, but the differences were not significant. Barkun et al. [7] used the Nottingham Health Profile (NHP) [50] and the VAS to compare laparoscopic transabdominal with open tension and nontension repair (1b). Ninety-two patients were followed over 3 months. One month after surgery, the laparoscopic group had better QoL scores on the NHP ($p = 0.035$), but there were no differences in pain.

Another RCT from the United Kingdom by Wellwood et al. [142] used the SF-36 to compare laparoscopic transabdominal with Lichtenstein repair (1b). The follow-up was 3 months and included 392 patients. One month after surgery the laparoscopic group had significantly better SF-36 scores for role-physical, bodily pain, vitality, social functioning, and mental health. At 3 months after surgery there were greater improvements in mean scores from baseline in the laparoscopic group for all scales except general health, but none of these differences reached significance. Tschudi et al. [125] compared laparoscopic abdominal with Shouldice repair (1b). They used an ad hoc questionnaire and followed 84 patients over 5 years. The laparoscopic group had less postoperative pain and returned to work earlier, but at 5 years post-surgery there was only 1 patient in each treatment arm who had persistent pain and impaired capability (not statistically different). In a three-armed RCT, Bringman et al. [15] compared TEP with Lichtenstein and open mesh-plug procedures (1b). There were 294 patients, who were followed for 3 months. They used the questionnaire developed by Kald and Nilsson [54] and the VAS for pain. The laparoscopic group returned to work earlier and had less postoperative pain. Fleming et al. [41] compared TEP and the Shouldice technique after enrolling 232 patients (1b). They employed a battery of standardized measures to assess QoL [22]. The follow-up was 12 months. The laparoscopic group had less postoperative pain and returned to full activity earlier. Sarli et al. [112] used an ad hoc questionnaire to compare bilateral laparoscopic transabdominal repair with bilateral Lichtenstein repair in 43 patients (1b). The laparoscopic group returned to work earlier and had less pain postoperatively. In the long term, at 36 months QoL was similar. Stengel and Lange [121] compared laparoscopic transabdominal with Lichtenstein and Shouldice repair in 269 patients (2b). They used the SF-36 and a VAS for pain and followed patients for 6 months. The laparoscopic group had less pain postoperatively and returned to work earlier than the open group. Jones et al. [53] analyzed return to work in 93 patients operated by one surgical group. In a bivariate analysis they showed that age, educational level, occupation, symptoms of depression, and expected time to work acounted for 61% of the variation in actual return to work. According to this evidence, the expert panel concluded that other factors besides the surgical technique used influence the return to work. To examine the impact of chronic pain and recurrence on QoL, annual long-term follow-up for 5 years is necessary. The details of different laparoscopic (endoscopic) techniques are beyond the scope of this article.

Nephrectomy for Malignancy

Key Points and Suggestion for QoL Assessment

No RCTs on QoL that compared laparoscopic and open nephrectomy either for benign or for malignant disease were identified. Laparoscopic nephrectomy (transabdominal or retroperitoneal) produces less pain in the postoperative period and enables earlier return to normal activities when compared to open surgery (EL 2b).

In addition to the use of a VAS for pain, we tentatively suggest the use of the SF-36 or the EORTC QLQ-C30 (generic measures). This recommendation for the generic measure has no basis in data. Because differences have been shown at 1 year after surgery, measurement of QoL in future trials should be done within this time frame.

Background and Evidence

Four nonrandomized trials compared laparoscopic and open nephrectomy with regard to postoperative QoL. McDougall et al. [78] compared radical laparoscopic transabdominal nephrectomy with its open counterpart (2b). Using an ad hoc questionnaire, it was shown in a sample of 24 patients that the laparoscopic group had significantly less postoperative pain. The laparoscopic group returned earlier to normal activities, and full recovery was also reached more rapidly. Gill et al. [43] compared radical laparoscopic (retroperitoneal) with open nephrectomy in 68 patients (2b). They used an ad hoc questionnaire. The laparoscopic group experienced less postoperative pain and returned to normal activities sooner. From a sample of 58 patients, Abbou et al. [3] showed that the laparoscopic (retroperitoneal) group experienced less pain in the postoperative period compared to the open nephrectomy group (2b). In the fourth study, Pace et al. [93] compared laparoscopic (transperitoneal) with open nephrectomy in a series of 61 patients (2b). They used the Postoperative Recovery Scale (PRS), which is based on the acute version of the SF-36 [136]. The laparoscopic group had significantly higher QoL scores at the 1-, 2-, 3-, and 6-month and 1-year postoperative assessments. This indicates a potential long-term benefit of laparoscopic nephrectomy.

Hysterectomy

Key Points and Suggestion for QoL Assessment

Laparoscopic-assisted hysterectomy improves QoL faster than abdominal hysterectomy (EL 1b). Long-term results of QoL status are similar (EL 1b).

For women undergoing a hysterectomy, the SF-36 (generic measure) may be used. Additional standardized questionnaires related to urinary and sexual function might be useful. Because differences have been shown at 6 months after surgery, measurement of QoL in future trials should be done at least 6 months.

Background and Evidence

Five randomized and four nonrandomized trials compared laparoscopic with open hysterectomy. Ellström et al. [30] administered the SF-36 to 76 patients (1b). Three weeks after operation, the laparoscopic group had significantly better scores in physical functioning, role-physical, bodily pain, and social functioning. At the end of follow-up, 12 weeks after surgery, there were no significant differences between the two patient groups. Lumsden et al. [74] used the Euroqol Health Questionnaire (Euroqol HQ) [34] for 166 hysterectomy patients (1b). The groups were compared 1, 6, and 12 months after surgery, but there were no significant differences in QoL. Schütz et al. [114] used an ad hoc questionnaire for QoL evaluation and the VAS for pain. A total of 35 patients were followed for 12 months (1b). The laparoscopic group had less postoperative pain and reported greater satisfaction with the operation. Falcone et al. [39] studied 48 patients using an ad hoc questionnaire and VASs for pain and activity (1b). Follow-up lasted 6 weeks. The laparoscopic group reported a shorter duration of fatigue and an earlier return to work. Eighty patients, randomized by Raju and Aold [101], were given an ad hoc questionnaire to evaluate return to normal activities over a 6-week postoperative period (1b). Laparoscopic hysterectomy with adnexectomy as opposed to open hysterectomy with adnexectomy resulted in an earlier return to normal activities.

In a similarly designed but nonrandomized study of 30 patients, Spirtos et al. [118] compared laparoscopic with open hysterectomy (2b). They used an ad hoc questionnaire to monitor the recovery of women over 17 weeks. Return to normal activity occurred earlier in the laparoscopic group. An ad hoc questionnaire was also used by Kolmorgen et al. [59], who studied 132 women over a 3-month follow-up period (2b). Again, less pain and an earlier return to normal activity were noted. In a small study of only 20 women, Nezhat et al. [89] confirmed that an earlier resumption of normal activities can be achieved by the use of laparoscopic hysterectomy (2b). Follow-up was 6 weeks. In the only study comparing QoL after open and laparoscopic hysterectomy for endometraial carcinoma, Eltabbakh et al. [31] followed 143 patients over a period of 17 months (2b). The laparoscopic group reported higher satisfaction with the procedure and returned earlier to full activity.

Prostatectomy

Key Points and Suggestion for QoL Assessment

Postoperative improvements in QoL are faster after laparoscopic than after open prostatectomy (EL 2b), but long-term results are similar (EL 2b).

Before and after prostatectomy, men should be assessed with the SF-36 or the EORTC QLQ-C30 questionnaire (generic measures). In addition, continence, sexual potency, and voiding symptoms may be evaluated separately, or they may be evaluated jointly with the new EORTC prostate-specific module. All QoL measurements should be done at least during the first 6 months.

Background and Evidence

Only one nonrandomized trail has compared laparoscopic with open prostatectomy with regard to QoL: Hara et al. [47] found no differences in QoL 6 months after surgery, but patient satisfaction was higher after laparoscopic surgery (2b). This study used a prostate-specific QoL questionnaire, which was under development by the EORTC. As symptom-specific instruments, the International Index of Erectile Function 5 (IIEF-5) and the International Continence Society Male (ICS_{male}) questionnaire were used to evaluate urinary and erectile function. Both instruments have been validated [26, 109]. Currently, the disease-specific EORTC module, the QLQ-PR25, is being tested for validity and reliability.

Discussion

The scope of this CDC was broad since we wanted to evaluate QoL after laparoscopic compared to open surgery for many different conditions. We have tried to include the most important diseases in laparoscopic surgery, for which evidence on QoL assessment is available. Although there are a large number of studies reporting QoL after laparoscopic surgery, only one third have compared laparoscopic with open surgery.

Here we provide some general remarks on QoL assessment in clinical and research settings. First, it should be kept in mind that no single QoL measure is ideal for all diseases or patient groups or settings. This implies that all instruments must be checked carefully for the psychometric properties in the context of endoscopic surgery. Occasionally, it may be necessary to extend existing instruments to fit the scope of a specific clinical problem or patient group, but only the reporting of standard measures allows readers to compare results across studies. Any modification of existing measures requires a new validation of the new measure. Second, it is often recommended to combine a generic instrument and a disease-specific instrument. For most diseases, the generic instruments have lower responsiveness compared to specific ones [145], but the generic measures are useful to compare the patient cohort against cohorts with other diseases or with the normal population. Third, the proof of superior QoL after one type of surgery is a strong but not a sufficient argument to use this type of surgery. Although QoL is a broad construct, it does not necessarily include all aspects that are relevant for clinical decision making. Therefore, we did not use grades of recommendations for the key statements.

With regard to choosing a QoL instrument, there is no hierarchy for grading the quality of QoL assessment tools. Since the different psychometric properties of an instrument are not a unidimensional issue, the choice of an instrument depends on the various practical and theoretical aspects of a study. Some projects on the development of such classifications are in progress and are the focus of experts in that field. A further methodologic problem is the difference between choosing a valid study design and a valid outcome measure: We think that a RCT should not automatically be considered high-level evidence, if the study does not report clinically relevant outcomes such as QoL via the use of standardized measures.

The overall quality of QoL research in endoscopic surgery compares well with other fields. In 1989, Guyatt et al. [46] found that less than half the RCTs in major journals examined QoL as an outcome, and two-thirds of these QoL measures had not been validated. Similarly, Gill and Feinstein [44] criticized that most clinical studies of QoL failed to define QoL, lacked a reliable QoL measure, and mixed up symptom checklists, proxy outcomes, QoL, and health-related QoL measures. Nevertheless, surgical researchers should increase the use of QoL measures in clinical trials. Since many validated instruments are obtainable free of charge from the primary investigators, there are no real obstacles to conduction more patient-centered research. For the well-known general instruments, further information can be found on the Internet.

Again, the importance of QoL assessment in laparoscopic surgery should be noted. QoL as an outcome is much more important to the patient than, for example, laboratory values and other traditional clinical end points. After biliary duct injury and successful repair of the injury, patients can have normal laboratory findings but permanently impaired QoL [45, 82]. This reinforces the question as to whether we are measuring what is relevant for the patients. Furthermore, the experts pointed out the importance of the preoperative QoL assessment for patient selection for laparoscopic surgery in specific diseases. This is especially true for GERD, for example, when deciding on surgery for depressed patients [55].

Evidence on QoL after laparoscopic compared to open surgery reported in this article represents all relevant data regarding this issue. Suggestions made for QoL assessment in different conditions are universal and can be used in every European country. We believe that the use of these suggestions will increase the quality of care in everyday practice as well as the quality of research. Implementation strategies and the evaluation of the impact of these guidelines need further discussion and will present a basis for further research.

Appendix: Information on Recommended Measures

Child Health Questionnaire

The CHQ, designed to measure the physical and psychological well-being of children 5 years or older, has several forms related to the age of the child and who completes the questionnaire [67]. There are three parent forms and a form to be completed by children aged 10 years or older (87 items). The questionnaires tap 14 concepts related to health and well-being. Item responses are on 4- to 6-point scales. Scale scores are transformed to range from 0 to 100. Higher scores reflect better health. Physical and psychological summary measures can be calculated. In addition to self-completion by child or parent, the forms may be administered in person or over the phone.

Psychometric performance is adequate in terms of internal consistency and test–retest reliability as well as content, criterion, and construct validity [67, 95, 139, 140]. The measure has been translated, adapted, and revalidated for use in a number of countries [68]. To obtain a manual and the questionnaire, contact J. M. Landgraf (Fax: +1-617-3757801).

European Organization for Research and Treatment of Cancer

The EORTC is a cancer-specific questionnaire that has a core component to be used in conjunction with one of a number of modules reflecting different sites of cancer [1, 2]. The core questionnaire EORTC QLQ-C30 contains 30 items that form seven subscales: physical functioning, role functioning, common physical symptoms of cancer and its treatment, emotional functioning, role functioning, financial impact, and overall perceived health status and global QoL. Most items are scored on a 4-point scale ranging from "not at all" to "very much"; the physical and role functioning subscales are scored dichotomously, and the global questions on health status and QoL have been expanded to a 7-point scale. The time frame of the questions is the past week. For the functional and global subscale, a higher score represents a higher QoL, whereas for the symptom subscales the reverse is true. The site-specific modules provide more detailed information on symptoms related to the specific tumor site and may tap additional areas.

A variety of studies attest to the adequate reliability and validity of the questionnaire. In particular, the symptom scales have shown sensitivity to clinical change. The questionnaire was developed by an international group of researchers. In consequence, careful attention was given to ensuring that the questions had a similar meaning across languages and cultures. The modules for colorectal and prostate cancer are forthcoming [120].

Fecal Incontinence Quality of Life Scale

The FIQL scale is a symptom-specific measure of QoL developed from input from both patients and caregivers [108]. It is composed of 29 items that form four scales: lifestyle (10), coping/behavior (9), depression/self-perception (7), and embarrassment (3). Each item has four to six response categories. Scale scores are the mean response to all items in a scale. A total score was not calculated by the developer, but one has been used by Jess and colleagues [52].

Confirmatory factor analysis supported use of four scales. Internal consistency estimates were 0.80 or greater for each scale. Mean scale scores of a test–retest situation were not significantly different, but agreement was not measured directly. Each scale was able to differentiate between a group of individuals with fecal incontinence and patients with other gastrointestinal problems. Convergent validity was demonstrated by significant correlations with selected scales of the SF-36. A Danish version of the measure has been developed, and the psychometric evaluation of this version produced results similar to those of the developers except that total scores were included [52]. The measure is included as an appendix in the original article [108].

Functional Assessment of Cancer Therapy

The FACT-G is a general measure of QoL for use with people who have cancer. It is the core instrument of the measurement system [16, 17]. FACT-G contains 29 items that constitute five subscales: physical well-being, social/family well-being, relationship with doctor, emotional well-being, and functional well-being. Items are scored on a 5-point scale and summed to provide subscale and total scores. The five subscales are included in the site-specific scales, and each has an additional subscale containing items related to the cancer, its symptoms, or its treatment. A number of site-specific scales, including the FACT-C (colorectal) [135] and the FACT-P (prostate), [33] are available.

Extensive documentation exists on the psychometric properties of FACT-G and its various versions. A manual is available [16] and the scales have been translated and adapted for use in different countries and cultures [11]. For information about using the measurement system, see http://www.facit.org.

Gastroesophageal Reflux Disease – Health-Related Quality of Life

The GERD-HRQL is a measure of symptom severity for use with individuals who have GERD [130, 133]. Ten common and distressing symptoms are listed. The first six are ordered in terms of their relative annoyance to patients. Each symptom is rated on a 6-point categorical scale that ranges from 0 (no symptoms) to 5 (symptoms are incapacitating – unable to do daily activities). The overall score is from 0 to 50, but there is an additional question asking about satisfaction with the patient's "present condition."

No data were found on test–retest reliability, but the developers reported evidence supporting construct validity and responsiveness to clinical change. When patients were grouped according to their level of satisfaction with their present condition, the median scores discriminated between those who were satisfied and those who were not. Sensitivity to the effects of both medical and surgical treatment provided preliminary evidence of responsiveness. A copy of the scale is provided in the article by Valanovich [130].

Gastrointestinal Quality of Life Index

The GIQLI is a self-reported, system-specific measure designed for use with people who have different gastrointestinal disorders [35, 37, 38]. The 36 items, reflecting physical, emotional, and social function as well as typical gastrointestinal symptoms, are each scored on a 5-point scale. Items are summed to produce a total score ranging from 0 to 176, with higher scores denoting better QoL. The measure was developed in German and English. French and Spanish GIQLI versions have been validated [100, 117].

A comprehensive process of development assured content validity. The internal consistency estimates were high, suggesting that the measure reflects an underlying dimension, QoL. Test–retest reliability was demonstrated in clinically stable patients (ICC = 0.92). Correlations between the GIQLI and appropriate measures supported construct validity. Scores on the measure were also able to differentiate groups of gastrointestinal patients with different levels of function, as well as between those with gastrointestinal disease and those who were ostensibly normal. Responsiveness is obviously highest in gastroesophageal disorders, but the GIQLI has also been used with variable responsiveness in other abdominal operations [14, 19, 42, 65, 73]. The GIQLI is available on the Quality of Life Database developed by the nonprofit Mapi Research Institute. This database can be found at http://www.qolid.org.

Gastrointestinal Symptom Rating Scale

The GSRS is a clinical symptom rating scale originally designed for patients with irritable bowel syndrome and peptic ulcer disease [122]. It has subsequently been evaluated in patients with GERD [105, 123]. GSRS for use with GERD patients contains 15 items, each assessed on a 1-point to 7-point scale, with 7 representing extreme discomfort. The items combine into five syndromes labeled reflux, abdominal pain, indigestion, diarrhea, and constipation. Mean scores are calculated from the items in each syndrome. The measure may be administered as a self-report or by an interviewer. The GSRS has been used in UK, Scandinavian, and US populations. It demonstrates acceptable reliability, both internal consistency and stability, evidence of construct and discriminative validity, as well as responsiveness to change. A copy of the US version of the GSRS is included in the article by Revicki and colleagues [105].

Impact of Weight on Quality of Life-Lite

The IWQOL-Lite is a 31-item version of its parent instrument, the Impact of Weight on Quality of Life (IWQOL) questionnaire [63, 64]. Data collected from 996 obese patients and controls were used to develop the shorter measure [61]. Items were selected by predefined criteria. The items are divided among five scales: physical function (11), self-esteem (7), public distress (5), sexual life (4), and work (4). Each item is scored on a 5-point scale (always true – never true). Lower scores indicate higher QoL. Exploratory factor analysis supported the scale structure.

Based on data from the cross-validation sample ($n=991$), individual scales and the total IWQOL-Lite questionnaire demonstrated strong measurement properties. Confirmatory factor analyses confirmed the adequacy of the scale structure. Internal consistency coefficients (alphas) ranged from 0.90 to 0.94 across the scales, with an overall alpha coefficient of 0.96. Correlations between appropriate IWQOL-Lite scales and appropriate standardized measures upheld construct validity. The measure also demonstrated the ability to differentiate between adjacent groups of obese individuals. Changes to scales over time correlated with changes in weight, verifying responsiveness to change. According to the authors, the IWQOL-Lite has been translated and pilot-tested for use in 23 countries [62]. To obtain further information, contact R.L. Kolotkin (1004 Norwood Avenue, Durham, NC, USA; e-mail: kolot001@mc.duke.edu).

Pediatric Quality of Life Inventory

The PedsQL is a generic instrument developed in modular format for measuring health-related QoL in children and adolescents aged 2–18 years [128, 129]. The PedsQL 4.0 Generic Core Scales assess functioning in four areas: physical (8), emotional (5), social (5), and school (5). Both parent and child versions of the inventory are available and use different response sets for scoring items. For parents and children aged 8–18, the inventory is generally self-administered, and for children aged 5–7 it is normally interviewer administered. Modules are available for a number of pediatric conditions, including cancer [127]. Higher PedsQL scores indicate better QoL.

The inventory has been extensively tested for reliability and validity. Internal consistency is adequate for group comparisons and the measure correlated moderately with measures of morbidity and illness burden as well as distinguishing between healthy children and those with a variety of acute and chronic illnesses. It is available in English and Spanish. Further information about the PedsQL is available at http://www.pedsql.org. To order the PedsQL, contact Caroline Anfray at the Mapi Research Institute (e-mail: canfray@mapi.fr).

Psychological General Well-Being Index

The PGWB index was developed as a measure of subjective well-being or distress [29]. This self-administered index contains 22 items, reflecting both positive and negative affect. These are divided into six dimensions: anxiety (5), depressed mood (3), positive well-being (4), self-control (3), general health (3), and vitality (4). Each item is scored on a 6-category scale (0–5 or 1– 6). The dimension scores combine for a total score ranging from 0–110 or 22–132.

Extensive tests of reliability and validity have been conducted, most often on the original version of the measure that contained 68 items and was referred to as the General Well-Being Schedule. These psychometric tests were carried out in a variety of normal populations and patient samples. Many have been reviewed by Dupuy [29]. Internal consistency estimates have most often been between 0.70 and 0.90, and test–retest reliability coefficients have ranged from moderate to strong. Construct validity has been shown by moderately strong correlations with a number of depression scales. Correlations with stressful life events and the use of health services were lower. Norms for the PSGWB index have been described for the Swedish population [25]. When used in a trial of patients with reflux disease, estimates of internal consistency were above 0.92 and decreased symptoms corresponded to an increase in PGWB scores [91]. Concurrent validity has also been confirmed in a variety of studies [85].

Quality of Life in Reflux and Dyspepsia Questionnaire

The QOLRAD is a disease-specific QoL questionnaire designed to address the health concerns of people with GERD or dyspepsia [146]. The measure contains 25 items encompassing five domains of importance to patients: emotional distress, sleep disturbance, eating and drinking issues, physical/social functioning, and vitality. Each item is scored on a 7-point scale and domain scores are calculated by averaging the item scores in that domain.

Good reliability in terms of both internal consistence and stability has been reported [123, 146]. Content, convergent, and discriminant validity as well as responsiveness to clinical change have been carefully documented, and results support the use of the measure in clinical studies [123, 146]. The measure was developed in English and French. For information on how to obtain the measure, contact Ingula Wiklund (Quality of Life Research, Astra Hassle AB, 431 83 MoIndal, Sweden).

Short Form 36

The SF-36 is a generic measure of perceived health status that incorporates behavioral functioning, subjective well-being, and perceptions of health by assessing eight health concepts: limitations in physical activities due to health problems, limitations in role activities due to physical health problems, pain, limitations in social activities due to health problems, general mental health, limitations in usual role activities due to, emotional problems, vitality (energy and fatigue), and general health perceptions [138]. The questionnaire is made up of 36 items that are divided into eight scales. The scores on all scales range from 0 to 100, with higher scores reflecting better health. The SF-36 takes 10–15 min to complete. It can be self-administered or used by a trained interviewer in person or over the telephone.

Reliability has been demonstrated, as have content, criterion, and construct validity [58, 79, 80, 138] and responsiveness to clinical change [58]. Recently, a method of scoring two components, physical and mental health, has been developed. Each component has been standardized to have a mean of 50 and a standard deviation of 10 [137]. There is also an acute version of the SF-36 that uses a 1-week recall, making it useful when treatment effects occur rapidly. As part of an international initiative that used a standard protocol, the SF-36 has been translated, culturally adapted, and revalidated in more than 50 languages. Norms for many countries are available [51].

For further information about the SF-36 and instructions for use, visit the SF-36 Web site (http://www.sf-36.com or http://www.qlmed.org/mot). The IQOLA Web site (http://www.iqola.org) provides information about the international project, and information on the availability of the translations can be found on the SF-36 Web site.

References

1. Aaronson N, Cull AM, Kaasa S, Sprangers MAJ (1996) The European Organization for Research and Treatment of Cancer (EORTC): modular approach to quality of life asessment in oncology. In: Spilker B (ed) Quality of life and pharmacoeconomics in clinical trials. Lippincott-Raven, Philadelphia, pp 179–189
2. Aaronson NK, Ahmedzai S, Bergman B, Bullinger M, Cull A, Duez NJ, Filiberti A, Fletchner H, Fleishman SB, de Haes JCJM, et al. (1993) The European Organization for Research and Treatment of Cancer QLQ-C30: a quality-of-life instrument for use in International Clinical Trials in Oncology. J Natl Cancer Inst 85:365–372
3. Abbou CC, Cicco A, Gasman D, Hoznek A, Antiphon P, Chopin DK, Salomon L (1999) Retroperitoneal laparoscopic versus open radical nephrectomy. J Urol 161:1776–1780
4. Aitken RCB (1969) Measurement of feelings using visual analogue scales. Proc R Soc Med 62:989–993
5. Bais JE, Bartelsman JF, Bonjer HJ, Cuesta MA, Go PM, Klinkenberg-Knol EC, van Lanschot JJ, Nadorp JH, Smout AJ, van der Graaf Y, Gooszen HG (2000) Laparoscopic or conventional Nissen fundoplication for gastro-oesophageal refluxdisease: randomised clinical trial. The Netherlands Antireflux Surgery Study Group. Lancet 355:170–174
6. Barkun JS, Barkun AN, Sampalis JS, Fried G, Taylor B, Wexler MJ, Goresky CA, Meakins JL (1992) Randomised controlled trial of laparoscopic versus mini cholecystectomy. The McGill Gallstone Treatment Group. Lancet 340:1116–1119
7. Barkun JS, Wexler MJ, Hinchey EJ, Thibeault D, Meakins JL (1995) Laparoscopic versus open inguinal herniorrhaphy: preliminary results of a randomized controlled trial. Surgery 118:703–710
8. Bergerer KP, Bobbit RA, Kressels S, Pollard WE, Gilson BS, Morris MR (1976) The sickness impact profile: conceptual formulation and methodology for the development of a health status measure. Int J Health Sci 6:343–415
9. Blomqvist A, Lonroth H, Dalenback J, Ruth M, Wiklund I, Lundell L (1996) Quality of life assessment after laparoscopic and open fundoplications. Results of a prospective, clinical study. Scand J Gastroenterol 31:1052–1058
10. Boerma D, Rauws EA, Keulemans YC, Bergman JJ, Obertop H, Huibregtse K, Gouma DJ (2001) Impaired quality of life 5 years after bile duct injury during laparoscopic cholecystectomy: a prospective analysis. Ann Surg 234:750–757
11. Bonomi AE, Cella DF, Hahn EA, Bjordal K, Sperner-Unterweger B, Gangeri L, Bergman B, Willems-Groot J, Hanquet P, Zittoun R (1996) Multilingual translation of the Functional Assessment of Cancer Therapy (FACT) quality of life measurement system. Qual Life Res 5:309–320
12. Bouillon B, Neugebauer E (1998) Outcome after polytrauma. Langenbeck's Arch Surg 383:228–234
13. Braga M, Vignali A, Gianotti L, Zuliani W, Radaelli G, Gruarin P, Dellabona P, Di Carlo V (2002) Laparoscopic versus open colorectal surgery: a randomized trial on short-term outcome. Ann Surg 236:759–767
14. Bremers AJ, Ringers J, Vijn A, Janss RA, Bemelman WA (2000) Laparoscopic adhesiolysis for chronic abdominal pain: an objective assessment. J Laparoendosc Adv Surg Tech A 10:199–202
15. Bringman S, Ramel S, Heikkinen TJ, Englund T, Westman B, Anderberg B (2003) Tension-free inguinal hernia repair: TEP versus mesh-plug versus Lichtenstein: a prospective randomized controlled trial. Ann Surg 237:142–147
16. Cella DF (1994) FACT manual: manual for the Function Assessment of Cancer Therapy (FACT) scales and the functional assessment of HIV infection (FAHI) scales. Rush–Presbyterian–St.Luke's Medical Center, Chicago
17. Cella DF, Tulsky DS, Gray G, Sarafian B, Linn E, Bonomi A, Silberman M, Yellen SB, Winicour P, Brannon J, et al. (1993) The Functional Assessment of Cancer Therapy scale: development and validation of the general measure. J Clin Oncol 11:570– 579
18. Cheek CM, Black NA, Devlin HB, Kingsnorth AN, Taylor RS, Watkin DF (1998) Groin hernia surgery: a systematic review. Ann R Coll Surg England 80:S1–S80

19. Chen L, Dai N, Shi X, Tao S, Zhang W (2002) Life quality of patients after cholecystectomy. Zhonghua Wai Ke Za Zhi 40:762–765
20. Chrysos E, Tsiaoussis J, Athanasakis E, Zoras O, Vassilakis JS, Xynos E (2002) Laparoscopic vs open approach for Nissen fundoplication. A comparative study. Surg Endosc 16:1679–1684
21. Chung RS, Rowland DY (1999) Meta-analyses of randomized controlled trials of laparoscopic vs conventional inguinal hernia repairs. Surg Endosc 13:689–694
22. Croog S, Levine S, Testa M, Brown B, Bulpitt C, Jenkins D, Klerman G, Williams G (1986) The effects of antihypertensive therapy on the quality of life. N Engl J Med 314:1657–1664
23. Decker G, Borie F, Bouamrirene D, Veyrac M, Guillon F, Fingerhut A, Millat B (2002) Gastrointestinal quality of life before and after laparoscopic Heller myotomy with partial posterior fundoplication. Ann Surg 236:750–758
24. Dempsey DT, Kalan MM, Gerson RS, Parkman HP, Maier WP (1999) Comparison of outcomes following open and laparoscopic esophagomyotomy for achalasia. Surg Endosc 13:747–750
25. Dimenas E, Carlsson G, Glise H, Israelsson B, Wiklund I (1996) Relevance of norm values as part of the documentation of quality of life instruments for use in upper gastrointestinal disease. Scand J Gastroenterol Suppl 221:8–13
26. Donovan JL, Peters TJ, Abrams P, Brookes ST, de la Rosette JJ, Schafer W (2000) Scoring the short form ICSmaleSF questionnaire. International Continence Society. J Urol 164:1948–1955
27. Dunker MS, Bemelman WA, Slors JF, van Duijvendijk P, Gouma DJ (2001) Functional outcome, quality of life, body image, and cosmesis in patients after laparoscopic-assisted and conventional restorative proctocolectomy: a comparative study. Dis Colon Rectum 44:1800–1807
28. Dunker MS, Stiggelbout AM, van Hogezand RA, Ringers J, Griffioen G, Bemelman WA (1998) Cosmesis and body image after laparoscopic-assisted and open ileocolic resection for Crohn's disease. Surg Endosc 12:1334–1340
29. Dupuy HJ (1984) The psychological General Well-being (PGWB) index. In: Wenger NK, Mattson ME, Furberg CF, Elinson J (eds) Assessments of quality of life in clinical trials of cardiovascular therapies. Le Jacq, pp 170–184
30. Ellström M, Ferraz-Nunes J, Hahlin M, Olsson JH (1998) A randomized trial with a cost–consequence analysis after laparoscopic and abdominal hysterectomy. Obstet Gynecol 91:30–34
31. Eltabbakh GH, Shamonki MI, Moody JM, Garafano LL (2001) Laparoscopy as the primary modality for the treatment of women with endometrial carcinoma. Cancer 91:378–387
32. Erickson P (1998) Evaluation of a population-based measure of quality of life: the Health and Activity Limitation Index (HALex). Qual Life Res 7:101–114
33. Esper P, Mo F, Chodak G, Sinner M, Cella D, Pienta KJ (1997) Measuring quality of life in men with prostate cancer using the functional assessment of cancer therapy–prostate instrument. Urology 50:920–928
34. EuroQuol Group (1990) EuroQoul – a new facility for the measurement of health related quality of life. Health Policy 16:199–208
35. Eypasch E, Troidl H, Wood-Dauphinée S, Williams JI, Reinecke K, Ure B, Neugebauer E (1990) Quality of life and gastrointestinal surgery: a clinimetric approach to developing an instrument for its measurement. Theor Surg 5:3–10
36. Eypasch E, Troidl H, Wood-Dauphinée S, Williams JI, Spangenberger W, Ure BM, Neugebauer E (1993) Immediate improval in quality of life after laparoscopic cholecystectomy. Minimally Invasive Therapy 2:139–146
37. Eypasch E, Williams JI, Wood-Dauphinée S, Ure BM, Schmulling C, Neugebauer E, Troidl H (1995) Gastrointestinal Quality of Life Index: development, validation and application of a new instrument. Br J Surg 82:216–222
38. Eypasch E, Wood-Dauphinée S, Williams JI, Ure B, Neugebauer E, Troidl H (1993) Der Gastrointestinale Lebensqualitätsindex (GLQI). Ein klinimetrischer Index zur Befindlichkeitsmessung in der gastroenterologischen Chirurgie. Chirurg 64:264–274

39. Falcone T, Paraiso MF, Mascha E (1999) Prospective randomized clinical trial of laparoscopically assisted vaginal hysterectomy versus total abdominal hysterectomy. Am J Obstet Gynecol 180:955–962
40. Filipi CJ, Gaston-Johansson F, McBride PJ, Murayama K, Gerhardt J, Cornet DA, Lund RJ, Hirai D, Graham R, Patil K, Fitzgibbons R Jr, Gaines RD (1996) An assessment of pain and return to normal activity. Laparoscopic herniorrhaphy vs open tension-free Lichtenstein repair. Surg Endosc 10:983–986
41. Fleming WR, Elliott TB, Jones RM, Hardy KJ (2001) Randomized clinical trial comparing totally extraperitoneal inguinal hernia repair with the Shouldice technique. Br J Surg 88:1183–1188
42. Freys SM, Tigges H, Heimbucher J, Fuchs KH, Fein M, Thiede A (2001) Quality of life following laparoscopic gastric banding in patients with morbid obesity. J Gastrointest Surg 5:401–407
43. Gill IS, Schweizer D, Hobart MG, Sung GT, Klein EA, Novick AC (2000) Retroperitoneal laparoscopic radical nephrectomy: the Cleveland clinic experience. J Urol 163:1665–1670
44. Gill TM, Feinstein AR (1994) A critical appraisal of the quality of quality-of-life measurements. J Am Med Assoc 272:619–626
45. Gouma DJ, Obertop H (2002) Quality of life after repair of bile duct injury. Br J Surg 89:385–386
46. Guyatt GH, Van Veldhuyzen Zanten SJO, Feeny DH, Patrick DL (1989) Measuring quality of life in clinical trials: a taxonomy and review. CMAJ 140:1441–1448
47. Hara I, Kawabata G, Miyake H, Nakamura I, Hara S, Okada H, Kamidono S (2003) Comparison of quality of life following laparoscopic and open prostatectomy for prostate cancer. J Urol 169:2045–2048
48. Heikkinen TJ, Haukipuro K, Bringman S, Ramel S, Sorasto A, Hulkko A (2000) Comparison of laparoscopic and open Nissen fundoplication 2 years after operation. A prospective randomized trial. Surg Endosc 14:1019–1023
49. Heikkinen TJ, Haukipuro K, Koivukangas P, Sorasto A, Autio R, Sodervik H, Makela H, Hulkko A (1999) Comparison of costs between laparoscopic and open Nissen fundoplication: a prospective randomized study with a 3-month follow-up. J Am Coll Surg 188:368–376
50. Hunt SM, McEwen J, McKenna SP (1985) Measuring health status: a new tool for clinicians and epidemiologists. J R Coll Gen Pract 35:185–188
51. IQOLA Project Group (1998) Special Issue on the International Quality of Life Assessment (IQOLA) Project. J Clin Epidemiol 51:891–1214
52. Jess P, Christiansen J, Bech P (2002) Quality of life after anterior resection versus abdominoperineal extirpation for rectal cancer. Scand J Gastroenterol 37:1201–1204
53. Jones KR, Burney RE, Peterson M, Christy B (2001) Return to work after inguinal hernia repair. Surgery 129:128–135
54. Kald A, Nilsson E (1991) Quality assessment in hernia surgery. Quality Assurance Health Care 3:205–210
55. Kamolz T, Granderath FA, Pointner R (2003) Does major depression in patients with gastroesophageal reflux disease affect the outcome of laparoscopic antireflux surgery? Surg Endosc 17:55–60
56. Kane RL, Lurie N, Borbas C, Morris N, Flood S, McLaughlin B, Nemanich G, Schultz A (1995) The outcomes of elective laparoscopic and open cholecystectomies. J Am Coll Surg 180:136–145
57. Katilius M, Velanovich V (2001) Heller myotomy for achalasia: quality of life comparison of laparoscopic and open approaches. JSLS 5:227–231
58. Katz JN, Larson MG, Phillips CB, Fossel AH, Liang MH (1992) Comparative measurement sensitivity of short and longer health status instruments. Med Care 30:917–925
59. Kolmorgen K, Beck H, Seidenschnur G (1991) Postoperatives Beschwerdebild und Arbeitsunfähigkeit nach Adnex-Operation per laparotomiam und nach pelviskopischen Operationen. Zentralbl Gynäkol 113:625–631

60. Kolotkin RL, Crosby RD (2002) Psychometric evaluation of the Impact of Weight on Quality of Life-Lite Questionnaire (IWQOL-lite) in a community sample. Quality Life Res 11:157–171
61. Kolotkin RL, Crosby RD, Kosloski KD, Williams GR (2001) Development of a brief measure to assess quality of life in obesity. Obes Res 9:102–111
62. Kolotkin RL, Crosby RD, Williams GR, Hartley GG, Nicol S (2001) The relationship between health-related quality of life and weight loss. Obes Res 9:564–571
63. Kolotkin RL, Head S, Brookhart A (1997) Construct validity of the Impact of Weight on Quality of Life Questionnaire. Obes Res 5:434–441
64. Kolotkin RL, Head S, Hamilton M, Tse CK (1995) Assessing Impact of Weight on Quality of Life. Obes Res 3:49–56
65. Korenkov M, Sauerland S, Arndt M, Bograd L, Neugebauer EAM, Troidl H (2002) Randomised clinical trial of suture repair, polypropylene mesh or autodermal hernioplasty for incisional hernia. Br J Surg 89:50–56
66. Laine S, Rantala A, Gullichsen R, Ovaska J (1997) Laparoscopic vs conventional Nissen fundoplication. A prospective randomized study. Surg Endosc 11:441–444
67. Landgraf JM, Abetz L, Ware JE (1996) The Child Health Questionnaire: a user's manual. Health Institute, New England Medical Center, Boston
68. Landgraf JM, Maunsell E, Speechley KN, Bullinger M, Campbell S, Abetz L, Ware JE (1998) Canadian–French, German and UK versions of the Child Health Questionnaire: methodology and preliminary item scaling results. Qual Life Res 7:433–445
69. Lawrence K, McWhinnie D, Goodwin A, Doll H, Gordon A, Gray A, Britton J, Collin J (1995) Randomised controlled trial of laparoscopic versus open repair of inguinal hernia: early results. Br Med J 311:981–985
70. Lawrence K, McWhinnie D, Jenkinson C, Coulter A (1997) Quality of life in patients undergoing inguinal hernia repair. Ann R Coll Surg Engl 79:40–45
71. Liang JT, Shieh MJ, Chen CN, Cheng YM, Chang KJ, Wang SM (2002) Prospective evaluation of laparoscopy-assisted colectomy versus laparotomy with resection for management of complex polyps of the sigmoid colon. World J Surg 26:377–383
72. Liem MS, Halsema JA, van der Graaf Y, Schrijvers AJ, van Vroonhoven TJ (1997) Cost-effectiveness of extraperitoneal laparoscopic inguinal hernia repair: a randomized comparison with conventional herniorrhaphy. Coala trial group. Ann Surg 226:668–676
73. Ludwig K, Patel K, Wilhelm L, Bernhardt J (2002) Prospektive Analyse zur Outcomebewertung nach laparoskopischer versus konventioneller Cholecystektomie. Zentralbl Chir 127:41–47
74. Lumsden MA, Twaddle S, Hawthorn R, Traynor I, Gilmore D, Davis J, Deeny M, Cameron IT, Walker JJ (2000) A randomised comparison and economic evaluation of laparoscopic-assisted hysterectomy and abdominal hysterectomy. BJOG 107:1386–1391
75. Mattioli G, Repetto P, Carlini C, Torre M, Pini Prato A, Mazzola C, Leggio S, Montobbio G, Gandullia P, Barabino A, Cagnazzo A, Sacco O, Jasonni V, Pini Prato A (2002) Laparoscopic vs open approach for the treatment of gastroesophageal reflux in children. Surg Endosc 16:750–752
76. McCorkle R, Quint-Benoliel J (1983) Symptom distress, current concerns and mood disturbance after diagnosis of life-threatening disease. Soc Sci Med 17:431–438
77. McCormack K, Scott NW, Go PMNYH, Ross S, Grant AM (2003) Laparoscopic techniques versus open techniques for inguinal hernia repair (Cochrane Review). In: Collaboration C (ed) The Cochrane database of systematic reviews, Vol. 1/2003 [CDROM]. Update Software, Oxford, UK
78. McDougall E, Clayman RV, Elashry OM (1996) Laparoscopic radical nephrectomy for renal tumor: the Washington University experience. J Urol 155:1180–1185
79. McHorney CA, Ware JE Jr, Lu JF, Sherbourne CD (1994) The MOS 36-item Short-Form Health Survey (SF-36): III. Tests of data quality, scaling assumptions, and reliability across diverse patient groups. Med Care 32:40–66

80. McHorney CA, Ware JE Jr, Raczek AE (1993) The MOS 36-Item Short-Form Health Survey (SF-36): II. Psychometric and clinical tests of validity in measuring physical and mental health constructs. Med Care 31:247-263

81. McMahon AJ, Russell IT, Baxter JN, Ross S, Anderson JR, Morran CG, Sunderland G, Galloway D, Ramsay G, O'Dwyer PJ (1994) Laparoscopic versus minilaparotomy cholecystectomy: a randomised trial. Lancet 343:135-138

82. Melton GB, Lillemoe KD, Cameron JL, Sauter PA, Coleman J, Yeo CJ (2002) Major bile duct injuries associated with laparoscopic cholecystectomy: effect of surgical repair on quality of life. Ann Surg 235:888-895

83. Meshkinpour H, Haghighat P, Meshkinpour A (1996) Quality of life among patients treated for achalasia. Dig Dis Sci 41:352-356

84. Muir Gray JA (1999) Evidence-based healthcare (2 edn) Churchill Livingstone, Edinburgh, UK

85. Naughton MJ, Wiklund I (1993) A critical review of dimension-specific measures of health-related quality of life in cross-cultural research. Qual Life Res 2:397-432

86. Neudecker J, Sauerland S, Neugebauer E, Bergamaschi R, Bonjer HJ, Cuschieri A, Fingerhut A, Fuchs KH, Jacobi C, Jansen FW, Koivusalo AM, Lacy A, McMahon MJ, Millat B, Schwenk W (2002) The European Association for Endoscopic Surgery clinical practice guideline on the pneumoperitoneum for laparoscopic surgery. Surg Endosc 16:1121-1143

87. In: Neugebauer E, Sauerland S, Troidl H (eds) (2000) Recommendations for evidence-based endoscopic surgery. The updated EAES consensus development conferences. Springer, Berlin Heidelberg New York

88. Neugebauer E, Troidl H, Wood-Dauphinee S, Eypasch E, Bullinger M (1991) Quality-of-life assessment in surgery: results of the Meran consensus development conference. Theor Surg 6:123-137

89. Nezhat F, Nezhat C, Gordon S, Wilkins E (1992) Laparoscopic versus abdominal hysterectomy. J Reproduct Med 37:247-250

90. Nguyen NT, Goldman C, Rosenquist CJ, Arango A, Cole CJ, Lee SJ, Wolfe BM (2001) Laparoscopic versus open gastric bypass: a randomized study of outcomes, quality of life, and costs. Ann Surg 234:279-291

91. Nilsson G, Larsson S, Johnsson F (2002) Randomized clinical trial of laparoscopic versus open fundoplication: evaluation of psychological well-being and changes in everyday life from a patient perspective. Scand J Gastroenterol 37:385-391

92. Oria HE, Moorehead MK (1998) Bariatric analysis and reporting outcome system (BAROS). Obes Surg 8:487-499

93. Pace KT, Dyer SJ, Stewart RJ, Honey RJ, Poulin EC, Schlachta CM, Mamazza J (2003) Health-related quality of life after laparoscopic and open nephrectomy. Surg Endosc 17:143-152

94. Pelgrims N, Closset J, Sperduto N, Gelin M, Houben JJ (2001) What did the laparoscopic Nissen approach of the gastrooesophageal reflux really change for the patients 8 years later? Acta Chir Belgium 101:68-72

95. Pencharz J, Young NL, Owen JL, Wright JG (2001) Comparison of three outcomes instruments in children. J Pediatr Orthop 21:425-432

96. Peters JH, Heimbucher J, Kauer WK, Incarbone R, Bremner CG, DeMeester TR (1995) Clinical and physiologic comparison of laparoscopic and open Nissen fundoplication. J Am Coll Surg 180:385-393

97. Pfeifer J, Wexner SD, Reissman P, Bernstein M, Nogueras JJ, Singh S, Weiss E (1995) Laparoscopic vs open colon surgery. Costs and outcome. Surg Endosc 9:1322-1326

98. Plaisier PW (1997) Incidence of persistent symptoms after laparoscopic cholecystectomy. Gut 41:579

99. Quintana JM, Cabriada J, Aróstegui I, de López Tejada I, Bilbao A (2003) Quality-of-life outcomes with laparoscopic vs open cholecystectomy. Surg Endosc

100. Quintana JM, Cabriada J, de López Tejada I, Varona M, Oribe V, Barriós B, Perdigo L, Bilbao A (2001) Translation and validation of the gastrointestinal Quality of Life Index (GIQLI). Rev Esp Enferm Dig 93:693-706

101. Raju KS, Auld BJ (1994) A randomised prospective study of laparoscopic vaginal hysterectomy versus abdominal hysterectomy each with bilateral salpingo-oophorectomy. BJOG 101:1068–1071
102. Rantanen TK, Salo JA, Salminen JT, Kellokumpu IH (1999) Functional outcome after laparoscopic or open Nissen fundoplication: a follow-up study. Arch Surg 134:240–244
103. Rattner DW, Brooks DC (1995) Patient satisfaction following laparoscopic and open antireflux surgery. Arch Surg 130:289–294
104. Reading AE (1989) Testing pain mechanisms in persons in pain. In: Wall P, Melzack R (eds) Textbook of pain (2 edn) Churchill Livingstone, New York, pp 269–280
105. Revicki DA, Wood M, Wiklund I, Crawley J (1998) Reliability and validity of the Gastrointestinal Symptom Rating Scale in patients with gastroesophageal reflux disease. Qual Life Res 7:75–83
106. Richards KF, Fisher KS, Flores JH, Christensen BJ (1996) Laparoscopic Nissen fundoplication: cost, morbidity, and outcome compared with open surgery. Surg Laparosc Endosc 6:140–143
107. Roblick UJ, Massmann A, Schwandner O, Sterk P, Krug F, Bruch HP, Schiedeck TH (2002) Lebensqualität nach chirurgischer Therapie einer Divertikulitis: Ergebnisse im Follow-up. Zentralbl Chir 127:31–35
108. RockwoodTH, ChurchJM, Fleshman JW, KaneRL, Mavrantonis C, Thorson AG, Wexner SD, Bliss D, Lowry AC (2000) Fecal Incontinence Quality of Life Scale: quality of life instrument for patients with fecal incontinence. Dis Colon Rectum 43:9–17
109. Rosen RC, Cappelleri JC, Smith MD, Lipsky J, Pena BM (1999) Development and evaluation of an abridged, 5-item version of the International Index of Erectile Function (IIEF-5) as a diagnostic tool for erectile dysfunction. Int J Impot Res 11:319–326
110. Sackett DL, Strauss DE, Richardson WS, Rosenberg W, Haynes RB (2000) Evidence-based medicine: how to practice and teach EBM (2 edn) Churchill Livingstone, London
111. Sanabria JR, Clavien PA, Cywes R, Strasberg SM (1993) Laparoscopic versus open cholecystectomy: a matched study. Can J Surg 36:330–336
112. Sarli L, Iusco DR, Sansebastiano G, Costi R (2001) Simultaneous repair of bilateral inguinal hernias: a prospective, randomized study of open, tension-free versus laparoscopic approach. Surg Laparosc Endosc Percutan Tech 11:262–267
113. Schmedt CG, Leibl BJ, Bittner R (2002) Endoscopic inguinal hernia repair in comparison with Shouldice and Lichtenstein repair: a systematic review of randomized trials. Dig Surg 19:511–517
114. Schütz K, Possover M, Merker A, Michels W, Schneider A (2002) Prospective randomized comparison of laparoscopic-assisted vaginal hysterectomy (LAVH) with abdominal hysterectomy (AH) for the treatment of the uterus weighing >200 g. Surg Endosc 16:121–125
115. Schwenk W, Böhm B, Müller JM (1998) Laparoskopische oder konventionelle kolorektale Resektionen: Beeinflusst die Operationstechnik die postoperative Lebensqualität? Zentralbl Chir 123:483–490
116. Scientific Advisory Committee of the Medical Outcomes Trust (2002) Assessing health status and quality-of-life: attributes and criteria. Qual Life Res 11:193–205
117. Slim K, Bousquet J, Kwiatkowski F, Lescure G, Pezet D, Chipponi J (1999) First validation of the French version of the Gastrointestinal Quality of Life Index (GIQLI). Gastroenterol Clin Biol 23:25–31
118. Spirtos NM, Schlaerth JB, Gross GM, Spirtos TW, Schlaerth AC, Ballon SC (1996) Cost and quality-of-life analyses of surgery for early endometrial cancer, laparotomy versus laparoscopy. Am J Obstet Gynecol 174:1795–1800
119. Spitzer WO, Dobson AJ, Hall J (1981) Measuring the quality of life of cancer patients: a concise QL-Index for use by physicians. J Chronic Dis 34:585–597
120. Sprangers MA, te Velde A, Aaronson NK (1999) The construction and testing of the EORTC coldrectal cancer-specific quality of life questionnaire module (QLQ-CR38). European Organization for Research and Treatment of Cancer Study Group on Quality of Life. Eur J Cancer 35:238–247

121. Stengel D, Lange V (1998) Lebensqualität nach Leistenhernienoperation — Ergebnisse einer prospektiven Studie (Shouldice, Lichtenstein, TAPP). Langenbecks Arch Chir Suppl Kongressbd 115:1020–1023

122. Svedlund J, Sjödin I, Dotevall G (1988) GSRS – a clinical rating scale for gastrointestinal symptoms in patients with irritable bowel syndrome and peptic ulcer disease. Dig Dis Sci 33:129–134

123. Talley N, Fullerton S, Junghard O, Wiklund I (2001) Quality of life in patients with endoscopy-negative heartburn: reliability and sensitivity of disease-specific instruments. Am J Gastroenterol 96:1998–2004

124. Topcu O, Karakayali F, Kuzu MA, Ozdemir S, Erverdi N, Elhan A, Aras N (2003) Comparison of long-term quality of life after laparoscopic and open cholecystectomy. Surg Endosc 17:291–295

125. Tschudi JF, Wagner M, Klaiber C, Brugger JJ, Frei E, Krahenbuhl L, Inderbitzi R, Boinski J, Hsu Schmitz SF, Husler J (2001) Randomized controlled trial of laparoscopic transabdominal preperitoneal hernioplasty vs Shouldice repair. Surg Endosc 15:1263–1266

126. Tsevat J, Dawson NV, Matchar DB (1990) Assessing quality of life and preferences in the seriously ill using utility theory. J Clin Epidemiol 43:73S–77S

127. Varni JW, Burwinkle TM, Katz ER, Meeske K, Dickinson P (2002) The PedsQL in pediatric cancer: reliability and validity of the Pediatric Quality of Life Inventory Generic Core Scales, Multidimensional Fatigue Scale, and Cancer Module. Cancer 94:2090–2106

128. Varni JW, Seid M, Kurtin PS (2001) PedsQL 4.0: reliability and validity of the Pediatric Quality of Life Inventory version 4.0 generic core scales in healthy and patient populations. Med Care 39:800–812

129. Varni JW, Seid M, Rode CA (1999) The PedsQL: measurement model for the Pediatric Quality of Life Inventory. Med Care 37:126–139

130. Velanovich V (1999) Comparison of symptomatic and quality of life outcomes of laparoscopic versus open antireflux surgery. Surgery 126:782–789

131. Velanovich V, Karmy-Jones R (2001) Surgical management of paraesophageal hernias: outcome and quality of life analysis. Dig Surg 18:432–438

132. Velanovich V, Shurafa MS (2001) Clinical and quality of life outcomes of laparoscopic and open splenectomy for haematological diseases. Eur J Surg 167:23–28

133. Velanovich V, Vallance SR, Gusz JR, Tapia FV, Harkabus MA (1996) Quality of life scale for gastroesophageal reflux disease. J Am Coll Surg 183:217–224

134. Visick A (1948) Measured radical gastrectomy: review of 505 operations for peptic ulcer. Lancet 1:505–510

135. Ward WL, Hahn EA, Mo F, Hernandez L, Tulsky DS, Cella D (1999) Reliability and validity of the Functional Assessment of Cancer Therapy-Colorectal (FACT-C) quality of life instrument. Qual Life Res 8:181–195

136. Ware J, Gandek B (1998) Overview of the SF-36 Health Survey and the International Quality of Life Assessment (IQOLA) Project. J Clin Epidemiol 51:903–912

137. Ware JE, Kosinski M, Keller SD (1999) SF-36 physical and mental health summary scales: a user's manual. Health Institute, New England Medical Center, Boston

138. Ware JE, Sherbourne CD (1992) The MOS 36-item short-form health survey (SF-36). I. Conceptual framework and item selection. Med Care 30:473–483

139. Waters EB, Salmon LA, Wake M (2000) The parent-form Child Health Questionnaire in Austalia: comparison of reliability, validity structure and norms. J Pediatr Psychol 25:381–391

140. Waters EB, Salmon LA, Wake M, Weight M, Hesketh KD (2001) The health and well-being of adolescents: a school-based population study of the self-report Child Health Questionnaire. J Adolesc Health 29:140–149

141. Weeks JC, Nelson H, Gelber S, Sargent D, Schroeder G (2002) Short-term quality-of-life outcomes following laparoscopic-assisted colectomy vs open colectomy for colon cancer: a randomized trial. J Am Med Assoc 287:321–328

142. Wellwood J, Sculpher MJ, Stoker D, Nicholls GJ, Geddes C, Whitehead A, Singh R, Spiegelhalter D (1998) Randomised controlled trial of laparoscopic versus open mesh repair for inguinal hernia: outcome and cost. Br Med J 317:103–110

143. Wenner J, Nilsson G, Oberg S, Melin T, Larsson S, Johnsson F (2001) Short-term outcome after laparoscopic and open 360 fundoplication. Surg Endosc 1124–1128
144. Westling A, Gustavsson S (2001) Laparoscopic vs open Roux-en-Y gastric bypass: aprospective, randomized trial. ObesSurg11:284–292
145. Wiebe S, Guyatt G, Weaver B, Matijevic S, Sidweli C (2003) Comparative responsiveness of generic and specific quality-of-life instruments. J Clin Epidemiol 56:52–60
146. Wiklund IK, Junghard O, Grace E, Talley NJ, Kamm M, van Veldhuyzen Zanten S, Pare P, Chiba N, Leddin DS, Bigard MA, Colin R, Schoenfeld P (1998) Quality of Life in Reflux and Dyspepsia patients. Psychometric documentation of a new disease-specific questionnaire (QOLRAD). Eur J Surg Suppl 583:41–49
147. Zigmond AS, Snaith RP (1983) The Hospital Anxiety and Depression Scale. Acta Psychiatr Scand 67:361–370

The EAES Clinical Practice Guidelines on the Pneumoperitoneum for Laparoscopic Surgery (2002)

Jens Neudecker, Stefan Sauerland, Edmund A. M. Neugebauer,
Roberto Bergamaschi, H. Jaap Bonjer, Alfred Cuschieri, Karl-Hermann Fuchs,
Christoph A. Jacobi, F. W. Jansen, A.-M. Koivusalo, Antonio M. Lacy,
M. J. McMahon, Bertrand Millat, Wolfgang Schwenk

Introduction

Only 15 years after the introduction of laparoscopic cholecystectomy, laparoscopic techniques (used either as a diagnostic tool or as a therapeutic access method) are among the most common procedures in surgery worldwide. However, concerns about higher surgical complications rates (such as vascular and intestinal injuries) compared to conventional techniques and anesthesiological risks have remained. Since the start of the laparoscopic era, numerous studies have described pathophysiological or clinical problems that are related to laparoscopy. Therefore, many technical innovations and modifications have been developed to improve safety and effectiveness of laparoscopy, but not all of them have been studied adequately before clinical use.

With these developments in mind, the European Association for Endoscopic Surgery (EAES) decided to develop authorative and evidence-based clinical practice guidelines on the pneumoperitoneum and its sequelae. The scope of these guidelines covers all important general surgical aspects of the pneumoperitoneum but not special laparoscopic procedures for defined pathologies. They address the pathophysiological basis for the clinical indications, aspects to establish the pneumoperitoneum, and perioperative aspects such as adhesions and pain. In addition, a clinical algorithm was formulated for practical use.

Methods

Under the mandate of the EAES Scientific Committee with the aim to set up evidence-based clinical practice guidelines, we combined the methodologies of a systematic review and a consensus development conference (CDC) because previous CDCs (both within and outside the EAES) had difficulties in identifying all relevant articles [218, 262, 280]. As a framework of the process, the key aspects pertaining to the pneumoperitoneum were precisely formulated in separate questions, which then were answered concurrently by the use of literature and expert evidence.

For the systematic review, one researcher (J.N.) performed comprehensive literature searches in Medline, Embase, and the Cochrane Library. We used the medical subject headings Laparoscopy and Pneumoperitoneum. Our primary intention was to identify all clinically relevant randomized controlled trials (RCTs). However, other trials using concurrent cohorts (CCTs), external or historical cohorts, population-based outcomes studies, case series, and case reports were accepted for a comprehensive evaluation of the pneumoperitoneum and its sequelae (Table 2.1). Included articles were scrutinized and classified by two reviewers (J.N. and S.S.). Furthermore, all panelists were asked to search the literature according to a list of defined questions. The reference lists of all relevant articles were also checked.

For the CDC, the conference organizers in Cologne, together with the scientific committee of the EAES, nominated a multidisciplinary expert panel. The criteria for selection were clinical and scientific expertise in the field of laparoscopy and geographical location within Europe.

Six months before the conference, the questions on laparoscopy were sent to the panelists. In parallel, the questions were answered by literature evidence found in systematic searches. One month before the conference, all answers from the panel and the literature searches were analyzed and subsequently combined into a provisional preconsensus statement and a clinical algorithm. Each panel member was also informed about the identities of the other members, which had not been previously disclosed.

In Maastricht, all panelists (except A.C. and H.J.B.) met for a first meeting on June 13, 2001. Here, the provisional bottom-line statements typed in bold and the clinical algorithm with the grades of recommendation were scrutinized word by word in a 5-h session in a nominal group process. For all statements, internal (expert opinion) and external evidence was compared. The following day the modified statement and the algorithm were presented to the conference audience by all panelists for public discussion (1.5-h session). During a postconsensus meeting on the same day, all suggestions from the audience were discussed again by the panelists, and the statement was further modified. The finalized statement as given later was mailed to all panelists for final approval (Delphi process) before publication.

To increase readability, a short version of the clinical practice guidelines with a clinical algorithm was prepared (Fig. 2.1). The extended version consists of a detailed appraisal of pathophysiologic background and clinical research evidence. Each recommendation is graded according to its reliability and the rigor of research evidence behind the statement (Table 2.1).

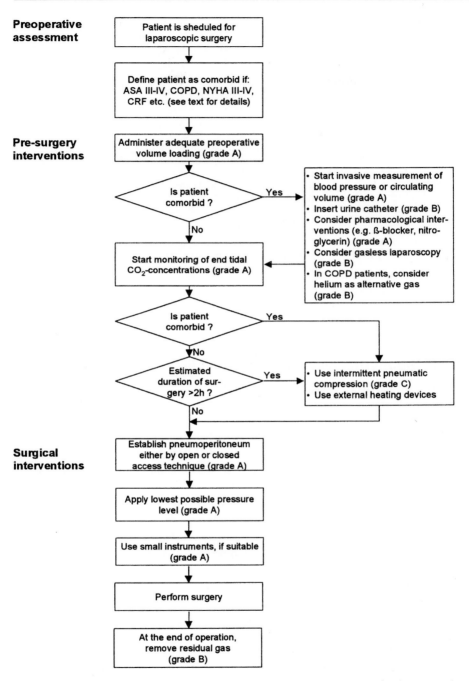

Fig. 2.1. Evidence-based clinical algorithm on the pneumoperitoneum for laparoscopic surgery. The recommendation is graded according to Table 2.1. *Diamond boxes* decision boxes, *square boxes* action boxes [255]

Table 2.1. A method for grading recommendations according to scientific evidence

Grade of recommendation	Level of evidence	Possible study designs for the evaluation of therapeutic interventions
A	1a	Systematic review (with homogeneity) of RCTs
	1b	Individual RCT (with narrow confidence interval)
	1c	All-or-none case series
B	2a	Systematic review (with homogeneity) of cohort studies
	2b	Individual cohort study (including low-quality RCT)
	2c	"Outcomes" research
	3a	Systematic review (with homogeneity) of case-control studies
	3b	Individual case-control study
C	4	Case series (and poor-quality cohort and case-control studies)
D	5	Expert opinion without explicity critical appraisal, or based on physiology, bench research, or "first principles"

From Sackett et al. [255]
RCT randomized controlled trial

Pathophysiological Basis for the Clinical Indications

Cardiovascular system

Cardiovascular effects of pneumoperitoneum occur most often during its induction, and this should be considered when initial pressure is increased for introduction of access devices. In ASA I and II patients, the hemodynamic and circulatory effects of a 12–14-mmHg capnoperitoneum are generally not clinically relevant (grade A). Due to the hemodynamic changes in ASA III and IV patients, however, invasive measurement of blood pressure or circulating volume should be considered (grade A). These patients should also receive adequate preoperative volume loading (grade A), beta-blockers (grade A), and intermittent sequential pneumatic compression of the lower limbs, especially in prolonged laparoscopic procedures (grade C). If technically feasible, gasless or low-pressure laparoscopy might be an alternative for patients with limited cardiac function (grade B). The use of other gases (e.g., helium) showed no clinically relevant hemodynamic advantages (grade A).

Pneumoperitoneum decreases venous return, preload, and cardiac output (CO) and increases heart rate (HR), mean arterial pressure (MAP), as well as systemic (SVR) and pulmonary vascular resistence (PVR). These hemodynamic and cardiovascular – changes mostly occur because of increased intraabdominal pressure (IAP) (1b [159, 221, 291]) and the stimulated neurohumoral vasoactive systems [vasopressin and rennin–aldosterone–angiotensine system (RAAS)] (1b [142, 158]), but are independent of type of gas (1b [28]). However, in otherwise healthy patients these changes are not dangerous when IAP does not exceed 15 mmHg (1b [27]).

Increased IAP, up to 12–15 mmHg, decreases venous return, which results in reduced preload and CO, without adequate intravascular volume loading (1b [63, 142, 162, 201, 221]). Additionally, changes in body position, especially head-up tilt position, intensify these negative effects of a pneumoperitoneum (2b [115, 116]), whereas head-down or Trendelenburg position has a positive effect on venous return (1b [162]). Furthermore, the use of positive end-expiratory pressure (PEEP) of 10 H_2O during pneumoperitoneum decreases preload and CO (4 [164]). Pneumoperitoneum increases sympathetic cardiac activity (1b [260]) and induces a hemodynamic stress response by activation of the neurohumoral vasoactive system (i.e., vasopressin and RAAS) resulting in increased HR, increased SVR and PVR, and increased arterial blood pressure (1b [142, 159]). This stress response leads to an increase in oxygen consumption, which might be deleterious for patients with compromised cardiac function. In clinical studies on ASA III and IV patients distinct intraoperative hemodynamic changes during pneumoperitoneum were described (4 [127]), but cardiovascular stability was unimpaired (4 [64, 83, 111, 322]) if appropriate invasive monitoring and pharmacologic interventions were used (4 [79, 292]). In contrast, there are reports of cardiovascular alterations persisting after release of the pneumoperitoneum (4 [108]). Most of these studies used an IAP of 12–15 mmHg without preoperatively volume loading. Without adequate intravascular volume loading a pneumoperitoneum in connection with head-up tilt position decreases CO significantly (up to 50%) (1b [142, 221]). In comorbid patients (ASA III and IV), RCTs with adequate sample size are missing.

In the majority of patients (ASA I and II), the hemodynamic effects of a pneumoperitoneum are without consequences and vanish after desufflation. Therefore, most patients without comorbidities (ASA I and II) do not need invasive hemodynamic monitoring. However, in ASA III and IV patients an invasive monitoring of blood pressure and circulating volume must be considered because only these measures allow early recognition and adequate treatment of severe cardiovascular changes (1b [162]). For intraoperative monitoring, a pulmonary artery catheter or COLD (cardiac oxygenation and lung water determination) monitoring should be applied, because transesophageal echocardiography in patients with cardiac disease has not been proven to be useful (4 [241]). For patients with severley compromised circulation, measurement of the pulmonary artery pressure (PAP) and CO can be necessary. However, interpreting changes in central venous pressure (CVP) and PAP may be difficult (4 [213]). Due to the consecutive increase in intrathoracic pressure during laparoscopy CVP and PAP also increase, but right arterial volume is not decreased. Therefore, CVP may only incorrectly describe the effective circulating blood volume and could be misinterpreted [162].

Since the effects of increased IAP on hemodynamics are volume dependent, adequate preoperative intravascular loading is essential, especially in patients with cardiac diseases, to prevent cardiovascular side effects of a pneumoperitoneum (1b [162]). Another intervention of proven effectiveness that also increases cardiac preload and thereby prevents hemodynamic changes (2b [6]) is intermittent sequential pneumatic compression of the lower extremities to augment venous blood return (1b [273, 274], 2b [273, 274]).

To minimize the effects of hemodynamic stress response on myocardial oxygen consumption, esmolol or clonidine can safely be used (1b [142, 163]) if volume depletion is not present. Intraoperative hemodynamic alterations in patients with underlying cardiopulmonary disease can be effectively controlled by appropriate pharmacological intervention (use of intravenous nitroglycerin) (2b [80]).

Hemodynamic and circulatory changes are independent from the used gas (CO_2 or helium) (1b [28]) but decreased during gasless laparoscopy (1b [5, 91, 159, 201, 22 1]). Therefore, gasless laparoscopy might be an alternative for patients with limited cardiac function. In summary, cardiac diseases are associated with an increased risk of general complications after laparoscopic surgery (and even higher risk after conventional surgery). Since various surgical and nonsurgical treatment options can be recommended to reduce these risks, the presence of heart disease does not principally contraindicate laparoscopic surgery (2b [239, 240]). There is a need for further trials in ASA III and IV patients.

Lung Physiology and Gas Exchange

Carbon dioxide pneumoperitoneum causes hypercapnia and respiratory acidosis. During laparoscopy, monitoring of end-tidal CO_2 concentration is mandatory (grade A) and minute volume of ventilation should be increased in order to maintain normocapnia. Increased intraabdominal pressure and head-down position reduce pulmonary compliance and lead to ventilation-perfusion mismatch (grade A). In patients with normal lung function, these intraoperative respiratory changes are usually not clinically relevant (grade A). In patients with limited pulmonary reserves, capnoperitoneum carries an increased risk of CO_2 retention, especially in the postoperative period (grade A). In patients with cardiopulmonary diseases, intra- and postoperative arterial blood gas monitoring is recommended (grade A). Lowering intraabdominal pressure and controlling hyperventilation reduce respiratory acidosis during pneumoperitoneum (grade A). Gasless laparoscopy, low-pressure capnoperitoneum, or the use of helium might be alternatives for patients with limited pul-

monary function (grade B). Laparoscopic surgery preserves postoperative pulmonary function better than open surgery (grade A).

The specifics of a capnoperitoneum, the IAP and the used gas, result in hypercapnia, respiratory acidosis, reduced pulmonary compliance, and increased airway resistance (1b [224, 307]). Additional changes in body position have minor influences (2b [68]) but could intensify these effects, especially in the head-down position (2b [114, 116]). Relaxation of the diaphragm caused by anesthesia in combination with increased intraabdominal pressure impairs excursion of the diaphragm and leads to compression of the lower lung lobes. These effects result in a decreased tidal volume, ventilation–perfusion mismatch, a decreased shunt volume, increased dead space, and decreased pulmonary compliance (1b [160], 2b [250]). Pulmonary gas exchange during laparoscopy can be optimized by the choice of the anesthetic procedure (1b [93]) and PEEP (5 [183]). Without hyperventilation P_aCO_2 will increase by 8–10 mmHg and pH will decrease (1b [315]) before a steady state is reached. Intraoperatively, pulmonary changes due to capnoperitoneum are compensated by otherwise healthy adults (1b [197]).

Various laparoscopic procedures have been shown to result in better postoperative pulmonary function when compared to their open-surgery counterparts (1b [38, 42, 48, 51, 74, 112, 149, 167, 197, 206, 275, 307]), but clinically more relevant end points such as postoperative pulmonary complications were rarely evaluated or found unchanged in ASA I and II patients (1b [205, 206]). These data generally prove that laparoscopy rather than conventional surgery should be advised for compromised patients, particularly those with obstructive lung disease. This superiority of laparoscopic surgery during the postoperative period is mostly related to its lesser extent of surgical trauma and pain, but laparoscopy has certain effects on ventilation that deserve special attention.

Capnoperitoneum with an IAP of more than 12 mmHg combined with head-down or Trendelenburg position should be avoided because it reduces pulmonary compliance by more than 30% and there is ventilation–perfusion impairment (1b [155, 159, 224] 2b [188, 250, 296]). Hypercapnia and respiratory acidosis can be avoided by controlled hyperventilation (1b [315]). CO_2 storage during pneumoperitoneum can result in postoperative hypercapnic hangover, which has to be particularly considered in cases, of accidential subcutaneous CO_2 insufflation. To recognize these changes intra- and postoperative arterial blood gas monitoring and continous capnometry are generally recommended for comorbid patients [161], particularly those with cardiopulmonary diseases (2b [314]). These patients may also benefit from prolonged postoperative mechanical ventilation [160]. From a more surgical standpoint, gasless laparoscopy or the use of other gases (e.g., helium and N_2O) may have clinically relevant advantages (1b [28, 155, 159, 224]), but the results of randomized trials are inconsistent (1b [92]) and need to be confirmed. Trocar positioning also has a relevant influence on pulmonary function, (1a [167]). Overall, most of the discussed randomized trials included only small numbers of patients, leading to an increased chance of type II error.

It should be mentioned that capnothorax can be a serious, albeit rare, complication that has been encountered in patients after capnoperitoneum (4 [7, 233]). Capnothorax occurs more often after laparoscopic esophageal or gastric surgery but has also been observed after lower abdominal procedures or even hernia repair. Because of the high solubility of CO_2, asymptomatic capnothorax diagnosed by postoperative chest X-ray may be treated conservatively. However, tension capnothorax may occur very rarely. Therefore, symptomatic capnothorax requires immediate drainage.

Venous Blood Return

During laparoscopy, both head-up position and elevated intraabdominal pressure independently reduce venous blood return from the lower extremities (grade A). Intraoperative sequential intermittent pneumatic compression of the lower extremities effectively reduces venous stasis during pneumoperitoneum (grade A/B) and is recommended for all prolonged laparoscopic procedures. The incidence of thromboembolic complications after pneumoperitoneum is not known.

Increased intraabdominal pressure together with reverse Trendelenburg position (head-up position) decreases venous return from the lower extremities by more than 40% (1b [273, 274], 2b [12, 99, 123, 204]) with a concomittant increase in femoral venous pressure (2b [12, 139]). However, it has been hypothesized that the systemic coagulation system is activated by laparoscopic surgery (1b [243], 2b [41, 178]), but controversial data exist (2b [67, 119, 192]). Due to the impairment of lower extremity circulation, the increased venous pressure, and the activation of the systemic fibrinolytic system, the potential risk for deep venous thrombosis (DVT) is increased. Although there are alarming reports about a high incidence of DVT after pneumoperitoneum (4 [230]), the rate of clinically evident postoperative thrombembolic complications after laparoscopic surgery remains unclear [10, 31, 184, 189]. The negative effects of elevated IAP and body position on venous blood return from the lower extremities can partly be counteracted by intermittent sequential compression of the lower limbs in laparoscopic cholecystectomy and colorectal surgery (1b [273, 274], 2b [273, 274]). Whether such compression does reduce thromboembolic event remains to be elucidated in larger trials.

The effects of a low-pressure pneumoperitoneum (5–7 mmHg) and abdominal wall lifting on thromboembolic complications have not been studied, although from a pathophysiologic standpoint a positive effect can be reasonably anticipated.

Perfusion of Intraabdominal Organs

Although in healthy subjects (ASA I and II), changes in kidney or liver perfusion (grade A) and also splanchnic perfusion (grade D) due to an intraabdominal pressure of 12–14 mmHg have no clinically relevant effects on organ function, this may not be the case in patients with already impaired perfusion. Especially in patients with impaired hepatic or renal function or atherosclerosis, intraabdominal pressure should be as low as possible to reduce microcirculatory disturbances (grade B). Patients with impaired renal function should be adequately volume loaded before and during elevated intraabdominal pressure (grade A).

Renal Effects

Randomized clinical trials showed a decrease in renal blood flow (RBF), glomerular filtration rate, and urine output in the initial phase of a pneumoperitoneum (1b [155, 221]). With increasing IAP renal function is gradually depressed (5 [146]). Elevated IAP causes renal dysfunction due to direct mechanical compression of renal parenchyma, renal arteries, and veins (5 [247]). The reduction in RBF and urine output is probably caused by a decrease in CO and/or the compression of the renal vein. In experimental studies, renal vein flow remained decreased for at least 2 h postoperatively (5 [195, 247]). Mediated by humoral factors, a sympathetic reaction induces a constriction of the renal artery. Pneumoperitoneum increases plasma renin activity (PRA) and consequently activates the RAAS, which promotes the renal vasoconstriction via angiotensin II. However, one prospective randomized trial found no signs of a clinically relevant impairment of renal function (1b [26]).

Hepatoportal Effects

When measured with laser Doppler, hepatoportal circulation is gradually decreased with increasing IAP (2b [69], 4 [136, 223]). In elderly patients, splanchnic circulation is very sensitive to elevated pressure (4 [261]). Experimental and clinical studies reported elevated liver enzymes after prolonged laparoscopic procedures and elevated intraabdominal pressure (1b [95], 2b [209]). However, in one RCT no signs of clinically relevant postoperative liver dysfunction were detected (1b [26]).

Splanchnic Effects

Elevated IAP mechanically compresses capillary beds, decreases splanchnic microcirculation, and thus impairs oxygen delivery to the intraabdominal organs. During pneumoperitoneum, a 24% reduction of blood flow in the superior mesenteric artery and the hepatic portal vein was reported (5 [125]). In healthy patients, a high vs low IAP (15 vs 10 mmHg) decreased blood flow into the stomach (54%), the jejunum (32%), the colon (4%), the parietal peritoneum (60%), and the duodenum (11%) (4 [266]). Furthermore, clinical and animal studies noted a decrease in gastric intramucosal pH (1b [157], 2b [69]), which may be the earliest indicator of alterated hemodynamic function compared to traditional measurements, such as CO, SVR, and lactate [154], but conflicting findings exist [69, 187, 223]. The clinical implications of these investigations remain unclear.

Otherwise healthy patients seem to compensate changes in intraabdominal organ perfusion without impairment of organ function. However, in patients with cardiovascular comorbidities or preexisting organ disorders, reduced alteration in organ perfusion could have detrimental effects. Therefore, for these patients careful observation and selection of surgical technique are required.

Several studies of different quality reported that in patients with limited hepatic or renal function, postoperative hepatic and renal function were better preserved by keeping IAP under 12 mmHg and by avoiding a prolonged pneumoperitoneum (1b–4 [69, 125, 154, 266]). Recently, one experimental study investigated the influence of different IAP levels on intra- and extraabdominal tissue blood flow by using color-labeled microspheres and reported, a nonimpaired tissue blood flow during capnoperitoneum of 10–12 mmHg (5 [317]). Esmolol inhibits the release of renin and blunts the pressor response to induction and maintenance of pneumoperitoneum. It may protect against renal ischemia during laparoscopy because urine output under, esmolol therapy was found to be higher (1b [162]). Nonsteroidal antiinflammatory drugs (NSAIDs), widely used in laparoscopic surgery, can cause renal medullary vasoconstriction. Because cases of renal failure after laparoscopic surgery and NSAID therapy were reported, NSAIDs should be replaced by other analgetics wherever possible (5; A.-M. Koivusalo, personal communication).

Stress Response and Immunologic Parameters

Changes in systemic inflammatory and antiinflammatory parameters (mainly cytokines) as well as in stress response parameters are less pronounced after laparoscopic surgery than after conventional surgery (grade A). Whether this leads to clinically relevant effects (e.g., less pain, fatigue, and complications) remains to be proven. There is no compelling clinical evidence that specific modifications of the pneumoperitoneum alter the immunological response.

The influence of pneumoperitoneum on the function of the immune system and stress response is poorly evaluated because most studies investigate surrogate parameters of the immunological function, such as cytokines and other cell products, and not the cell function itself (e.g., account, ratio, concentration, and activity of immunological cells). The essential clinical outcomes after surgery concerning immunological functions are infections (e.g., sepsis, pneumonia, urinary tract infection, and local wound-related infections) and cancer growth (e.g., metastasis and local tumor spread). However, there is no study in the field of laparoscopic surgery demonstrating an association between changes of intra- and postoperative immune function and the occurrence of clinical complications.

Clinical controlled trials of laparoscopic versus conventional surgery have mostly focused on changes of cytokine levels to describe the influence of pneumoperitoneum on systemic immunological functions. These studies showed differences in serum cytokine levels between laparoscopic and conventional surgery for IL-1(1b [174]), IL-6 (1b [36, 135, 165, 176, 254, 320, 322]), CRP (1b [135, 140, 176, 235, 254, 320], CRP (1b [133, 138, 174, 233, 252, 318]) and cell-mediated immunity (1b [224]) that have not been confirmed by other authors (1b [17, 198], 2b [89]). In RCTs, postoperative immunological functions seemed to be better preserved after laparoscopic compared to conventional procedures (1b [13, 45, 151, 176, 235, 276, 284, 308, 321]); however, some trials found no differences (1b [73, 113, 173, 203, 226, 248, 270, 289, 295]) and one trial even reported a more pronounced immunodepression after laparoscopy (1b [290]). Additional RCTs examined perioperative stress response and found adrenaline (1b [150]), noradrenaline (1b [150]), and cortisol (1b [150, 174, 303]) decreased to a lesser extent after laparoscopic than after conventional procedures, although one study did not confirm this result (1b [112]). By comparisons carbon dioxide insufflation with gasless laparoscopy, similar courses of stress response parameters were found (1b [158, 162]), but conflicting data exist (1b [126]). Since all these studies compared laparoscopic and open surgery, the immunological effects of the pneumoperitoneum and the surgical procedure overlap each other, precluding the quantification of any specific effects.

The influence of the specifics of the pneumoperitoneum (e.g., IAP, gas, and warming and humidified surrounding) on immunological function has only partly been studied in experimental settings. Helium seems to preserve cell-mediated intraperitoneal immunity better than CO_2 (5 [47, 219]) and causes a less pronounced cytokine response and bacterial translocation (5 [194]). In clinical trials, postoperative intraperitoneal cytokine response after warming the insufflation gas was attenuated (1b [244]). Another study suggested a similar stress response (IL-6, CRP, neutrophil elastase, and white cell count) after pneumoperitoneum or abdominal wall lifting (1b [221]). It is questionable whether the specifics of the pneumoperitoneum have clinically relevant effects or even benefits on postoperative immunological function and outcome (e.g., less pain, fatigue, and complications). Thus, additional clinical trials with adequate end points and sample sizes have to be performed to confirm the hypothesis of better preservation of the immune function by minimally invasive surgery.

Peritonitis

Presupposing appropriate perioperative measures (e.g., adequate preoperative volume loading) and hemodynamic stability, there are no contraindications to create a pneumoperitoneum when laparoscopic surgery is applicable in cases of peritonitis (grade B). The results from animal studies on the influence of pneumoperitoneum bacteremia and endotoxemia are controversial.

In experimental studies, a penumoperitoneum seems to increase the risk of bacteremia and endotoxemia [23–25, 77, 101, 214]. Other animal studies demonstrated that the systemic inflammation is higher after laparotomy than after laparoscopy, causing a transient decrease in immunologic defense and possibly leading to sepsis (5 [131, 180]).

With regard to the specifics of a pneumoperitoneum, any increase in IAP seems to further promote bacteraemia (2b [77]), but data are inconsistent. The used gas seems to play only a minor role (5 [105]). A clinical RCT found no difference in the acute phase response and endotoxemia between laparoscopic and conventional gastric surgery in cases of peritonitis (1b [173]). Furthermore, laparoscopic compared to conventional cholecystectomy for acute and gangrenous cholecystitis does not increase the mortality rate (1b [153]), and the morbidity rate seems to be even lower after laparoscopy (1b [153, 182]). Two small conflicting RCTs assessed bacteremia during appendectomy and found 0/11 versus 6/12 and 5/14 versus 5/13 positive blood cultures after open and laparoscopic access, respectively (1b [222, 279]). The hypothesis that in cases of peritonitis laparoscopy leads to a lesser depression of the systemic immune response with better postoperative outcome is unproven.

In conclusion, the decision to perform a laparoscopic procedure in case of peritonitis depends on the extent of peritonitis, the onset of disease, and the general clinical state of the patient. No clinical trials have found any contraindication to perform laparoscopy in case of beginning peritonitis (e.g., perforated appendicitis).

Risk of Tumor Spreading

There is no strong clinical evidence (except case reports) that pneumoperitoneum in patients with intraabdominal malignant disease increases the risk of tumor spread (grade D). The panel considers that there is no reason to contraindicate pneumoperitoneum in these patients, given the fact that an appropriate operative technique is used (grade C). The type of insufflation gas seems to affect intraabdominal tumor growth, whereas intraabdominal pressure is of little im-

portance (grade D). Due to the low level of evidence, patients undergoing laparoscopic surgery for malignant disease should be included in randomized controlled trials or at least in quality registries.

Several animal studies have been conducted to evaluate the pathogenesis of portsite metastasis in laparoscopic surgery, but the experimental models and tumor cell techniques vary considerably (5 [32, 33, 132, 134, 151, 219]). Port-site recurrence is common in small animal models after inoculation of high numbers of tumor cells and more pronounced after capnoperitoneum compared to laparotomy or gasless laparoscopy (5 [132, 134, 219]). IAP has little influence on intraperitoneal tumor growth or the incidence of port-site metastasis, whereas insufflation with helium may decrease subcutaneous tumor growth (5 [132, 134, 219]). In contrast to these findings, intraperitoneal tumor growth is stimulated more by laparotomy than by laparoscopy, gasless laparoscopy, or anesthesia alone without any operative procedure (5[130]).

Port dislocations should be avoided and ports should be irrigated intraperitoneally before they are retracted from the abdominal cavity. Before the tumor is extracted, the incision has to be protected against direct tumor cell contamination. The risk of tumor cell dissemination may be reduced by intraabdominal instillation of cytotoxic solutions at the end of the operation (5 [34]).

Prospective clinical trials failed to show a higher incidence of free intraperitoneal tumor cells (5 [37]) or recurrence in the skin incision (2a [304], 5 [37]) for laparoscopic compared to conventional surgery. A systematic review of clinical trials found no significant differences in overall survival, disease-free survival, cancer-related death, locoregional tumor recurrences, port-site metastasis, or distant metastasis in patients undergoing laparoscopic or conventional colorectal resections (2a [304]). Perioperatively, mobilization of neoplastic cells occurs frequently in patients with colorectal cancer, but the surgical approach does not seem to be a determining factor (16 [18]). Randomized trials with low quality found no wound or port-site metastasis in 91 patients during a mean follow-up of 21.4 months and in 43 patients after long-term 5-year follow-up (2b [57, 169]). Adequately powered RCTs on laparoscopic and conventional resections of colorectal carcinoma are missing, but such trials are currently being performed in Europe, the USA, and Australia. Results of these trials will be available in 2004–2006.

Establishing the Pneumoperitoneum

Creation of a Pneumoperitoneum

For severe complications (vessel perforation) it is impossible to prove a difference between closed- and open-access technique in RCTs; therefore, large outcome studies should be considered. In the RCTs, the rate of major and minor complications is surprisingly high, which may be due to the definition of a complication or surgical learning curve. Insertion of the first trocar with the open technique is faster as compared to the Veress needle (grade A). The randomized controlled trials comparing closed (Veress plus trocar) versus open approach have inadequate sample sizes to find a difference in serious complications. In large outcome studies there were less complications in the closed group (grade B). Although RCTs found the open approach faster and associated with a lower incidence of minor complications (grade A), the panel cannot favor the use of either access technique. However, the use of either technique may have advantages in specific patient subgroups (grade B).

Among the various techniques for achieving a pneumoperitoneum and introducing the first trocar, two common methods are usually performed. The first, so-called closed technique requires the Veress needle, which is inserted in the abdominal cavity for CO_2 insufflation followed by blind introduction of the first trocar. The second, so-called open technique was first described by Hasson [110]. This technique begins with a small incision at the umbilical site and subsequently all layers of the abdominal wall are incised. The first trocar is then inserted under direct vision followed by gas insuation.

Table 2.2. Randomized clinical trials of Veress needle or open approach

Reference/ year	No. of patients	Procedure	Access time (min)	Complications	Results
Gullà et al. [103]/2000	262	Diagnostic and operative laparoscopy	Not mentioned	Needle: 11/101 Open: 0/161	Open technique is safer
Saunders et al. [262]/ 1998	176	Diagnostic laparoscopy in abdominal trauma	Needle: 2.7 Open: 7.3	Needle: 0/98 Open: 0/78	Veress technique is faster
Cogliandolo et al. [50]/ 1998	150	Laparoscopic cholecystectomy	Needle: 4.5 Open: 3.2	Needle: 5/75 Open: 5/75	Open technique is faster
Peitgen et al. [231]/1997	50	Diagnostic and operative laparoscopy	Needle: 3.8 Open: 1.8	Needle: 0/25 Open: 0/25	Open technique is faster
Byron et al. [39]/1993	252	Diagnostic and operative laparoscopy	Needle: 5.9 Open: 2.2	Needle: 19/141 Open: 4/111	Open technique is safer and faster
Nezhat et al. [219]/1991	200	Diagnostic and operative laparoscopy	Not mentioned	Needle: 22/100 Open: 3/100	Open technique has fewer complications
Borgatta et al. [30]/ 1990	212	Laparoscopic tubal sterilization	Needle: 9.6 Open: 7.5	Needle: 7/110 Open: 4/102	Open technique is safer and faster

The morbidity associated with the establishment of the pneumoperitoneum and the insertion of the first trocar is estimated to be less than 1% (4 [29, 109, 264]), but the true incidence of visceral and vascular injury for both techniques is unknown. However, major vascular injuries occur most often with the Veress needle (2c [44, 236]). Several RCTs found that the open technique on average causes less complications and is cheaper and faster than the Veress needle technique (1b [30, 39, 50, 104, 220, 232]) (Table 2.2). However, one study on the access technique for percutaneous diagnostic peritoneal lavage in blunt trauma patients showed that the Veress needle technique was faster compared to the open technique (1b [263]). A recent three-armed RCT found it easier to establish the pneumoperitoneum with a new access device (TrocDoc) than with the open technique or the Veress needle (1b [14]). The choice between reusable and single-use instruments was outside our scope. In specific patient subgroups, the access technique has to be chosen according to the patients characteristics (e.g., pregnancy, obesity, and trauma).

Gas Embolism and Its Prevention

Clinically relevant gas embolism is very rare, but if it occurs, it may be a fatal complication (grade C). The true incidence of clinically inapparent gas embolism is not known. Most described cases of gas embolism have been caused by accidental vessel punction with a Veress needle at the induction of pneumoperitoneum. Low intraabdominal pressure, low insufflation rates, as well as careful surgical technique may reduce the incidence of gas embolism (grade D). A sudden decrease in end-tidal CO_2 concentration and blood pressure during abdominal insufflation should be considered a sign of gas embolism (grade C). Due to the low incidence of clinically relevant gas embolism, advanced invasive monitoring (transesophageal Doppler sonography) cannot be recommended for clinical routine (grade B).

The incidence of gas embolism during pneumoperitoneum is estimated to be less than 0.6% (2 [282], 4 [122, 144]). Many case reports have detailed fatal or near-fatal coronary, cerebral, or other gas embolism (4 [102, 152, 172, 231, 238]). In more than 60% of cases, gas embolism occurred during the creation of a pneumoperitoneum.

The usual cause leading to gas embolism was the accidental displacement of a needle or trocar into a blood vessel. Similarly, any injury to the veins of parenchymal organs can result in direct gas flow into systemic circulation. CO_2 bubbles are capable of reaching the right heart (2b–5 [61, 66, 79, 267]). This is best detectable when patients are studied with transesophageal echocardiography (2b–5 [61, 66]. Transcranial Doppler has shown that CO_2 bubbles may even reach the cerebral circulation (4 [267]). Furthermore, gas emboli are able to escape from venous to arterial circulation through pulmonary arteriovenous shunts (5 [306]) or an open Foramen ovale (4 [190]).

Experimental animal studies have induced gas embolism by infusing air directly into a vein or by lacerating a large intraabdominal vein during a pneumoperitoneum (5 [66, 145, 147]). Increased IAP of more than 20 mmHg in connection with an insoluble gas (helium or argon) enhanced the risk of gas embolism during pneumoperitoneum (5 [146, 148, 251]), suggesting that caution should be exerted when laparoscopic surgery is performed close to large veins (5 [66]). Furthermore, the use of nitrious oxide for anesthesia may increase the risk of developing gas embolism during laparoscopy (4 [200, 242], 5 [147]).

In clinical practice, there are few technical options available to reduce the risk of gas embolism. It is therefore very important that especially the surgeon who creates the pneumoperitoneum be experienced in laparoscopic access techniques. It can be assumed that blunt trocars reduce the risk of accidental vessel puncture (1b [14]).

The most sensitive method to detect gas embolism is transesophageal Doppler monitoring (TEE) (2b [283, 316]). Simple measures to detect clinically relevant gas embolism are electrocardiogram (ECG) and $EtCO_2$ monitoring, which have low costs and require low personal effort. During surgery, decreasing $EtCO_2$ values of more than 3 mmHg could be related with gas embolism and should be clarified immediately (4 [52], 5 [147]). In case of injury of larger veins during abdominal insufflation, ECG and $EtCO_2$ should be closely monitored, especially when gases with low solubility are used. Because of the low incidence of gas embolism, special perioperative monitoring (e.g., TEE) is not indicated.

Choice of Insufflation Pressure

The panel recommends use of the lowest IAP allowing adequate exposure of the operative field rather than using a routine pressure (grade B). An IAP lower than 14 mmHg is considered safe in a healthy patient (grade A). Abdominal wall-lifting devices have no clinically relevant advantages compared to low-pressure (5–7 mmHg) pneumoperitoneum (grade B).

Normal and low laparoscopic insufflation pressure are defined as 12–15 and 5–7 mmHg, respectively. It is important to differentiate between the pressure at induction of the pneumoperitoneum and that during the operation. Initially, the IAP might be increased up to 15 mmHg to reduce the risk of trocar injuries. As already stated, IAP affects the physiology of heart, lung, and circulation. In order to attenuate these possible side effects of high IAP, the intravascular volume should be adequately filled preoperatively (1b [159]) and the insufflation pressure should be selected according to the planned laparoscopic procedure and the patient characteristics. In ASA I and II patients, a low-pressure pneumoper-

Table 2.3. Randomized clinic trials comparing low- and high-pressure pneumoperitoneum

Refrenence/ year	No. of patients/ASA	Pressures compared	Results	Conclusions
Wallace et al. [308]/1997	40/ASA I–II	7.5 vs 15 mmHg CO_2	CI↓, MAP↑, HR↓, end-tidal CO_2↑, pain scores↓	Cardiac changes in both groups similar; postop pain in low-pressure group reduced
Pier et al. [236]/1994	33/ASA I–II	8 vs 15 vs 19 mmHg CO_2	No differences in pain, analgesic use, FEV_1, or VC	Pressure has little effect on pain
Dexter et al. [63]/1999	20/ASA I–II	7 vs 15 mmHg CO_2	MAP↑, HR↑, SV↓, CO↓	High pressure reduces SV and CO more than low PP

All trials were performed on laparoscopic cholecystectomy
CO cardiac output, *HR* heart rate, *MAP* mean arterial pressure

itoneum reduces adverse effects on physiology without compromising laparoscopic feasibility (1b [63, 237, 309]) (Table 2.3). It remains questionable whether these physiologic changes are associated with clinically relevant side effects.

In older and compromised patients (ASA III and IV), the effects of a high vs low IAP have only been studied in nonrandomized clinical trials (2b [64, 83, 111], 4 [257]). In these studies, an elevated IAP (12–15 mmHg) showed considerable cardiac alterations. With the use of invasive monitoring, adequate volume loading, and vasoactive drug, it was possible to keep the hemodynamic and cardiac function stable. Therefore, in ASA III and IV patients, gasless or low-pressure laparoscopy could be alternatives, which should be further tested.

Warming and Humidifying of Insufflation Gas

Warming and humidifying insufflation gas is intended to decrease heat loss. However, compared to external heating devices, the clinical effects of warmed, humidified insufflation gas are minor (grade B). Data on its influence on postoperative pain are contradictory (grade A).

Perioperative hypothermia is related to increased catecholamine and cortisol levels leading to peripheral vasoconstriction and higher arterial blood pressures (2b [86]). Maintaining normothermia generally decreases postoperative cardiovascular morbidity (1b [84, 85]).

General and regional anesthesia essentially determine body core temperature by downregulation of the internal temperature level. Once vasoconstric-

Table 2.4. Pneumoperitoneum and hypothermia; randomized clinical trials

Reference/year	No. of patients, operations	Treatments	Temperature measurement	Pathophysiological results	Clinical results
Dietterle et al. [323]/1998	100 vs 100 operative or diagnostic pelviscopic procedures	Body vs room temperature, pressure and humidifying not mentioned	None	None	Gas warming lowers the intensity of diaphragm and shoulder pain and reduces the use of analgesics
Saad et al. [254]/2000	10 vs 10 lap. CCE	37 vs 21°C, CO_2 IAP 15 mm Hg, humidifying not mentioned	Esophageal thermotip catheter	No differences in body and intraabdominal temperatures and pain scores	Gas warming has no clinically relevant effect
Slim et al. [284]/1999	Double-blind 49 warm vs 51 cold gas, different upper abdominal lap. procedures	37 vs 21°C, CO_2 IAP 14 mmHg humidifying not mentioned, 20°RT	Subdiaphramatic thermometric probe	Subdiaphramatic temperature equal VAS score for shoulder tip pain higher in the warm group	Gas warming increases postoperative pain (VAS)
Mouton et al. [209]/1999	20 vs 20, lap. CCE	34–37 vs 21–25°C	Esophagus	No difference in core temperature; pain score less in humidified group	Humidified heated gas reduces pain but preserves no heat loss
Nelskylä et al. [215]/1999	18 vs 19 women, lap, HE end point: heart rate variability	37 vs 24°C, CO_2 IAP 12–14 mmHg, humidifying not mentioned	Tympanic and nasopharyngeal	Body core temperature decreases more in the warming group	Heating of insufflation gas does not prevent decrease of body temperature
Puttick et al. [243]/1999	15 vs 15, ASA I–II, lap. CCE	37 vs 21°C, CO_2, mean duration of surgery 32 min	Esophagus	Body core temperature decreases more in room temperature group	Higher cytokine levels in room temperature group; pain scores and consumption not different

Bäcklund et al. [11]/1998	13 vs 13 prolonged lap. Procedures >90 min	37 vs 21 °C, CO_2, IAP 11–15 mmHg, humidifing not mentioned	Swan–Ganz catheter	Core temperature and urine output higher in warm PP	Warm insufflation increases urine output
Ott et al. [226]/1998	Double-blinded multicenter (7) study, 72 women	36°C and humidified vs 23 °C, CO_2 IAP?	Endotracheal	Warm insufflation: less intraoperative hypothermia, postoperative stay and pain	Gas warming reduces lap. induced hypothermia
Korell et al. [162]/1996	50 vs 53 women, div. laparoscopic procedures	Heated CO_2 (30–32 °C) vs normal CO_2 (23–24 °C)	Flow therme	VAS scores reduced for shoulder and subdiaphragmatic pain	Warm CO_2 reduces postoperative pain
Semm et al. [277]/1994	30 vs 30 lap. pelviscopy	37 °C PP vs 21 °C PP, CO_2 IAP 12 mmHg, humidifying not mentioned	Intraabdominal and rectal probe	37 °C group shoulder tip pain; pain medication and incidence of tachycardia reduced	Warm insufflation reduces shoulder tip pain; pain medication

IAP intraabdominal pressure

tion has occurred, application of warming systems is less effective in compensating heat loss (1b [245]). Therefore, forced-air warmer systems should be applied before heat loss occurs. In contrast, warming and humidifying of the insufflation gas is less important than application of external warming devices before and during anesthesia.

Warming of the insufflation gas reduces postoperative intraperitoneal cytokine response (1b [243]) and reduces postoperative hospital stay (1b [226]) and pain (1b [226, 277, 323]) (Table 2.4). In contrast, a double-blind RCT found an increase in shoulder tip pain after warming the insufflation gas (1b [284]). Other groups found no clinically relevant effects of warming the insufflation gas (1b [198, 215, 254, 311]). Additional humidifying of warmed insufflation gas seems to reduce postoperative pain but has no heat-preserving effect in brief laparoscopic procedures (1b [209]). Since most of the studies have small sample sizes with possible type II error, no firm conclusions can be drawn. Given their possible small effects, the costs of these devices have also to be considered.

Abdominal Wall-Lifting Devices

Abdominal wall lifting as compared to capnoperitoneum results in less impairment of hemodynamic, pulmonary, and renal function (grade A). In ASA and I and II patients, the magnitude of these benefits is too small to recommend abdominal wall lifting (grade D). In patients with limited cardiac, pulmonary, or renal function, abdominal wall lifting combined with low-pressure pneumoperitoneum might be an alternative (grade C). Nevertheless, surgical handling and operative view were impaired in most surgical procedures (grade A).

Gasless laparoscopy has been developed to avoid the pathophysiological side effects of elevated IAP and CO2 insufflation, especially in patients with comorbities (ASA III and IV). However, most RCTs on gasless laparoscopy vs pneumoperitoneum have been performed in healthy ASA I and II patients (Tables 2.5, 2.6). In these patients, gasless laparoscopy results in a more stable hemodynamic and pulmonary function (1b [155, 220, 223]), a concomitant increase in urine output (1b [156, 223]), reduced hormonal stress responses (1b, [156, 223]), less postoperative pain (1b [131, 153]), and less drowsiness (1b [155, 178]). Contrarily, other RCTs found no differences in postoperative pain (1b [102]) and cardiorespiratory functions (1b [200]). Many surgeons encountered technical difficulties due to inadequate visualization (1b [136, 184, 200]). This led to high conversion rates in these trials, one of which was even terminated prematurely [136]. Although gasless laparoscopy may have hemodynamic and cardiovascular advantages in ASA III and IV patients, clinical trials in this group of patients have not been per-

Table 2.5. Randomized clinical trials comparing gasless to low- or high-pressure pneumoperitoneum

Reference/year	No. of patients, ASA	Pressures compared	Results in experimental group	Conclusions
Lubkan et al. [184]/2000	30, single blind	Laparolift vs 15 mmHg	VAS score for visualization less in gasless patients	Conventional PP provides better view
Ogihara et al. [223]/1999	12, ASA I–II	Gasless vs 13 mmHg CO_2 (Trendelenburg position 15–20° in both groups)	CO_2 group: pulmonary compliance↓, epinephrine↑, norepinephrine↑, dopamine↑, ADH↑, urine output↓	Gasless: lesser hormonal stress responses; better pulmonary function; higher urine output
Schulze et al. [271]/1999	17	Gasless vs 12 mmHg CO_2 (thPDA in both groups)	CO_2 group Blood flow↓, HR↑, MAP↑, CVP↑	No clinically relevant differences; CO_2 group less pain and more fatigue
Vezakis et al. [304]/1999	36, ASA I–II	Gasless vs 8 mmHg CO_2	No changes in postop pain and analgesic consumption	Shoulder pain more frequent
Cravello et al. [53]/1999	103	Gasless vs CO_2 PP (IAP unknown) (8 conversions)	No differences in complication pain medication hospital stay	Gasless technique needs further evaluation
Guido et al. [102]/1999	54	Gasless vs 15 mmHg CO_2	No differences in shoulder, pelvic, and periumbilical pain	Similar pain scores compared to conventional PP
Meijer et al. [200]/1997	20, ASA I–II	Gasless (AWL) +5 vs 15 mmHg CO_2	Gasless surgery lasted longer; CO, RR, and HR equal in both groups	AWL is not recommended for laparoscopic cholecystectomy; view impaired
Koivusalo et al. [156]/1997	30, ASA I–II	IAP 12–13 mmHg CO_2 vs gasless	CO_2 group: MAP↑, pulmonary compliance↓, urine output↓, U-NAG↑, intramucosal pH↓	Gasless: more stable in hemodynamics; protects renal and splanchnic ischemia
Koivusalo et al. [155]/1997	25, ASA I–II	IAP 12–15 mmHg CO_2 vs gasless AWL	Drowsiness shorter	Avoiding CO_2 reduces drowsiness
Johnson and Sibert [136]/1997	18	Gasless vs CO_2 PP (IAP not mentioned)	Increased technical difficulty – poor visualization	CO_2 PP is preferable for routine LTC

Table 2.5 (continued)

Reference/year	No. of patients, ASA	Pressures compared	Results in experimental group	Conclusions
Casati et al. [42]/1997	20	Gasless vs 12 mmHg CO_2	Better pulmonary compliance: oxigenation unchanged	Better lung compliance
Goldberg and Maurser [96]/1997	57	Gasless (laparolift) vs 15 mmHg CO_2; 9/28 converted because of inadequate exposure	Technically difficult; no differences in cardiopulmonary parameters and pain scores	No clinical benefit
Koivusalo et al. [154, 157]/1996	26, ASA I–II	IAP 12–15 mmHg vs laparolift	Maddox–Wing deviation higher in conventional PP group gasless: plasma renin activity↓, diuresis higher	Less right shoulder pain, nausea, and vomiting; smaller neuroendocrine responses; better renal function
Lindgren et al. [178]/1995	25, ASA I–II	PP (IAP 12–15 mmHg + CO_2) vs AWL	CO_2 group MAP↑, HR↑, pulmonary compliance↓	MAP lower; postoperative nausea, vomiting, and right shoulder pain less often

AWL abdominal wall lifting

Table 2.6. Cross-tabulation of current research on the effects of technical modifications of laparoscopy on pathophysiologic and medical outcomes

	Open-acces technique	Smaller trocars (3.5 mm)	Warmed insufflation gas	Helium, argon, or NO_2	Low-pressure laparoscopy	Gasless laparoscopy	Intraperitoneal anaesthetics
Pathophysioloical effects							
Circulatory	(0)	(0)	++ [277]	0 [28]	++ [63, 158, 236, 308]	++ [96, 156, 158, 178, 200, 220, 223]	(0)
Pulmonary	(0)	(0)	?	0 [28]	+ [236]	++ [155, 158, 200, 220, 223]	?
Renal/hepatic/intestinal	(0)	(0)	++ [11]		+	++ [156, 158, 223]	(0)
Immunological	(0)	?	++ [243]	(0)	(0)	+/0 [220]	?
Hormonal	(0)	?	?	(0)	(0)	++ [156, 223]	?
Body core temperature	(0)	(0)	+/0 [11, 215, 226, 243, 254]	?	(0)	+	(0)
Technical effects	++ [262]	– [276]	(0)	(0)	–/0 [63, 158, 308]	– [96, 136, 184, 200]	(0)
Clinical effects							
Intraoperative surgical incidents	+++ [30, 39, 50, 103, –219, –231]	+ [276]	+	(0)	(0)	?	(0)
Heart and lung complications	(0)	+ [276]	?	(0)	-10	+/0	?
Kidney and liver complications	(0)	(0)	?	(0)	-10	+/0	?
Pain	(0)	++ [22, 35, 276]	+/0 [162, 243, 254, 277, 284]	0 [236]	++ [258, 308]	+/0 [53, 102, 154, 178, 271, 304]	+++ [3, 40, 49, 55, 69, 70, 93, 211, 214, 227, 228, 293, 297, 309]

Table 2.6 (continued)

	Open-acces technique	Smaller trocars (3.5 mm)	Warmed insufflation gas	Helium, argon, or NO_2	Low-pressure laparoscopy	Gasless laparoscopy	Intraperitoneal anaesthetics
Drowsiness and fatigue	(0)	0 [276]	?	(0)	(0)	++ [155, 178, 271]	?
Cosmetic results	?	++ [276]	(0)	(0)	(0)	(0)	(0)
Incisional hernia	?	++	(0)	(0)	(0)	(0)	(0)
Adhesions	(0)	+	(0)	(0)	+	(0)	(0)
Infections	(0)	?	(0)	(0)	(0)	(0)	(0)

+++strong RCT evidence in favour of intervention; ++, some RCT evidence in favour of intervention; + non-RCT evidence in favour of intervention; +/0, conflicting RCT evidence in favour of intervention; 0 some RCT evidence for no effect of intervention; (0) non-RCT evidence for no effect of intervention; – non-RCT evidence against intervention; -/0 conflicting RCT evidence against intervention; – some RCT evidence against intervention; – strong RCT evidence against intervention; ? no valid research evidence available formed. Since gasless laparoscopy also requires excellent surgical expertise, its use should be restricted to certain subgroups of surgeons and patients.

Size of Access Devices

Smaller access devices (≤ 5 mm) in laparoscopy are only feasible in selected group of patients. The use of 2–5-mm instead of 5–10-mm access devices improves cosmetic result and postoperative pain marginally in laparoscopic cholecystectomy (grade A).

Although it has been assumed that smaller access devices may markedly improve the patients outcome of laparoscopic surgery, this has not been shown in valid RCTs (1b [22]). Merely modest advantages have been reported concerning a better cosmetic result (1b [276]) and less postoperative pain (1b [22, 35, 46, 276], 4 [192]) after laparoscopic cholecystectomy. Postoperative pulmonary function and fatigue were unchanged (1b [276]). Other clinical trials found a shorter convalescence by using smaller access devices in laparoscopic procedures (4 [192]). The incidence of postlaparoscopic incisional hernia is less than 1% (4 [165, 169]). Whether smaller access devices prevent incisional hernia has not been clarified (4 [165]). To prove a difference would require a large sample size and an extensive postoperative observation period. Currently, the general use of smaller trocars cannot be recommended due to difficulties in handling and reduced optical quality, especially when using smaller laparoscopes (1b [22, 276], 4 [168]). Recently published RCTs reported a reduction in postlaparoscopic pain when a radially expanding access device was compared to the conventional cutting trocar (1b [19, 80, 170, 318]). No data are available on other clinical effects.

Perioperative Aspects

Adhesions

Some laparoscopic procedures may cause less postoperative adhesions compared to their conventional counterparts (grade B). However, the specifics of a pneumoperitoneum (gas, pressure, temperature, and humidity) seem to have no major effect on the development of postsurgical adhesions (grade D).

Two RCTs found less postsurgical adhesions after laparoscopic compared to conventional surgery (2b [61, 62, 185]), but these studies have methodological flaws (small sample size, unclear allocation concealment, no intention-to-treat analysis, and losses to follow-up). Furthermore, since postsurgical adhesions are usually assessed by means of different scoring systems, it is difficult to compare the results of the trials in between or to rule out observer bias in these unblinded trials.

Pathophysiologically, a reduced peritoneal fibrinolytic activity seems to be the main cause for postsurgical adhesions (4 [116]). Experimental studies indicate that adhesion rates also depend on intraabdominal pressure (5 [317]) and the type of gas used (5 [132, 213]). However, one clinical RCT found no difference in peritoneal fibrinolytic activity in elective laparoscopic compared to conventional colorectal resections (1b [216]). It seems that the specifics of a pneumoperitoneum do not influence generally the peritoneal fibrinolytic activity and the development of postoperative adhesions. Therefore, avoiding local peritoneal damage seems to be the most significant factor to prevent postsurgical adhesions.

Pain, Nausea, and Vomiting

Pain after laparoscopic surgery is multifactorial and should be treated with a multimodal approach (grade A). Shape and size of access devices have to be considered (grade A). Low-pressure pneumoperitoneum, heated and humidified insufflation gas, incisional and intraperitoneal instillation of local anesthetics, intraperitoneal instillation of saline, and removal of residual gas all reduce postlaparoscopic pain (grade B). Inconclusive data and small effect sizes of singular approaches make it difficult to recommend these treatments in general (grade D). No evidence exists that the specifics of a pneumoperitoneum have any effect on postoperative nausea and vomiting.

Although pain after laparoscopic surgery is less severe and of shorter duration than that after open surgery, it still causes considerable discomfort and increased stress response. The etiology of postlaparoscopic pain can be classified into at least three aspects: visceral, incisional, and shoulder pain [21, 140, 300]. Although visceral pain may also depend on the extent of intraabdominal surgery, incisional pain is related to the number and size of access devices and also to the technique of incision closure and drainage. The origin of shoulder pain is only partly understood, but it is commonly assumed that the continual stretching of the peritoneum during and after the pneumoperitoneum is responsible. Clinically, incisional and deep abdominal pain dominate over shoulder pain. However, shoulder pain is specific for laparoscopic surgery. After different abdominal laparoscopic procedures, shoulder pain was noted in 30–50% of cases, which is significantly higher than after the corresponding open procedures (1b [43, 55, 174, 297]). It was suggested that shoulder tip pain is caused mechanically by stretching the diaphragmatic ligaments (1b [308]). The hypothesis of a chemical effect of the pneumoperitoneum with a decrease in intraperitoneal pH could not be verified [233].

The incidence of postoperative nausea and vomiting after laparoscopic procedures ranges from 10 to 60% [81, 201, 312]. After laparoscopic cholecystectomy, nausea and vomiting persisted up to 14 days in some patients [296]. The pathogenesis of postoperative nausea and vomiting is multifactorial, depending on anesthesia, surgery, gender, and perioperative administration of opioids. Several RCTs examined the influence of antiemetics and analgesics on postoperative nausea and vomiting, but this was beyond the scope of this guideline.

Within the past few years, various modifications of the pneumoperitoneum have been developed and clinically tested in order to reduce peritoneal pain after laparoscopic surgery [21, 310]. Here, we focus on those interventions that are directly related to the pneumoperitoneum, thus excluding oral, intravenous, or epidural drug administration and other nonlocal treatments. The intensity of postoperative pain varies largely among different cultures, settings, and individuals.

The following interventions were all shown in RCTs to effectively reduce pain after laparoscopy:
- Reducing IAP (1b [178, 236, 299, 308])
- Using other insufflation gases, such as N_2O, helium, or argon (1b [2, 180, 206, 236, 280])
- Lowering the insufflation rate (1b [16])
- Warming and humidifying the insufflation gas (1b [162, 209, 210, 226, Removal of residual intraabdominal gas at the end of operation (1b [86, 137, 298], 2b [4, 128], 4 [4, 128])
- Intraperitoneal instillation of fluids (1b [233])
- Intraperitoneal instillation of anesthetics (1b [3, 40, 49, 55, 69, 70, 93, 211, 214, 227, 228, 293, 297, 309])
- Reducing the size of trocars (1b [22, 35, 97, 166])
- Injecting anesthetics into the trocar sites (1b [3, 21, 257, 301])
- Omitting drains (which is beyond the scope of this recommendation, since it depends on the type of operation)

The intraperitoneal instillation of anesthetics is well studied. Most RCTs found a significant decrease in postlaparoscopic pain, including shoulder tip pain (1b [3, 40, 49, 55, 69, 70, 93, 211, 214, 227, 228, 293, 297, 309]), whereas other trials found no effect (1b [21, 87, 140, 244, 264, 270]). Since there is also evidence that postlaparoscopic instillation of normal saline or Ringers lactate reduces pain (1b [233]), it is important to distinguish between trials that used placebo controls from those that did not.

Humidifying the insufflation gas reduced postoperative pain in one trial (1b [211]) but increased it in another (1b [284]). After gasless laparoscopy, one double-blind RCT showed that shoulder tip pain (as primary end point) was more frequent than after conventional pneumoperitoneum (1b [304]), a second RCT with a smaller sample size reported the contrary (1b [154]), and a third found no difference (1b [101]).

On the basis of these contradictory results, the panel is not able to favor one treatment option over another. For the multifactorial pathogenesis of postlaparoscopic pain, we assume that a combined therapeutic approach is most effective ([20, 201]). Surgical awareness of this significant patient problem needs to be improved.

Pregnancy

Presupposing obstetrical consultation, laparoscopic procedures during pregnancy should be performed in the second trimester if possible (grade C). Perioperatively, maternal end-tidal CO_2 concentration and arterial blood gases must be monitored to control maternal hyperventilation and to prevent fetal acidosis (grade C). For the establishment of the pneumoperitoneum the open technique should be preferred (grade C). During laparoscopy intraabdominal pressure should be kept as low as possible and body positioning should be considered in order to avoid inferior vena cava compression by the uterus (grade C). Furthermore, pneumatic compression devices are recommended (grade D).

Surgery during pregnancy always carries an increased risk of fetal loss. Therefore, the indication for surgical intervention during pregnancy is generally limited to urgent situations such as acute appendicitis [268] or acute cholecystitis [99, 287]. The incidence of acute appendicitis and acute cholecystitis during pregnancy is similar to that of nongravid females and is estimated to be less than (0.1% (4 [195, 248]). The treatment of acute cholecystitis in gravid women should consider effective nonsurgical therapeutic options (4 [292]). Today, pregnancy should not be seen as an absolute but a relative contraindication for laparoscopic procedures. Because of increased risk for postoperative abortion in the first trimester and hindrance of operation due to the enlarged uterus, surgery during pregnancy should be performed during the second trimester (4 [190, 286]). During pregnancy laparoscopic compared to conventional surgery is preferred because of possibly less fetal impairment due to less postoperative analgetic requirements (4 [176]) and less postoperative maternal respiratory depression (4 [56]). However, increased intraabdominal pressure may decrease maternal respiratory compliance (5 [9, 58]), uterine blood flow (5 [58]), or preterm labor (5 [58, 96]). Furthermore, the use of carbon dioxide seems to increase fetal acidosis (5 [54, 59, 120]), to enhance the risk for fetal loss (4 [8]), and may lead to detrimental side effects if hyperventilation fails (5 [54]). Most of these concerns are based on experimental studies and case reports and should be confirmed by randomized controlled trials. Due to the low incidence of surgical interventions during pregnancy, these studies have to be performed as multicenter trials.

Intracranial Pressure

Increased IAP and head-down position increase intracranial pressure (ICP) (grade A). Therefore, elevated IAP, head-down position, and hypoventilation should be avoided (grade D). In patients with head injury or neurological disorders, perioperative monitoring of ICP should be considered (grade C). Gasless laparoscopy might be an alternative to prevent ICP peaks (grade D).

During pneumoperitoneum, IAP and head-down position increase ICP (5 [75, 117, 142, 207, 252], 4 [123]), enhance cerebral blood flow velocity (4 [1]), and diminish cerebrospinal fluid absorption (5 [106]). Elevated ICP values during laparoscopic surgery return to baseline after desufflation (5 [75]). There is no evidence that elevated ICP during pneumoperitoneum is clinically relevant.

Pathophysiological studies suggested that an increased intraabdominal pressure hinders venous drainage of the lumbar venous plexus followed by a decline in cerebrospinal fluid absorption during abdominal CO_2 insufflation (5 [105, 106]). Furthermore, it was hypothesized that this mechanical effect leads to an increase in ICP and a central nervous system response causing systemic hypertension (5 [15, 251]). However, the exact pathophysiology of increasing ICP during pneumoperitoneum remains unclear. Experimental and clinical studies showed that hemodynamic changes are directly related to the increase in ICP (4 [89, 123], 5 [142, 251]). Therefore, in patients with severe head injuries or conditions associated with elevated ICP, intraabdominal pressure should be as low as possible, sudden IAP peaks should be avoided, and intraoperative ICP monitoring should be considered (4 [127]). Furthermore, gasless laparoscopy could be an option to avoid the effects of IAP on ICP (5 [75, 117]).

The use of carbon dioxide as insufflation gas leads to hypercarbia and acidosis, which possibly influence the intracerebral circulation by vascular autoregulation. CO_2 increases ICP more than do helium and nitric oxide (5 [267]). Hypoventilation and hypercarbia increase ICP compared to hyperventilation and hypocarbia, but during acute elevations of ICP hyperventilation did not decrease ICP effectively (5 [251]). The insufflation gas has fewer effects on ICP than on IAP (4 [74], 5 [60]).

Abdominal Trauma

There are no prospective studies evaluating the specifics of a pneumoperitoneum (type of gas, IAP, and temperature) in patients with blunt or penetrating abdominal trauma (grade D).

Laparoscopy is used as a diagnostic tool in hemodynamically stable patients after blunt or penetrating trauma in order to detect those injuries that require laparotomy or laparoscopic repair (2b [71, 77, 285]). In rare cases of penetrating trauma, the establishment of a pneumoperitoneum led to an insufflation of injured organs or cavities ([119]). Nevertheless, the panel agrees that there is no reason to contraindicate pneumoperitoneum in stable trauma patients.

The use of different intraabdominal pressures, different types of gas, or even gasless laparoscopy has not been evaluated in patients with blunt or penetrating abdominal trauma. Thus, no recommendations are reasonably justifiable. However, one clinical RCT tested which access technique is faster and safer, and found advantages for the closed technique (1b [262]), thus refuting data from nontrauma surgery.

Discussion

After a 2-year break, the EAES has continued its guideline activities, now on an even more evidence-based level and with much more advanced preparation than in the past. We believe that the result of this endeavor can be considered to be a milestone in the societys responsibility of being a bridge-tender between primary research and clinical practice and vice versa.

We hope that the reader understands the importance of guideline methodology. In a European survey 2 years ago, many members complained that the EAES consensus panels had always been consisting of the same clique of people. The panel for this guideline still contains many well-known names from the EAES simply because the number of experts in endoscopic surgery is limited, as are resources for guideline development. Wherever interdisciplinary coworking was necessary, experts from other fields were invited to join the panel, although this guideline could have received further benefit from the input of a pediatric surgeon.

The scope of this guideline is broad since the pneumoperitoneum is the key issue in laparoscopic surgery. However, it is impossible for a guideline to answer all relevant points in detail or to discuss the role of the pneumoperitoneum separately for every disease entity. The panel tried to formulate the statements as concise as possible. However, for those issues, for which no strong evidence was found, it was often impossible to recommend any specific option. Those who find such broad statements disappointing should remember that the panel can only judge on the basis of clinical experience and published evidence. Often, a treatment is widely held to be evidence based, although not a single study has ever been performed.

Therefore, one of our aims was to define some implications for future research. A fair amount of RCTs were retrievable to answer the various issues. We consider it unlikely that important studies were missed by our literature searches because we combined various techniques to capture all relevant studies. However, the available studies mostly focused on those questions which can be answered already using a small sample size and short-term observation. Some other statements did not receive grade A because the existing RCTs had methodological flaws. What is of general concern is that such a large proportion of trials assessed pathophysiological rather than clinical outcomes. These trials, albeit randomized, are usually insufficient to answer the clinical questions we had posed. Therefore, the plea for clinically relevant RCTs cannot be reiterated too often. It is a future task to check whether the recommendations have to be modified on the basis of new data.

Developing guidelines is only worthwhile if they are used clinically. Guideline use hinges upon guideline awareness and knowledge. Therefore, the format and dissemination of the current guideline goes beyond simple publication. Since guidelines created on a European level cannot address the local circumstances in every European country or even hospital, the EAES scientific committee recommends the use of the current guideline as a basis for a locally adapted and translated guideline, which could then be implemented at any given level.

The most important factors that have to be considered before adapting this guideline for local use are individual surgical expertise and health care setting. Some surgical techniques that are discussed or even recommended here are probably not practical or affordable for every European surgeon. This is why we decided not to include cost comparisons in this guideline.

References

1. Abe K, Hashimoto N, Taniguchi A, Yoshiya I (1998) Middle cerebral artery blood flow velocity during laparoscopic surgery in head-down position. Surg Laparosc Endosc 8:1–4
2. Aitola P, Airo I, Kaukinen S, Ylitalo P (1998) Comparison of N_2O and CO_2 pneumoperitoneums during laparoscopic cholecystectomy with special reference to postoperative pain. Surg Laparosc Endosc 8:140–144
3. Alexander DJ, Ngoi SS, Lee L, So J, Mak K, Chan S, Goh PM (1996) Randomized trial of periportal peritoneal bupivacaine for pain relief after laparoscopic cholecystectomy. Br J Surg 83:1223–1225
4. Alexander JI, Hull MGR (1987) Abdominal pain after laparoscopy: the value of a gas drain. Br J Obstet Gynaecol 94:267–269
5. Alijani A, Hanna GB, Cuschieri A (2001) Cardiac function during conventional pneumoperitoneum versus mechanical abdominal wall lift in laparoscopic cholecystectomy [abstract] Br J Surg 88:743–744
6. Alishahi S, Francis N, Crofts S, Duncan L, Bickel A, Cuschieri A (2001) Central and peripheral adverse hemodynamic changes during laparoscopic surgery and their reversal with a novel intermittent sequential pneumatic compression device. Ann Surg 233:176–182
7. Altarac S, Janetschek G, Eder E, Bartsch G (1996) Pneumothorax complicating laparoscopic ureterolysis. J Laparoendosc Surg 6:193–196
8. Amos JD, Schorr SJ, Norman PF, Poole GV, Thomae KR, Mancino AT, Hall TJ, Scott-Conner CEH (1996) Laparoscopy during pregnancy. Am J Surg 171:435–437
9. Andreoli M, Servakov M, Meyers P, Mann Jr. WJ (1999) Laparoscopic surgery during pregnancy. J Am Assoc Gynecol Laparosc 6:229–233
10. Baca I, Schneider B, Koehler T, Misselwitz F, Zehle A, Muehe F (1997) Thromboembolieprophylaxe bei minimal-invasiven Eingriffen und kurzstationärer Behandlung. Ergebnisse einer, multi-centrischen, prospektiven, randomisierten, kontrollierten Studie mit einem niedermolekularen Heparin. Chirurg 68:1275–1280

11. Bäcklund M, Kellokumpu I, Scheinin T, von Smitten K, Tikkanen I, Lindgren L (1998) Effect of temperature of insufflated CO_2 during and after prolonged laparoscopic surgery. Surg Endosc 12:1126–1130
12. Beebe DS, McNevin MP, Crain JM, Letourneau JG, Belani KG, Abrams JA, Goodale RL (1993) Evidence of venous stasis after abdominal insufflation for laparoscopic cholecystectomy. Surg Gynecol Obstet 176:443–447
13. Bellón JM, Manzano L, Bernardos L, Ga-Honduvilla N, Larrad A, Buján J, Alvarez-Mon M (1997) Cytokine levels after open and laparoscopic cholecystectomy. Eur Surg Res 29:27–34
14. Bemelman WA, Dunker MS, Busch OR, Den Boer KT, de Wit LT, Gouma DJ (2000) Efficacy of establishment of pneumoperitoneum with the Veress needle, Hasson trocar, and modified blunt trocar (TrocDoc): a randomized study. J Laparoendosc Adv Surg Tech A 10:325–330
15. Ben-Haim M, Mandeli J, Friedman RL, Rosenthal RJ (2000) Mechanisms of systemic hypertension during acute elevation of intraabdominal pressure. J Surg Res 91:101–105
16. Berberoglu M, Dilek ON, Ercan F, Kati I, Özmen M (1998) The effect of CO_2 insufflation rate on the postlaparoscopic shoulder pain. J Laparoendosc Adv Surg Tech A 8:273–277
17. Berggren U, Gordh T, Grama D, Haglund U, Rastad J, Arvidsson D (1994) Laparoscopic versus open cholecystectomy: hospitalization, sick leave, analgesia and trauma responses. Br J Surg 81:1362–1365
18. Bessa X, Castells A, Lacy AM, Elizalde I, Delgado S, Boix L, Pinoi V, Pellisé M, García-Valdecasas JC, Piqué JM (2001) Laparoscopic-assisted vs open colectomy for colorectal cancer: influence on neoplastic cell mobilization. J Gastrointest Surg 5:66–73
19. Bhoyrul S, Payne J, Stees B, Swanstrom L, Way LW (2000) A randomized prospective study of radially expanding trocars in laparoscopic surgery. J Gastrointest Surg 4:392–397
20. Bisgaard T, Kehlet H, Rosenberg J (2001) Pain and convalescence after laparoscopic cholecystectomy. Eur J Surg 167:84–96
21. Bisgaard T, Klarskov B, Kristiansen VB, Callesen T, Schulze S, Kehlet H, Rosenberg J (1999) Multi-regional local anesthetic in-filtration during laparoscopic cholecystectomy in patients receiving prophylactic multi-modal analgesia: a randomized, double- blinded, placebo-controlled study. Anesth Analg 89:1017–1024
22. Bisgaard T, Klarskov B, Trap R, Kehlet H, Rosenberg J (2000) Pain after microlaparoscopic cholecystectomy. A randomized double-blind controlled study. Surg Endosc 14:340–344
23. Bloechle C, Emmermann A, Strate T, Scheurlen UJ, Schneider C, Achilles E, Wolf M, Mack D, Zornig C, Broelsch CE (1998) Laparoscopic vs open repair of gastric perforation and abdominal lavage of associated peritonitis in pigs. Surg Endosc 12:212–218
24. Bloechle C, Emmermann A, Treu H, Achilles E, Mack D, Zornig C, Broelsch CE (1995) Effect of a pneumoperitoneum on the extent and severity of peritonitis induced by gastric ulcer perforation in the rat. Surg Endosc 9:898–901
25. Bloechle C, Kluth D, Holstein AF, Emmermann A, Strate T, Zomig C, Izbicki JR (1999) A pneumoperitoneum perpetuates severe damage to the ultrastructural integrity of parietal peritoneum in gastric perforation-induced peritonitis in rats. Surg Endosc 13:683–688
26. Böhm B, Junghans T, Neudecker J, Schwenk W (1999) Leber und Nierenfunktion nach laparoskopischer und konventioneller Resektion kolorektaler Tumore—Ergebnisse aus einer prospektiv randomisierten Studie. Visceralchirurgie 34:20–24
27. Böhm B, Schwenk W, Junghans T (2000) Das pneumoperitoneum. Springer, Berlin Heidelberg New York pp 42–46
28. Bongard FS, Pianim NA, Leighton TA, Dubecz S, Davis IP, Lippmann M, Klein S, Liu SY (1993) Helium insufflation for laparoscopic operation. Surg Gynecol Obstet 177:140–146
29. Bonjer HJ, Hazebroek EJ, Kazemier G, Giu rida MC, Meijer WS, Lange JF (1997) Open versus closed establishment of pneumoperitoneum in laparoscopic surgery. Br J Surg 84:599–602
30. Borgatta L, Gruss L, Barad D, Kaali SG (1990) Direct trocar insertion vs Verres needle use for laparoscopic sterilization. J Reprod Med 35:891–894

31. Bounameaux H, Didier D, Polat O, Desmarais S, de Moerloose P, Huber O (1997) Antithrombotic prophylaxis in patients undergoing laparoscopic cholecystectomy. Thromb Res 86:271–273

32. Bouvy ND, Giu rida MC, Tseng LN, Steyerberg EW, Marquet RL, Jeekel H, Bonjer HJ (1998) Effects of carbon dioxide pneumoperitoneum, air pneumoperitoneum, and gasless laparoscopy on body weight and tumor growth. Arch Surg 133:652–656

33. Bouvy ND, Marquet RL, Jeekel H, Bonjer HJ (1996) Impact of gas(less) laparoscopy and laparotomy on peritoneal tumor growth and abdominal wall metastases. Ann Surg 224:694–701

34. Braumann C, Jacobi CA, Ordemann J, Stößlein R, Müller JW (2000) Einfluß der intraoperativen, intravenösen und intraperitonealen Gabe von Taurolidin/Heparin in der laparoskopischen Chirurgie auf das intra – und – xtraperitoneale Tumorwachstum. In: Encke A (ed) Chirurgisches Forum 2000 für experimentelle und klinische Forschung, Band, pp 29

35. Bresadola F, Pasqualucci A, Donini A, Chiarandini P, Anania G, Terrosu G, Sistu MA, Pasetto A (1999) Elective transumbilical compared with standard laparoscopic cholecystectomy. Eur J Surg 165:29–34

36. Bruce DM, Smith M, Walker CB, Heys SD, Binnie NR, Gough DB, Broom J, Eremin O (1999) Minimal access surgery for cholelithiasis induces an attenuated acute phase response. Am J Surg 178:232–234

37. Buchmann P, Christen D, Moll C, Flury R, Sartoretti C (1996) Tumorzellen in der peritonealen Spülflüssigkeit bei konventionellen und laparoskopischen Operationen wegen kolorektaler Karzinome. Swiss Surg Suppl 4:45–49

38. Byrne J, Timon D, Armstrong C, Horgan PG, Quill DS (1994) A comparison of analgesic requitements and pulmonary function in open versus laparoscopic cholecystectomy. Minimally Invasive Ther 3:3–6

39. Byron JW, Markenson G, Miyazawa K (1993) A randomized comparison of Verres needle and direct trocar insertion for laparoscopy. Surg Gynecol Obstet 177:259–262

40. Callesen T, Hjort D, Mogensen T, Schouenborg L, Nielsen D, Reventlid H, Kehlet H (1999) Combined field block and i.p. instillation of ropivacaine for pain management after laparoscopic sterilization. Br J Anaesth 82:586–590

41. Caprini JA, Arcelus JI, Laubach M, Size G, Ho man KN, Coats RW, Blattner S (1995) Postoperative hypercoagulability and deepvein thrombosis after taparoscopic cholecystectomy. Surg Endosc 9:304–309

42. Casati A, Valentini G, Ferrari S, Senatore R, Zangrillo A, Torri G(1997) Cardiorespiratory changes during gynaecological laparoscopy by abdominal wall elevation: comparison with carbon dioxide pneumoperitoneum. Br J Anaesth 78:51–54

43. Cason CL, Seidel SL, Bushmaier M (1996) Recovery from laparoscopic cholecystectomy procedures. AORN J 63:1099–1116

44. Chandler JG, Corson SL, Way LW (2001) Three spectra of laparoscopic entry access injuries. J Am Coll Surg 192:478–491

45. Chaudhary D, Verma GR, Gupta R, Bose SM, Ganguly NK(1999) Comparative evaluation of the inflammatory mediators in patients undergoing laparoscopic versus conventional cholecy stectomy. Aust N Z J Surg 69:369–372

46. Cheah WK, Lenzi JE, So JBY, Kum CK, Goh PMY (2001) Randomized trial of needlescopic versus laparoscopic cholecystectomy. Br J Surg 88:45–47

47. Chekan EG, Nataraj C, Clary EM, Haywati TZ, Brody FJ, Stamat JC, Fina MC, Eubanks WS, Westcott CJ (1999) Intraperitoneal immunity and pneumoperitoneum. Surg Endosc 13:1135–1138

48. Chumillas S, Ponce JL, Delgado F, Viciano V (1998) Pulmonary function and complications after laparoscopic cholecystectomy. Eur J Surg 164:433–437

49. Chundrigar T, Hedges AR, Morris R, Stamatakis JD (1993) Intraperitoneal bupivacaine for effective pain relief after laparoscopic cholecystectomy. Ann R Coll Surg England 75:437–439

50. Cogliandolo A, Manganaro T, Saitta FP, Micali B (1998) Blind versus open approach to laparoscopic cholecystectomy: a randomized study. Surg Laparosc Endosc 8:353–355

51. Coskun I, Hatipoglu AR, Topaloglu A, Yoruk Y, Yalcinkaya S, Caglar T (2000) Laparoscopic versus open cholecystectomy: effect on pulmonary function tests. Hepatogastroenterology 47:341–342

52. Cottin V, Delafosse B, Viale JP (1996) Gas embolism during laparoscopy: a report of seven cases in patients with previous abdominal surgical history. Surg Endosc 10:166–169

53. Cravello L, DErcole C, Roger V, Samson D, Blanc B (1999) Laparoscopic surgery in gynecology: randomized prospective study comparing pneumoperitoneum and abdominal wall suspension. Eur J Obstet Gynecol Reprod Biol 83:9–14

54. Cruz AM, Southerland LC, Duke T, Townsend HG, Ferguson JG, Crone LA (1996) Intraabdominal carbon dioxide insufflation in the pregnant ewe. Uterine blood flow, intraamniotic pressure, and cardiopulmonary effects. Anesthesiology 85:1395–1402

55. Cunniffe MG, McAnena OJ, Dar MA, Calleary J, Flynn N (1998) A prospective randomized trial of intraoperative bupivacaine irrigation for management of shoulder-tip pain following laparoscopy. Am J Surg 176:258–261

56. Curet MJ, Allen D, Joslo RK, Pitcher DE, Curet LB, Miscall BG, Zucker KA (1996) Laparoscopy during pregnancy. Arch Surg 131:546–551

57. Curet MJ, Putrakul K, Pitcher DE, Joslo RK, Zucker KA (2000) Laparoscopically assisted colon resection for colon carcinoma: perioperative results and long-term outcome. Surg Endosc 14:1062–1066

58. Curet MJ, Vogt DA, Schob O, Quails C, Izquierdto LA, Zucker KA (1996) Effects of CO_2 pneumoperitoneum in pregnant ewes. J Surg Res 63:339–344

59. Curet MJ, Weber DM, Sae A, Lopez J (2001) Effects of helium pneumoperitoneum in pregnant ewes. Surg Endosc 15:710–714

60. De Cosmo G, Iannace E, Primieri P, Valente MR, Proietti R, Matteis M, Silvestrini M (2001) Changes in cerebral hemodynamics during laparoscopic cholecystectomy. Neurol Res 21:658–660

61. Derouin M, Couture P, Boudreault D, Girard D, Gravel D (1996) Detection of gas embolism by transesophageal echocardiography during laparoscopic cholecystectomy. Anesth Analg 82:119–124

62. de Wilde RL (1991) Goodbye to late bowel obstruction after appendicectomy. Lancet 338:1012

63. Dexter SP, Vucevic M, Gibson J, McMahon MJ (1999) Hemodynamic consequences of high- and low-pressure capnoperitoneum during laparoscopic cholecystectomy. Surg Endosc 13:376–381

64. Dhoste K, Lacoste L, Karayan J, Lehuede MS, Thomas D, Fusciardi J (1996) Haemodynamic and ventilatory changes during laparoscopic cholecystectomy in elderly ASA III patients. Can J Anaesth 43:783–788

65. Dion YM, Levesque C, Doillon CJ (1995) Experimental carbon dioxide pulmonary embolization after vena cava laceration under pneumoperitoneum. Surg Endosc 9:1065–1069

66. Di Vita G, Sciume C, Lauria Lauria G, Stella C, Raimondo D, Leo P (2000) Il sistema fibrinolitico dopo colecistectomia laparoscopica. Minerva Chir 55:587–592

67. Drummond GB, Martin LV (1978) Pressure–volume relationships in the lung during laparoscopy. Br J Anaesth 50:261–270

68. Eleftheriadis E, Kotzampassi K, Botsios D, Tzartinoglou E, Farmakis H, Dadoukis J (1996) Splanchnic ischemia during laparoscopic cholecystectomy. Surg Endosc 10:324–326

69. Elhakim M, Amine H, Kamel S, Saad F (2000) Effects of intraperitoneal lidocaine combined with intravenous or intraperitoneal tenoxicam on pain relief and bowel recovery after laparoscopic cholecystectomy. Acta Anaesthesiol Scand 44:929–933

70. Elhakim M, Elkott M, Ali NM, Tahoun HM (2000) Intraperitoneal lidocaine for postoperative pain after laparoscopy. Acta Anaesthesiol Scand 44:280–284

71. Elliott DC, Rodriguez A, Moncure M, Myers RA, Shillinglaw W, Davis F, Goldberg A, Mitchell K, McRitchie D (1998) The accuracy of diagnostic laparoscopy in trauma patients: a prospective, controlled study. Int Surg 83:294–298

72. Ellström M, Bengtsson A, Tylman M, Haeger M, Olsson JH, Hahlin M (1996) Evaluation of tissue trauma after laparoscopic and abdominal hysterectomy: measurements of neutrophil activation and release of interteukin-6, cortisol, and C-reactive protein. J Am Coll Surg 182:423–430

73. Ellström M, Olsén MF, Olsson JH, Nordberg G, Bengtsson A, Hahlin M (1998) Pain and pulmonary function following laparoscopic and abdominal hysterectomy: a randomized study. Acta Obstet Gynecol Scand 77:923–928

74. Emeljanov SI, Fedenko W, Levite EM, Panfilov SA, Bobrinskaya IG, Fedorov AV, Matveev NL, Evdoshenko W, Luosev SV, Bokarev W, Musaeva SR (1998) Pneumoperitoneum risk prognosis and correction of venous circulation disturbances in laparoscopic surgery. A pilot study. Surg Endosc 12:1224–1231

75. Este-McDonald JR, Josephs LG, Birkett DH, Hirsch EF (1995) Changes in intracranial pressure associated with apneumic retractors. Arch Surg 130:362–366

76. Evasovich MR, Clark TC, Horattas MC, Holda S, Treen L (1996) Does pneumoperitoneum during laparoscopy increase bacterial translocation? Surg Endosc 10:1176–1179

77. Fabian TC, Croce MA, Stewart RM, Pritchard FE, Minard G, Kudsk KA (1993) A prospective analysis of diagnostic laparoscopy in trauma. Ann Surg 217:557–565

78. Fahy BG, Hasnain JU, Flowers JL, Plotkin JS, Odonkor P, Ferguson MK (1999) Transesophageal echocardiographic detection of gas embolism and cardiac valvular dysfunction during laparoscopic nephrectomy. Anesth Analg 88:500–504

79. Feig BW, Berger DH, Dougherty TB, Dupuis JF, Hsi B, Hickey RC, Ota DM (1994) Pharmacologic intervention can reestablish baseline hemodynamic parameters during laparoscopy. Surgery 116:733–741

80. Feste JR, Bojahr B, Turner DJ (2000) Randomized trial comparing a radially expandable needle system with cutting trocars. JSLS 4:11–45

81. Fleisher LA, Yee K, Lillemoe KD, Talamini MA, Yeo CJ, Heath R, Bass E, Snyder DS, Parker SD (1999) Is outpatient laparoscopic cholecystectomy safe and cost-effective? A model to study transition of care. Anesthesiology 90:1746–1755

82. Fleming RY, Dougherty TB, Feig BW (1997) The safety of helium for abdominal insufflation. Surg Endosc 11:230–234

83. Frank SM, Fleisher LA, Breslow MJ, Higgins MS, Olson KF, Kelly S, Beattie C (1997) Perioperative maintenance of normothermia reduces the incidence of morbid cardiac events. A randomized clinical trial. J Am Med Assoc 277:1127–1134

84. Frank SM, Higgins MS, Breslow MJ, Fleisher LA, Gorman RB, Sitzmann JV, Ra H, Beattie C (1995) The catecholamine, cortisol, and hemodynamic responses to mild perioperative hypothermia. A randomized clinical trial. Anesthesiology 82:83–93

85. Frank SM, Higgins MS, Fleisher LA, Sitzmann JV, Ra H, Breslow MJ (1997) Adrenergic, respiratory, and cardiovascular effects of core cooling in humans. Am J Physiol 272:R557–R562

86. Fredman B, Jedeikin R, Olsfanger D, Flor P, Gruzman A (1994) Residual pneumoperitoneum: a cause of postoperative pain after laparoscopic cholecystectomy. Anesth Analg 79:152–154

87. Fuhrer Y, Charpentier C, Boulanger G, Menu N, Grosdidier G, Laxenaire MC (1996) Analgésie après cholécystectomie par voie coelioscopique par administration intrapéritonéale de bupivacaine. Ann Fr Anesth Reanim 15:128–134

88. Fujii Y, Tanaka H, Tsuruoka S, Toyooka H, Amaha K (1994) Middle cerebral arterial blood flow velocity increases during laparoscopic cholecystectomy. Anesth Analg 78:80–83

89. Fukushima R, Kawamura YJ, Saito H, Saito Y, Hashiguchi Y, Sawada T, Muto T (1996) Interleukin-6 and stress hormone responses after uncomplicated gasless laparoscopic-assisted and open sigmoid colectomy. Dis Colon Rectum 39:S29–S34

90. Galizia G, Prizio G, Lieto E, Castellano P, Pelosio L, Imperatore V, Ferrara A, Pignatelli C (2001) Hemodynamic and pulmonary changes during open, carbon dioxide pneumoperitoneum and abdominal wall-lifting cholecystectomy. Surg Endosc 15:477–483

91. Gándara MV, de Vega DS, Escri N, Olmedilla C, Pèrez-Mencia MT, Zueras R, López A (1997) Alterationes respiratorias durante la colecistectomía laparoscópica. Estudio comparativo de tres técnicas anestésicas. Rev Esp Anestesiol Reanim 44:177–181

92. Gehring H, Kuhmann K, Klotz KF, Ocklitz E, Roth-lsigkeit A, Sedemund-Adib B, Schmucker P (1998) Effects of propofol vs isoflurane on respiratory gas exchange during laparoscopic cholecystectomy. Acta Anaesthesiol Scand 42:189–194

93. Gharaibeh KL, Al-Jaberi TM (2000) Bupivacaine instillation into gallbladder bed after laparoscopic cholecystectomy: does it decrease shoulder pain? J Laparoendosc Adv Surg Tech A 10:137–141

94. Giraudo G, Brachet Contul R, Caccetta M, Morino M, Glasgow RE, Visser BC, Harris HW, Patti MG, Kilpatrick SJ, Mulvihill SJ (2001) Gasless laparoscopy could avoid alterations in hepatic function. Surg Endosc 15:741–746

95. Glasgow RE, Visser BC, Harris HW, Patti MG, Kilpatrick SJ, Mulvihill SJ (1998) Changing management of gallstone disease during pregnancy. Surg Endosc 12:241–246

96. Goldberg JM, Maurer WG (1997) A randomized comparison of gasless laparoscopy and CO_2 pneumoperitoneum. Obstet Gynecol 90:416–420

97. Golder M, Rhodes M (1998) Prospective randomized trial of 5- and 10-mm epigastric ports in laparoscopic cholecystectomy. Br J Surg 85:1066–1067

98. Goodale RL, Beebe DS, McNevin MP, Boyle M, Letourneau JG, Abrams JH, Cerra FB (1993) Hemodynamic, respiratory, and metabolic effects of laparoscopic cholecystectomy. Am J Surg 166:533–537

99. Gouldman JW, Sticca RP, Rippon MB, McAlhany Jr JC (1998) Laparoscopic cholecystectomy in pregnancy. Am Surg 64:93–98

100. Greif WM, Forse RA (1998) Hemodynamic effects of the laparoscopic pneumopentoneum during sepsis in a porcine endotoxic shock model. Ann Surg 227:474–480

101. Gueugniaud PY, Bertin-Maghit M, Petit P, Muchada R (1995) Diagnostic par surveillance du débit aortique et du capnogramme d'un arrét circulatoire par embolie de CO_2 au cours de la chirurgie laparoscopique. Ann Fr Anesth Reanim 14:417–420

102. Guido RS, Brooks K, McKenzie R, Gruss J, Krohn MA (1998) A randomized, prospective comparison of pain after gasless laparoscopy and traditional laparoscopy. J Am Assoc Gynecol Laparosc 5:148–153

103. Gulla N, Patriti A, Lazzarini F, Tristaino B (2000) Accesso anteriore transperitoneale nella surrenalectomia videolaparoscopica. Minerva Chir 55:371–375

104. Gurtner GC, Robertson CS, Chung SC, Ling TK, Ip SM, Li AK (1995) Effect of carbon dioxide pneumopentoneum on bacteraemia and endotoxaemia in an animal model of peritonitis. Br J Surg 82:844–848

105. Halverson A, Buchanan R, Jacobs L, Shayani V, Hunt T, Riedel C, Sackier J (1998) Evaluation of mechanism of increased intracranial pressure with insufflation. Surg Endosc 12:266–269

106. Halverson AL, Barrett WL, Iglesias AR, Lee WT, Garber SM, Sackier JM (1999) Decreased cerebrospinal fluid absorption during abdominal insufflation. Surg Endosc 13:797–800

107. Harris SN, Ballantyne GH, Luther MA, Perrino AC (1996) Alterations of cardiovascular performance during laparoscopic colectomy: a combined hemodynamic and echocardiographic analysis. Anesth Analg 83:482–487

108. Hashizume M, Sugimachi K (1997) Needle and trocar injury during laparoscopic surgery in Japan. Surg Endosc 11:1198–1201

109. Hasson HM (1971) A modified instrument and method for laparoscopy. Am J Obstet Gynecol 110:886–870

110. Hein HAT, Joshi GP, Ramsay MAE, Fox LG, Gawey BJ, Hellman CL, Arnold JC (1997) Hemodynamic changes during laparoscopic cholecystectomy in patients with severe cardiac disease. J Clin Anesth 9:261–265

111. Hendolin HI, Pääkönen ME, Alhava EM, Tarvainen R, Kemppinen T, Lahtinen P (2000) Laparoscopic or open cholecystectomy: a prospective randomised trial to compare postoperative pain, pulmonary function, and stress response. Eur J Surg 166:394–399

112. Hewitt PM, Ip SM, Kwok SPY, Somers SS, Li K, Leung KL, Lau WY, Li AKC (1998) Laparoscopic-assisted vs open surgery for colorectal cancer: comparative study of immune effects. Dis Colon Rectum 41:901–909
113. Hirvonen EA, Nuutinen LS, Kauko M (1995) Hemodynamic changes due to Trendelenburg positioning and pneumoperitoneum during laparoscopic hysterectomy. Acta Anaesthesiol Scand 39:949–955
114. Hirvonen EA, Nuutinen LS, Vuolteenaho O (1997) Hormonal responses and cardiac filling pressures in head-up or head-down position and pneumoperitoneum in patients undergoing operative laparoscopy. Br J Anaesth 78:128–133
115. Hirvonen EA, Poikolainen EO, Pääkkönen ME, Nuutinen LS(2000) The adverse hemodynamic effects of anesthesia, head-up tilt, and carbon dioxide pneumoperitoneum during laparoscopic cholecystectomy. Surg Endosc 14:272–277
116. Holmdahl L, Eriksson E, Eriksson Bl, Risberg B (1998) Depression of peritoneal fibrinolysis during operation is a local response to trauma. Surgery 123:539–544
117. Holthausen UH, Razek TSA, Hinchey EJ, Oung CM, Chiu RC-J, Nagelschmidt M, Troidl H (1997) Monitoring des intrakraniellen Druckes im Modell eines "Schädeltraumas": Kohlendioxid (CO_2)-Pneumoperitoneum versus Laparolift-Verfahren. Langenbecks Arch Chir Kongressbd 114:257–260
118. Horzic M, Korusic A, Bunoza D, Maric K (1998) The influence of increased intra-abdominal pressure on blood coagulation values. Hepatogastroenterology 45:1519–1521
119. Howells GA, Uzieblo MR, Bair H, Boyer MD (2000) Tension pneumopericardium during laparoscopy for trauma. Surg Laparosc Endosc Percutan Tech 10:44–46
120. Hunter JG, Swanstrom L, Thornburg K (1995) Carbon dioxide pneumoperitoneum induces fetal acidosis in a pregnant ewe model. Surg Endosc 9:272–279
121. Hynes SR, Marshall RL (1992) Venous gas embolism during gynaecological laparoscopy. Can J Anaesth 39:748–749
122. Ido K, Suzuki T, Kimura K, Taniguchi Y, Kawamoto C, Isoda N, Nagamine N, Ioka T, Kumagai M, Hirayama Y (1995) Lower-extremity venous stasis during laparoscopic cholecystectomy as assessed using color Doppler ultrasound. Surg Endosc 9:310–313
123. Irgau I, Koyfman Y, Tikellis JI (1995) Elective intraoperative intracranial pressure monitoring during laparoscopic cholecystectomy. Arch Surg 130:1011–1013
124. Ishizaki Y, Bandai Y, Shimomura K, Abe H, Ohtomo Y, Idezuki Y (1993) Safe intraabdominal pressure of carbon dioxide pneumoperitoneum during laparoscopic surgery. Surgery 114:549–554
125. Ishizuka B, Kuribayashi Y, Kobayashi Y, Hamada N, Abe Y, Amemiya A, Aoki T, Satoh T (2000) Stress response during laparoscopy with CO_2 insufflation and with mechanical elevation of the abdominal wall. J Am Assoc Gynecol Laparosc 3:363–371
126. Iwase K, Takenaka H, Yagura A, Ishizaka T, Ohata T, Takagaki M, Oshima S (1992) Hemodynamic changes during laparoscopic cholecystectomy in patients with heart disease. Endoscopy 24:771–773
127. Jackman SV, Weingart JD, Kinsman SL, Docimo SG (2000) Laparoscopic surgery in patients with ventriculoperitoneal shunts: safety and monitoring. J Urol 164:1352–1354
128. Jackson SA, Laurence AS, Hill JC (1996) Does post-laparoscopy pain relate to residual carbon dioxide? Anaesthesia 51:485–487
129. Jacobi CA, Ordemann J, Böhm B, Zieren HU, Volk HD, Lorenz W, Halle E, Müller JM (1997) Does laparoscopy increase bacteremia and endotoxemia in a peritonitis model? Surg Endosc 11:235–238
130. Jacobi CA, Ordemann J, Zieren HU, Volk HD, Bauhofer A, Halle E, Müller JM (1998) Increased systemic inflammation after laparotomy vs laparoscopy in an animal model of peritonitis. Arch Surg 133:258–262
131. Jacobi CA, Sabat R, Ordemann J, Wenger F, Volk HD, Müller JM (1997) Peritoneale Instillation von Taurolidin und Heparin zur Verhinderung von intraperitonealem Tumorwachstum und Trokarmetastasen bei laparoskopischen Operationen im Rattenmodell. Langenbecks Arch Chir 382:S31–S36

132. Jacobi CA, Sterzel A, Braumann C, Halle E, Stösslein R, Krähenbühl L, Müller JM (2001) The impact of conventional and laparoscopic colon resection (CO_2 or helium) on intraperitoneal adhesion formation in a rat peritonitis model. Surg Endosc 15:380–386

133. Jacobi CA, Wenger F, Sabat R, Volk T, Ordemann J, Müller JM (1998) The impact of laparoscopy with carbon dioxide versus helium on immunologic function and tumor growth in a rat model. Dig Surg 15:110–116

134. Jakeways MSR, Mitchell V, Hashim IA, Chadwick SJD, Shenkin A, Green CJ, Carii F (1994) Metabolic and inflammatory responses after open or laparoscopic cholecystectomy. Br J Surg 81:127–131

135. Jakimowicz J, Stultiens G, Smulders F (1998) Laparoscopic insufflation of the abdomen reduces portal venous flow. Surg Endosc 12:129–132

136. Johnson PL, Sibert KS (1997) Laparoscopy. Gasless vs CO_2 pneumoperitoneum. J Reprod Med 42:255–259

137. Jorgensen JO, Gillies RB, Hunt DR, Caplehom JRM, Lumley T(1995) A simple and effective way to reduce postoperative pain after laparoscopic cholecystectomy. Aust N Z J Surg 65:466–469

138. Jorgensen JO, Lalak NJ, North L, Hanel K, Hunt DR, Morris DL (1994) Venous stasis during laparoscopic cholecystectomy. Surg Laparosc Endosc 4:128–133

139. Joris J, Cigarini I, Legrand M, Jacquet N, De Groote D, Franchimont P, Lamy M (1992) Metabolic and respiratory changes after cholecystectomy performed via laparotomy or laparoscopy. Br J Anaesth 69:341–345

140. Joris J, Thiry E, Paris P, Weerts J, Lamy M (1995) Pain after laparoscopic cholecystectomy: characteristics and effect of intraperitoneal bupivacaine. Anesth Analg 81:379–384

141. Joris JL, Chiche JD, Canivet JLM, Jacquet NJ, Legros JJ, Lamy ML (1998) Hemodynamic changes induced by laparoscopy and their endocrine correlates: effects of clonidine. J Am Coll Cardiol 32:1389–1396

142. Josephs LG, Este-McDonald JR, Birkett DH, Hirsch EF (1994) Diagnostic laparoscopy increases intracranial pressure. J Trauma 36:815–819

143. Joshi GP (2001) Complications of laparoscopy. Anesthesiol Clin North Am 19:89–105

144. Junghans T, Böhm B, Gründel K, Scheiba-Zörron R, Muller JM (1999) Effects of induced intravenous helium and CO_2 embolism on the cardiovascular system. Minimal Invasive Chirurgie 8:52–56

145. Jungharls T, Böhm B, Gründel K, Schwenk W, Müller JM (1997) Does pneumoperitoneum with different gases, body positions, and intraperitoneal pressures influence renal and hepatic blood flow? Surgery 121:206–211

146. Junghans T, Böhm B, Meyer E (2000) Influence of nitrous oxide anesthesia on venous embolism with carbon dioxide and helium during pneumoperitoneum. Surg Endosc 14:1167–1170

147. Junghans T, Böhm B, Neudecker J, Mansmann U, Gründel K (1999) Auswirkungen von Argon-Gasembolien während eines Pneumoperitoneums. Chirurg 70:184–189

148. Kanellos I, Zarogilidis K, Ziogas E, Dadoukis I (1994) Prospektiv-vergleichende Studie der Lungenfunktion nach laparoskopischer, Mini-Lap- oder konventioneller Cholezystectomie. Minimal Invasive Chirurgie 4:169–171

149. Karayiannakis AJ, Makri GG, Mantzioka A, Karousos D, Karatzas G (1997) Systemic stress response after laparoscopic or open cholecystectomy: a randomized trial. Br J Surg 84:467–471

150. Kazemier G, Berends FJ, Bouvy ND, Lange JF, Bonjer HJ (1997) The influence of pneumoperitoneum on the peritoneal implantation of free intraperitoneal cancer cells. Surg Endosc 11:698–699

151. Khan AU, Pandya K, Clifton MA (1995) Near fatal gas embolism during laparoscopic cholecystectomy. Ann R Coll Surg Engl 77:67–68

152. Kiviluoto T, Sirén J, Luukkonen P, Kivilaakso E (1998) Randomised trial of laparoscopic versus open cholecystectomy for acute and gangrenous cholecystitis. Lancet 351:321–325

153. Knolmayer TJ, Bowyer MW, Egan JC, Asbun HJ (1998) The effects of pneumoperitoneum on gastric blood flow and traditional hemodynamic measurements. Surg Endosc 12:115–118
154. Koivusalo AM, Kellokumpu I, Lindgren L (1996) Gasless laparoscopic cholecystectomy: comparison of postoperative recovery with conventional technique. Br J Anaesth 77:576–580
155. Koivusalo AM, Kellokumpu I, Lindgren L (1997) Postoperative drowsiness and emetic sequelae correlate to total amount of carbon dioxide used during laparoscopic cholecystectomy. Surg Endosc 11:42–44
156. Koivusalo AM, Kellokumpu I, Ristkari S, Lindgren L (1997) Splanchnic and renal deterioration during and after laparoscopic cholecystectomy: a comparison of the carbon dioxide pneumoperitoneum and the abdominal wall lift method. Anesth Analg 85:886–891
157. Koivusalo AM, Kellokumpu I, Scheinin M, Tikkanen I, Halme L, Lindgren L (1996) Randomized comparison of the neuroendocrine response to laparoscopic cholecystectomy using either conventional or abdominal wall lift techniques. Br J Surg 83:1532–1536
158. Koivusalo AM, Kellokumpu I, Scheinin M, Tikkanen I, Mäkisalo H, Lindgren L (1998) A comparison of gasless mechanical and conventional carbon dioxide pneumoperitoneum methods for laparoscopic cholecystectomy. Anesth Analg 86:153–158
159. Koivusalo AM, Lindgren L (1999) Respiratory mechanics during laparoscopic cholecystectomy. Anesth Analg 89:800
160. Koivusalo AM, Lindgren L (2000) Effects of carbon dioxide pneumoperitoneum for laparoscopic cholecystectomy. Acta Anaesthesiol Scand 44:834–841
161. Koivusalo AM, Scheinin M, Tikkanen I, Yli-Suomu T, Ristkari S, Laakso J, Lindgren L (1998) Effects of esmolol on haemodynamic response to CO_2 pneumoperitoneum for laparoscopic surgery. Acta Anaesthesiol Scand 42:510–517
162. Korell M, Schmaus F, Strowitzki T, Schneeweiss SG, Hepp H (1996) Pain intensity following laparoscopy. Surg Laparosc Endosc 6:375–379
163. Kraut EJ, Anderson JT, Safwat A, Barbosa R, Wolfe BM (1999) Impairment of cardiac performance by laparoscopy in patients receiving positive end-expiratory pressure. Arch Surg 134:76–80
164. Kristiansson M, Saraste L, Soop M, Sundqvist KG, Thörne A(1999) Diminished interleukin-6 and C-reactive protein responses to laparoscopic versus open cholecystectomy. Acta Anaesthesiol Scand 43:146–152
165. Krug F, Herald A, Wenk H, Bruch HP (1995) Narbenhernien nach laparoskopischen Eingriffen. Chirurg 66:419–423
166. Kum CK, Eypasch E, Aljaziri A, Troidl H (1996) Randomized comparison of pulmonary function after the "French" and "American" techniques of laparoscopic cholecystectomy. Br J Surg 83:938–941
167. Kuthe A, Tamme C, Saemann T, Schneider C, Kockeriing F (1999) Die laparoskopische Cholezystektomie mit Mini-Instrumentarium. Zentralbl Chir 124:749–753
168. Lacy AM, Delgado S, Garcfa-Valdecasas JC, Castells A, Piqué JM, Grande L, Fuster J, Tararona EM, Pera M, Visa J (1998) Port site metastases and recurrence after laparoscopic colectomy. A randomized trial. Surg Endosc 12:1039–1042
169. Lajer H, Widecrantz S, Heisterberg L (1997) Hernias in trocar ports following abdominal laparoscopy. A review. Acta Obstet Gynecol Scand 76:389–393
170. Lam TYD, Lee SW, So HS, Kwok SPY (2000) Radially expanding trocar: a less painful alternative for laparoscopic surgery. J Laparoendosc Adv Surg Tech A 10:269–273
171. Lantz PE, Smith JD (1994) Fatal carbon dioxide embolism complicating attempted laparoscopic cholecystectomy–case report and literature review. J Forensic Sci 39:1468–1480
172. Lau JYW, Lo SY, Ng EKW, Lee DWH, Lam YH, Chung SCS (1998) A randomized comparison of acute phase response and endotoxemia in patients with perforated peptic ulcers receiving laparoscopic or open patch repair. Am J Surg 175:325–327

173. Le Blanc-Louvry I, Coquerel A, Koning E, Maillot C, Ducrotte P(2000) Operative stress response is reduced after laparoscopic compared to open cholecystectomy: the relationship with postoperative pain and ileus. Dig Dis Sci 45:1703–1713

174. Lejus C, Delile L, Plattner V, Baron M, Guillou S, Héloury Y, Souron R (1996) Randomized, single-blinded trial of laparoscopic versus open appendectomy in children: effects on postoperative analgesia. Anesthesiology 84:801–806

175. Leung KL, Lai PBS, Ho RLK, Meng WCS, Yiu RYC, Lee JFY, Lau WY (2000) Systemic cytokine response after laparoscopic-assisted resection of rectosigmoid carcinoma: A prospective randomized trial. Ann Surg 231:506–511

176. Levy T, Dicker D, Shalev J, Dekel A, Farhi J, Peleg D, Ben-Rafael Z (1995) Laparoscopic unwinding of hyperstimulated ischaemic ovaries during the second trimester of pregnancy. Hum Reprod 10:1478–1480

177. Lindberg F, Rasmussen I, Siegbahn A, Bergqvist D (2000) Coagulation activation after laparoscopic cholecystectomy in spite of thromboembolism prophylaxis. Surg Endosc 14:858–861

178. Lindgren L, Koivusalo AM, Kellokumpu I (1995) Conventional pneumoperitoneum compared with abdominal wall lift for laparoscopic cholecystectomy. Br J Anaesth 75:567–572

179. Linhares L, Jeanpierre H, Borie F, Fingerhut A, Millat B (2001) Lavage by laparoscopy fares better than lavage by laparotomy: experimental evidence. Surg Endosc 15:85–89

180. Lipscomb GH, Summitt RL, McCord ML, Ling FW (1994) The effect of nitrous oxide and carbon dioxide pneumoperitoneum on operative and postoperative pain during laparoscopic sterilization under local anesthesia. J Am Assoc Gynecol Laparosc 2:57–60

181. Lo CM, Liu CL, Fan ST, Lai ECS, Wong J (1998) Prospective randomized study of early versus delayed laparoscopic cholecystectomy for acute cholecystitis. Ann Surg 227:461–467

182. Loeckinger A, Kleinsasser A, Hoermann C, Gassner M, Keller C, Lindner KH (2000) Inert gas exchange during pneumoperitoneum at incremental values of positive end-expiratory pressure. Anesth Analg 90:466–471

183. Lord RV, Ling JJ, Hugh TB, Coleman MJ, Doust BD, Nivison- Smith I (1998) Incidence of deep vein thrombosis after laparoscopic vs minilaparotomy cholecystectomy. Arch Surg 133:967–973

184. Lukban JC, Jaeger J, Hammond KC, LoBraico DA, Gordon AMC, Graebe RA (2000) Gasless versus conventional laparoscopy. N J Med 97:29–34

185. Lundor P, Thorburn J, Hahlin M, Kallfelt B, Lindblom B (1991) Laparoscopic surgery in ectopic pregnancy. A randomized trial versus laparotomy. Acta Obstet Gynecol Scand 70:343–348

186. Mäkinen MT, Heinonen PO, Klemola UM, Yli-Hankala A (2001) Gastric air tonometry during laparoscopic cholecystectomy: a comparison of two $PaCO_2$ levels. Can J Anaesth 48:121–128

187. Mäkinen MT, Yli-Hankala A (1996) The effect of laparoscopic cholecystectomy on respiratory compliance as determined by continuous spirometry. J Clin Anesth 8:119–122

188. Mall JW, Schwenk W, Rödiger O, Zippel K, Pollmann C, Müller JM (2001) Blinded prospective study of the incidence of deep venous thrombosis following conventional or laparoscopic colcrectal resection. Br J Surg 88:99–105

189. Marquez J, Sladen A, Gendell H, Boehnke M, Mendelow H (1981) Paradoxical cerebral air embolism without an intracardiac septal defect. Case report. J Neurosurg 55:997–1000

190. Martin IG, Dexter SPL, McMahon MJ (1996) Laparoscopic cholecystectomy in pregnancy. Surg Endosc 10:508–510

191. Martinez-Ramos C, Lopez-Pastor A, Nunez-Pena JR, Gopegui M, Sanz-Lopez R, Jorgensen T, Pastor L, Fernandez-Chacon JL, Tamames-Escobar S (1999) Changes in hemostasis after laparoscopic cholecystectomy. Surg Endosc 13:476–479

192. Matsuda T, Ogura K, Uchida J, Fujita I, Terachi T, Yoshida O (1995) Smaller ports result in shorter convalescence after laparoscopic varicocelectomy. J Urol 153:1175–1177

193. Matsumoto T, Tsuboi S, Dolgor B, Bandoh T, Yoshida T, Kitano S (2001) The effect of gases in the intraperitoneal space on cytokine response and bacterial translocation in a rat model. Surg Endosc 15:80–84
194. McDougall EM, Monk TG, Wolf JS, Hicks M, Clayman RV, Gardner S, Humphrey PA, Sharp T, Martin K (1996) The effect of prolonged pneumoperitoneum on renal function in an animal model. J Am Coll Surg 182:317–328
195. McKellar DP, Anderson CT, Boynton CJ, Peoples JB (1992) Cholecystectomy during pregnancy without fetal loss. Surg Gynecol Obstet 174:465–468
196. McMahon AJ, Baxter JN, Kenny G, O'Dwyer PJ (1993) Ventilatory and blood gas changes during laparoscopic and open cholecystectomy. Br J Surg 80:1252–1254
197. McMahon AJ, O'Dwyer PJ, Cruikshank AM, McMillan DC, O'Reilly DS, Lowe GD, Rumley A, Logan RW, Baxter JN (1993) Comparison of metabolic responses to laparoscopic and minilaparotomy cholecystectomy. Br J Surg 80:1255–1258
198. Mecke H, Kroll K (1999) Postlaparoskopisches Schmerzsyndrom nach Pneumoperitoneum mit angewärmten und kaltem CO_2-Gas. Geburtshilfe Frauenheilkunde 59:611–615
199. Mehta M, Sokoll MD, Gergis SD (1984) Effects of venous air embolism on the cardiovascular system and acid base balance in the presence and absence of nitrous oxide. Acta Anaesthesiol Scand 28:226–231
200. Meijer DW, Rademaker BPM, Schlooz S, Bemelman WA, de Wit LT, Bannenberg JJG, Stijnen T, Gouma DF (1997) Laparoscopic cholecystectomy using abdominal wall retraction. Hemodynamics and gas exchange, a comparison with conventional pneumoperitoneum. Surg dosc 11:645–649
201. Michaloliakou C, Chung F, Sharma S (1996) Preoperative muttimodal analgesia facilitates recovery after ambulatory laparoscopic cholecystectomy. Anesth Analg 82:44–51
202. Milheiro A, Sousa FC, Manso EC, Leitao F (1994) Metabolic responses to cholecystectomy: open vs laparoscopic approach. J Laparoendosc Surg 4:311–317
203. Millard JA, Hill BB, Cook PS, Fenoglio ME, Stahlgren LH (1993) Intermittent sequential pneumatic compression in prevention of venous stasis associated with pneumoperitoneum during laparoscopic cholecystectomy. Arch Surg 128:914–919
204. Milsom JW, Böhm B, Hammerhofer KA, Fazio V, Steiger E, Elson P (1998) A prospective, randomized trial comparing laparoscopic versus conventional techniques in colorectal cancer surgery: a preliminary report. J Am Coll Surg 187:46–55
205. Mimica Z, Biocic M, Bacic A, Banovic I, Tocilj J, Radonic V, Ilic N, Petricevic A (2000) Laparoscopic and laparotomic cholecystectomy: a randomized trial comparing postoperative respiratory function. Respiration 67:153–158
206. Minoli G, Terruzzi V, Spinzi GC, Benvenuti C, Rossini A (1982) The influence of carbon dioxide and nitrous oxide on pain during laparoscopy: a double-blind, controlled trial. Gastrointest Endosc 28:173–175
207. Moncure M, Salem R, Moncure K, Testaiuti M, Marburger R, Ye X, Brathwaite C, Ross SE (1999) Central nervous system metabolic and physiologic effects of laparoscopy. Am Surg 65:168–172
208. Morino M, Giraudo G, Festa V (1998) Alterations in hepatic function during laparoscopic surgery. An experimental clinical study. Surg Endosc 12:968–972
209. Mouton WG, Bessell JR, Millard SH, Baxter PS, Maddern GJ (1999) A randomized controlled trial assessing the benefit of humidified insufflation gas during laparoscopic surgery. Surg Endosc 13:106–108
210. Mouton WG, Naef M, Bessell JR, Wagner HE, Maddern GJ (2001) A randomized controlled trial to determine the effect of humidified carbon dioxide (CO_2) insufflation on postoperative pain following thoracoscopic procedures. Surg Endosc 15:579–581
211. Mraovic B, Jurisic T, Kogler-Majeric V, Sustic A (1997) Intraperitoneal bupivacaine for analgesia after laparoscopic cholecystectomy. Acta Anaesthesiol Scand 41:193–196
212. Myre K, Buanes T, Smith G, Stokland O (1997) Simultaneous hemodynamic and echocardiographic changes during abdominal gas insufflation. Surg Laparosc Endosc 7:415–419

213. Nagelschmidt M, Holthausen U, Goost H, Fu ZX, Minor T, Troidl H, Neugebauer E (2000) Evaluation of the effects of a pneumoperitoneum with carbon dioxide or helium in a porcine model of endotoxemia. Langenbecks Arch Surg 385:199–206

214. Narchi P, Benhamou D, Fernandez H (1991) Intraperitoneal local anaesthetic for shoulder pain after day-case laparoscopy. Lancet 338:1569–1570

215. Nelskyla K, Yli-Hankala A, Sjoberg J, Korhonen I, Korttila K (1999) Wanning of insufflation gas during laparoscopic hysterectomy: e ect on body temperature and the autonomic nervous system. Acta Anaesthesiol Scand 43:974–978

216. Neudecker J, Junghans T, Ziemer H, Schwenk W (2001) Einfluß der Operationstechnik auf das fibrinolytische Potential des Peritoneums und der Peritonealflüssigkeit bei laparoskopischen und konventionellen kolorektalen Resektionen – Eine prospektiv randomisierte Studie. In: Schönleben K (ed) Chirurgisches Forum 2001 für experimentelle und klinische Forschung: Band 30. Springer, Berlin Heidelberg New York, p 539

217. Neugebauer E, Sauerland S, Troidl H (2000) Recommendations for evidence-based, endoscopic surgery. The updated EAES consensus development conferences. Springer, Berlin Heidelberg New York

218. Neuhaus SJ, Watson Dl, Ellis T, Rofe AM, Mathew G, Jamieson GG (2000) Influence of gases on intraperitoneal immunity during laparoscopy in tumor-bearing rats. World J Surg 24:1227–1231

219. Nezhat FR, Silfen SL, Evans D, Nezhat C (1991) Comparison of direct insertion of disposable and standard reusable laparoscopic trocars and previous pneumoperitoneum with Veress needle. Obstet Gynecol 78:148–150

220. Ninomiya K, Kitano S, Yoshida T, Bandoh T, Baatar D, Matsumoto T (1998) Comparison of pneumoperitoneum and abdominal wall lifting as to hemodynamics and surgical stress response during laparoscopic cholecystectomy. Surg Endosc 12:124–128

221. Nordentoft T, Bringstrup FA, Bremmelgaard A, Stage JG (2000) Effect of laparoscopy on bacteremia in acute appendicitis: a randomized controlled study. Surg Laparosc Endosc Percutan Tech 10:302–304

222. Odeberg S, Ljungqvist O, Sollevi A (1998) Pneumoperitoneum for laparoscopic cholecystectomy is not associated with compromised splanchnic circulation. Eur J Surg 164:843–848

223. Ogihara Y, Isshiki A, Kindscher JD, Goto H (1999) Abdominal wall lift versus carbon dioxide insufflation for laparoscopic resection of ovarian tumors. J Clin Anesth 11:406–412

224. Ordemann J, Jacobi C, Schwenk W, Stösslein R, Müller JM (2001) Cellular and humoral inflammatory response after laparoscopic and conventional colorectal resections–results of a prospective randomized trial. Surg Endosc 15:600–608

225. Ortega AE, Peters JH, Incarbone R, Estrada L, Ehsan A, Kwan Y, Spencer CJ, Moore-Jeries E, Kuchta K, Nicolo JT (1996) A prospective randomized comparison of the metabolic and stress hormonal responses of laparoscopic and open cholecystectomy. J Am Coll Surg 183:249–256

226. Ott DE, Rejch H, Love B, McCorvey R, Toledo A, Liu CY, Syed R, Kumar K (1998) Reduction of laparoscopic-induced hypothermia, postoperative pain and recovery room length of stay by pre-conditioning gas with the Insuflow device: a prospective randomized controlled multicenter study. JSLS 2:321–329

227. Pasqualucci A, Contardo R, Da Broi U, Colo F, Terrosu G, Donini A, Sorrentino M, Pasetto A, Bresadola F (1994) The effects of intraperitoneal local anesthetic on analgesic requirements and endocrine response after laparoscopic cholecystectomy: a randomized double-blind controlled study. J Laparoendosc Surg 4:405–412

228. Pasqualucci A, de Angelis V, Contardo R, Colo F, Terrosu G, Donini A, Pasetto A, Bresadola F (1996) Preemptive analgesia: intraperitoneal local anesthetic in laparoscopic cholecystectomy. A randomized, double-blind, placebo-controlled study. Anesthesiology 85:11–20

229. Patel MI, Hardman DTA, Nicholls D, Fisher CM, Appleberg M (1996) The incidence of deep venous thrombosis after laparoscopic cholecystectomy. Med J Aust 164:652–654, 656

230. Péchinot M, Rapenne T, Galloux Y, Vérain C (1996) Embolie gazeuse au cours d'une chotecystectomie par coelioscopie. Cah Anesthesiol 44:365–367
231. Peitgen K, Nimtz K, Hellinger A, Walz MK (1997) Offener Zugang oder Veress-Nadel bei laparoskopischen Eingriffen? Ergebnisse einer prospektiv randomisierten Studie. Chirurg 68:910–913
232. Perez JE, Alberts WM, Mamel JJ (1997) Delayed tension pneumothorax after laparoscopy. Surg Laparosc Endosc 7:70–72
233. Perry CP, Tombrello R (1993) Effect of fluid instillation on postlaparoscopy pain. J Reprod Med 38:768–770
234. Perttilä J, Salo M, Ovaska J, Grönroos J, Lavonius M, Katila A, Lähteenmäki M, Pulkki K (1999) Immune response after laparoscopic and conventional Nissen fundopfication. Eur J Surg 165:21–28
235. Philips PA, Amaral JF (2001) Abdominal access complications in laparoscopic surgery. J Am Coll Surg 192:525–536
236. Pier A, Benedic M, Mann B, Buck V (1994) Das postlaparoskopische Schmerzsyndrom: Ergebnisse einer prospektiven, randomisierten Studie. Chirurg 65:200–208
237. Popesco D, Le MiéAre E, Maitre B, Darchy B, Domart Y (1997) Embolie gazeuse coronaire lors de la chirurgie coelioscopique. Ann Fr Anesth Reanim 16:381–385
238. Popken F, Küchle R, Heintz A, Junginger T (1997) Die laparoskopische Cholecystektomie beim Hochrisikopatienten. Chirurg 68:801–805
239. Popken F, Kuchle R, Heintz A, Junginger T (1998) Die Cholecystektomie beim Hochrisikopatienten: Ein Vergleich zwischen konventionellem und laparoskopischen Verfahren. Chirurg 69:61–65
240. Popken CA, Compton RP, Walter DN, Browder IW (1995) Benefits of pulmonary artery catheter and transesophageal echocardiographic monitoring in laparoscopic cholecytectomy patients with cardiac disease. Am J Surg 169:202–207
241. Presson RG, Kirk KR, Haselby KA, Wagner WW (1991) Effect of ventilation with soluble and diffusible gases on the size of air emboli. J Appl Physiol 70:1068–1074
242. Prisco D, De Gaudio AR, Caria R, Gori AM, Fedi S, Cella AP, Gensini GF, Abbate R (2000) Videolaparoscopic cholecystectomy induces a hemostasis activation of lower grade than does open surgery. Surg Endosc 14:170–174
243. Puttick MI, Scott-Coombes DM, Dye J, Nduka CC, Menzies-Gow NM, Mansfield AO, Darzi A (1999) Comparison of immunologic and physiologic effects of CO_2 pneumoperitoneum at room and body temperatures. Surg Endosc 13:572–575
244. Rademaker BMP, Kalkman CJ, Odoom JA, de Wit L, Ringers J(1994) Intraperitoneal local anaesthetics after laparoscopic cholecystectomy: effects on postoperative pain, metabolic responses and lung function. Br J Anaesth 72:263–266
245. Rasmussen YH, Leikersfeldt G, Drenck NE (1998) Forced-air surface warming versus oesophageal heat exchanger in the prevention of peroperative hypothermia. Acta Anaesthesiol Scand 42:348–352
246. Razvi HA, Fields D, Vargas JC, Vaughan ED, Vukasin A, Sosa RE (1996) Oliguria during laparoscopic surgery: evidence for direct renal parenchymal compression as an etiologic factor. J Endouro 10:1–4
247. Redmond HP, Watson RWG, Houghton T, Condron C, Watson RGK, Bouchier-Hayes D (1994) Immune function in patients undergoing open vs laparoscopic cholecystectomy. Arch Surg 129:1240–1246
248. Retzke U, Graf H, Schmidt M (1998) Appendizitis in graviditate. Zentralbl Chir 123:61–65
249. Rishimani ASM, Gautam SC (1996) Hemodynamic and respiratory changes during laparoscopic cholecystectomy with high and reduced intraabdominal pressure. Surg Laparosc Endosc 6:201–204
250. Roberts MW, Mathiesen KA, Ho HS, Wolfe BM (1997) Cardiopulmonary responses to intravenous infusion of soluble and relatively insoluble gases. Surg Endosc 11:341–346
251. Rosenthal RJ, Friedman RL, Kahn AM, Martz J, Thiagarajah S, Cohen D, Shi Q, Nussbaum M (1998) Reasons for intracranial hypertension and hemodynamic instability

during acute elevations of intra-abdominal pressure: observations in a large animal model. J Gastrointest Surg 2:415–425

252. Rosenthal RJ, Hiatt JR, Phillips EH, Hewitt W, Demetriou AA, Grode M (1997) Intracranial pressure. Effects of pneumoperitoneum in a large-animal model. Surg Endosc 11:376–380

253. Roumen RMH, van Meurs PA, Kuypers HHC, Kraak WAG, Sauerwein RW (1992) Serum interleukin-6 and C reactive protein responses in patients after laparoscopic or conventional cholecystectomy. Eur J Surg 158:541–544

254. Saad S, Minor I, Mohri T, Nagelschmidt M (2000) The clinical impact of warmed insufflation carbon dioxide gas for laparoscopic cholecystectomy. Surg Endosc 14:787–790

255. Sackett DL, Straus SE, Richardson WS, Rosenberg W, Haynes RB (2000) Evidence-based medicine: How to practice and teach EBM, 2nd edn. Churchill Livingston, London

256. Safran D, Sgambati S, Orlando R (1993) Laparoscopy in high-risk cardiac patients. Surg Gynecol Obstet 176:548–554

257. Sarac AM, Aktan AÖ, Baykan N, Yegen C, Yalin R (1996) The effect and timing of local anesthesia in laparoscopic cholecystectomy. Surg Laparosc Endosc 6:362–366

258. Sarli L, Costi R, Sansebastiano G, Trivelli M, Roncoroni L (2000) Prospective randomized trial of low-pressure pneumoperitoneum for reduction of shoulder-tip pain following laparoscopy. Br J Surg 87:1161–1165

259. Sato N, Kawamoto M, Yuge O, Suyama H, Sanuki M, Matsumoto C, Inoue K (2000) Effects of pneumoperitoneum on cardiac autonomic nervousactivity evaluated by heart rate variability analysis during sevoflurane, isoflurane, or propofol anesthesia. Surg Endosc 14:362–366

260. Sato K, Kawamura T, Wakusawa R (2000) Hepatic blood flow and function in elderly patients undergoing laparoscopic cholecystectomy. Anesth Analg 90:1198–1202

261. Sauerland S, Neugebauer E (2000) Consensus conferences must include a systematic search and categorization of the evidence. Surg Endosc 14:908–910

262. Saunders C, Battistella F, Whetzel T, Stokes R (1998) Percutaneous diagnostic peritoneal lavage using a Veress needle versus an open technique: A prospective randomized trial. J Trauma 44:883–888

263. Schäfer M, Lauper M, Krähenbühl L (2001) Trocar and Veress needle injuries during laparoscopy. Surg Endosc 15:275–280

264. Scheinin B, Kellokumpu I, Lindgren L, Haglund C, Rosenberg PH (1995) Effect of intraperitoneal bupivacaine on pain after laparoscopic cholecystectomy. Acta Anaesthesiol Scand 39:195–198

265. Schilling MK, Redaelli C, Krähenbühl L, Signer C, Büchler MW (1997) Splanchnic microcirculatory changes during CO_2 laparoscopy. J Am Coll Surg 184:378–383

266. Schindler E, Muller M, Kelm C (1995) Cerebral carbon dioxide embolism during laparoscopic cholecystectomy. Anesth Analg 81:643–645

267. Schob OM, Alien DC, Benzel E, Curet MJ, Adams MS, Baldwin NG, Largiader F, Zucker KA (1996) A comparison of the pathophysiologic effects of carbon dioxide, nitrous oxide, and helium pneumoperitoneum on intracranial pressure. Am J Surg172:248–253

268. Schreiber JH (1990) Laparoscopic appendectomy in pregnancy. Surg Endosc 4:100–102

269. Schrenk P, Bettelheim P, Woisetschlager R, Rieger R, Wayand WU (1996) Metabolic responses after laparoscopic or open hernia repair. Surg Endosc 10:628–632

270. Schulte-Steinberg H, Weninger E, Jokisch D, Hofstetter B, Misera A, Lange V, Stein C (1995) Intraperitoneal versus interpleural morphine or bupivacaine for pain after laparoscopic cholecystectomy. Anesthesiology 82:634–640

271. Schulze S, Lyng KM, Bugge K, Perner A, Bendtsen A, Thorup J, Nielsen HJ, Rasmussen V, Rosenberg J (1999) Cardiovascular and respiratory changes and convalescence in laparoscopic colonic surgery: comparison between carbon dioxide pneumoperitoneum and gasless laparoscopy. Arch Surg 134:1112–1118

272. Schwenk W, Böhm B, Fugener A, Müller JM (1998) Intermittent pneumatic sequential compression (ISC) of the lower extremities prevents venous stasis during laparoscopic cholecystectomy. A prospective randomized study. Surg Endosc 12:7–11
273. Schwenk W, Böhm B, Junghans T, Hofmann H, Müller JM (1997) Intermittent sequential compression of the lower limbs prevents venous stasis in laparoscopic and conventional colorectal surgery. Dis Colon Rectum 40:1056–1062
274. Schwenk W, Böhm B, Witt C, Junghans T, Gründel K, Müller JM (1999) Pulmonary function following laparoscopic or conventional colorectal resection: a randomized controlled evaluation. Arch Surg 134:6–13
275. Schwenk W, Jacobi C, Mansmann U, Böhm B, Müller JM (2000) Inflammatory response after laparoscopic and conventional colorectal resections-results of a prospective randomized trial. Langenbecks Arch Surg 385:2–9
276. Schwenk W, Neudecker J, Mall J, Böhm B, Müller JM (2000) Prospective randomized blinded trial of pulmonary function, pain, and cosmetic results after laparoscopic vs microlaparoscopic cholecystectomy. Surg Endosc 14:345–348
277. Semm K, Arp WD, Trappe M, Kube D (1994) Schmerzreduzierung nach pelvi-/laparoskopischen Eingriffen durch Einblasen von körperwarmem CO_2-gas (Flow-Therme). Geburtshilfe Frauenheilkunde 54:300–304
278. Sezeur A, Bure-Rossier AM, Rio D, Savigny B, Tricot C, Martel P, Baubion O (1997) La coelioscopie augmente-t-elle le risque bactériologique de l'appendicectomie? Résultats d'une étude prospective randomisée. Ann Chir 51:243–247
279. Shaneyfelt TM, Mayo-Smith MF, Rothwangl J (1999) Are guidelines following guidelines? The methodological quality of clinical practice guidelines in the peer-reviewed medical literature. J Am Med Assoc 281:1900–1905
280. Sharp JR, Pierson WP, Brady CE (1982) Comparison of CO_2- and N_2O-induced discomfort during peritoneoscopy under local anesthesia. Gastroenterology 82:453–456
281. Shea JA, Healey MJ, Berlin JA, Clarke JR, Malet PF, Staroscik RN, Schwartz JS, Williams SV (1996) Mortality and complications associated with laparoscopic cholecystectomy. A meta analysis. Ann Surg 224:609–620
282. Shulman D, Aronson HB (1984) Capnography in the early diagnosis of carbon dioxide embolism during laparoscopy. Can Anaesth Soc J 31:455–459
283. Sietses C, Wiezer MJ, Eijsbouts QAJ, Beelen RH, van Leeuwen PAM, von Blomberg BME, Meijer S, Cuesta MA (1999) A prospective randomized study of the systemic immune response after laparoscopic and conventional Nissen fundoplication. Surgery 126:5–9
284. Slim K, Bousquet J, Kwiatkowski F, Lescure G, Pezet D, Chipponi J (1999) E ect of CO_2 gas warming on pain after laparoscopic surgery: a randomized double-blind controlled trial. Surg Endosc 13:1110–1114
285. Smith RS, Fry WR, Morabito DJ, Koehler RH, Organ Jr CH(1995) Therapeutic laparoscopy in trauma. Am J Surg 170:632–637
286. Society of American Gastrointestinal Endoscopic Surgeons (1998) Guidelines for laparoscopic surgery during pregnancy. Surg Endosc 12:189–190
287. Soper NJ, Hunter JG, Petrie RH (1992) Laparoscopic cholecystectomy during pregnancy. Surg Endosc 6:115–117
288. Squirrell DM, Majeed AW, Troy G, Peacock JE, Nicholl JP, Johnson AG (1998) A randomized, prospective, blinded comparison of postoperative pain, metabolic response, and perceived health after laparoscopic and small incision cholecystectomy. Surgery 123:485–495
289. Stage JG, Schulze S, Moller P, Overgaard H, Andersen M, Rebsdorf-Pedersen VB, Nielsen HJ (1997) Prospective randomized study of laparoscopic versus open colonic resection for adenocarcinoma. Br J Surg 84:391–396
290. Stone J, Dyke L, Fritz P, Reigle M, Verrill H, Bhakta K, Boike G, Graham J, Gerbasi F (1998) Hemodynamic and hormonal changes during pneumoperitoneum and Trendelenburg positioning for operative gynecologic laparoscopy surgery. Prim Care Update Ob Gyns 5:155

291. Stuttmann R, Vogt C, Eypasch E, Doehn M (1995) Haemodynamic changes during laparoscopic cholecystectomy in the high-risk patient. Endosc Surg Allied Technol 3:174–179

292. Sungler P, Heinerman PM, Steiner H, Waclawiczek HW, Holzinger J, Mayer F, Heuberger A, Boeckl O (2000) Laparoscopic cholecystectomy and interventional endoscopy for gallstone complications during pregnancy. Surg Endosc 14:267–271

293. Szem JW, Hydo L, Barie PS (1996) A double-blinded evaluation of intraperitoneal bupivacaine vs saline for the reduction of postoperative pain and nausea after laparoscopic cholecystectomy. Surg Endosc 10:44–48

294. Tang C-L, Eu K-W, Tai B-C, Soh JGS, Machin D, Seow-Choen F (2001) Randomized clinical trial of the e ect of open versus laparoscopically assisted colectomy on systemic immunity in patients with colorectal cancer. Br J Surg 88:801–807

295. Tang CS, Tsai LK, Lee TH, Su YC, Wu YJ, Chang CH, Tseng CK (1993) The hemodynamic and ventilatory effects between Trendelenburg and reverse Trendelenburg position during laparoscopy with CO_2 insufflation. Ma Zui Xue Za Zhi 31:217–224

296. Troidl H, Spangenberger W, Langen R, al-Jaziri A, Eypasch E, Neugebauer E, Dietrich J (1992) Laparoscopic cholecystectomy: technical performance, safety and patient's benefit. Endoscopy 24:252–261

297. Tsimoyiannis EC, Glantzounis G, Lekkas ET, Siakas P, Jabarin M, Tzourou H (1998) Intraperitoneal normal saline and bupivacaine infusion for reduction of postoperative pain after laparoscopic cholecystectomy. Surg Laparosc Endosc 8:416–420

298. Tsimoyiannis EC, Siakas P, Tassis A, Lekkas ET, Tzourou H, Kambili M (1998) Intraperitoneal normal saline infusion for postoperative pain after laparoscopic cholecystectomy. World J Surg 22:824–828

299. Unbehaun N, Feussner H, Slewert J (1995) Niederdruckinsuationstechnik in der laparoskopischen Cholezystektomie. Minimal Invasive Chirurgie 4:10–15

300. Ure BM, Troidl H, Spangenberger W, Dietrich A, Lefering R, Neugebauer E (1994) Pain after laparoscopic cholecystectomy. Intensity and localization of pain and analysis of predictors in preoperative symptoms and intraoperative events. Surg Endosc 8:90–96

301. Ure BM, Troidl H, Spangenberger W, Neugebauer E, Lefering R, Ullmann K, Bende J (1993) Preincisional local anesthesia with bupivacaine and pain after laparoscopic cholecystectomy. A double-blind randomized clinical trial. Surg Endosc 7:482–488

302. Uzunkoy A, Coskun A, Akinci OF, Kocyigit A (2000) Systemic stress responses after laparoscopic or open hernia repair. Eur J Surg 166:467–471

303. Vardulaki KA, Bennett-Loyd BD, Parfitt J, Normond C, Paisley S, Darzi A, Reeves BC (2000) A systematic review of the effectiveness and cost-effectiveness of laparoscopic surgery for colorectal cancer. A systematic review of the effectiveness and cost-effectiveness of laparoscopic surgery for colorectal cancer. National Institute for Clinical Excellence, London

304. Vezakis A, Davides D, Gibson JS, Moore MR, Shah H, Larvin M, McMahon MJ (1999) Randomized comparison between low-pressure laparoscopic cholecystectomy and gasless laparoscopic cholecystectomy. Surg Endosc 13:890–893

305. Vik A, Jenssen BM, Brubakk AO (1991) Effect of aminophylline on transpulmonary passage of venous air emboli in pigs. J Appl Physiol 71:1780–1786

306. Volpino P, Cangemi V, D'Andrea N, Cangemi B, Piat G (1998) Hemodynamic and pulmonary changes during and after laparoscopic cholecystectomy. A comparison with traditional surgery. Surg Endosc 12:119–123

307. Walker CBJ, Bruce DM, Heys SD, Gough DB, Binnie NR, Eremin O (1999) Minimal modulation of lymphocyte and natural killer cell subsets following minimal access surgery. Am J Surg177:48–54

308. Wallace DH, Serpell MG, Baxter JN, O'Dwyer PJ (1997) Randomized trial of different insufflation pressures for laparoscopic cholecystectomy. Br J Surg 84:455–458

309. Weber A, Munoz J, Garteiz D, Cueto J (1997) Use of subdiaphragmatic bupivacaine instillation to control postoperative pain after laparoscopic surgery. Surg Laparosc Endosc 7:6–8

310. Wills VL, Hunt DR (2000) Pain after laparoscopic cholecystectomy. Br J Surg 87:273–284

311. Wills VL, Hunt DR, Armstrong A (2001) A randomized controlled trial assessing the effect of heated carbon dioxide for insufflation on pain and recovery after laparoscopic fundoplication. Surg Endosc 15:166–170

312. Wilson EB, Bass CS, Abrameit W, Roberson R, Smith RW (2001) Metoclopramide versus ondansetron in prophylaxis of nausea and vomiting for laparoscopic cholecystectomy. Am J Surg 181:138–141

313. Wittgen CM, Andrus CH, Fitzgerald SD, Baudendistel LJ, Dahms TE, Kaminski DL (1991) Analysis of the hemodynamic and ventilator effects of laparoscopic cholecystectomy. Arch Surg 126:997–1001

314. Wurst H, Schulte-Steinberg H, Finsterer U (1995) Zur Frage der CO_2-Speicherung bei laparoskopischer Cholezystektomie mit CO_2-Pneumoperitoneum. Anaesthesist 44:147–153

315. Yacoub OF, Cardona I, Coveler LA, Dodson MG (1982) Carbon dioxide embolism during laparoscopy. Anesthesiology 57:533–535

316. Yavuz Y, Ronning K, Lyng O, Marvik R, Gronbech JE (2001) E ect of increased intraabdominal pressure on cardiac output and tissue bloodflow assessed by color-labeled microspheres in the pig. Surg Endosc 15:149–155

317. Yesildaglar N, Koninckx PR (2000) Adhesion formation in intubated rabbits increases with high insufflation pressure during endoscopic surgery. Hum Reprod 15:687–691

318. Yim SF, Yuen PM (2001) Randomized double-masked comparison of radially expanding access device and conventional cutting tip trocar in laparoscopy. Obstet Gynecol 97:435–438

319. Yoshida S, Ohta J, Yamasaki K, Kamei H, Harada Y, Yahara T, Kaibara A, Ozaki K, Tajiri T, Shirouzu K (2000) Effect of surgical stress on endogenous morphine and cytokine levels in the plasma after laparoscopoic or open cholecystectomy. Surg Endosc 14:137–140

320. Yoshida T, Kobayashi E, Suminaga Y, Yamauchi H, Kai T, Toyama N, Kiyozaki H, Fujimura A, Miyata M (1997) Hormone-cytokine response. Pneumoperitoneum vs abdominal wall- lifting in laparoscopic cholecystectomy. Surg Endosc 11:907–910

321. Zieren J, Jacobi CA, Wenger FA, Volk HD, Müller JM (2000) Fundoplication: a model for immunologic aspects of laparoscopic and conventional surgery. J Laparoendosc Adv Surg Tech A 10:35–40

322. Zollinger A, Krayer S, Singer T, Seifert B, Heinzelmann M, Schlumpf R, Pasch T (1997) Haemodynamic effects of pneumoperitoneum in elderly patients with an increased cardiac risk. Eur J Anaesthesiol 14:266–275

323. Dietterle S, Pott C, Arnold A, Riedel HH (1998) The influence of insufflated carbon dioxide gas temperature on the pain intensity after pelviscopic procedures. Min Invas Chir 7:103–105

Pneumoperitoneum – Update 2006

Ann-Cathrin Moberg, Agneta Montgomery

Introduction

The European Association for Endoscopic Surgery (EAES) published guidelines concerning pneumoperitoneum for laparoscopic surgery in 2002 [14]. This extensive documentation concerns evidence-based clinical practice guidelines focussing on the pathophysiological basis for clinical indications, establishing pneumoperitoneum and perioperative aspects. Technique-specific complications are of great concern and most of these are related to the access of the abdominal cavity and the creation of pneumoperitoneum in laparoscopic surgery.

Under the mandate of the EAES Scientific Committee, an update concerning the access technique, insufflation pressure and warming of the insufflation gas has been performed. The pathophysiological bases for the clinical indications and perioperative aspects are not discussed in this update.

Methods

For this update a systematic review was performed by searches (as of March 2006) in Medline, the Cochrane Library and reference lists. The update includes studies published between 1999 and 2006 that have not been referred to in the previous guidelines. The medical subject headings used were laparoscopy, pneumoperitoneum in combination with access, Veress, open, insufflation, warming, humidified and randomised. The primary intention was to identify clinically relevant randomised controlled trials (RCTs). Systematic reviews and large individual cohort studies were also included. No animal studies were included. Only studies written in English were considered. All studies were graded according to the scientific-evidence level described by Sackett et al. [16] also used in the previous EAES guidelines.

The tables of RCTs have been updated from the previous guidelines and summarised in three settings: clinical trials of different access techniques, low- and high-pressure pneumoperitoneum, and hypothermia.

Access Techniques

Consensus 2002: For severe complications (e.g. vessel perforation) it is impossible to show a difference between closed- and open-access techniques in RCTs; therefore, large-outcome studies should be considered. In the RCTs, the rate of major and minor complications is surprisingly high, which may be due to the surgical learning curve or to how "complication" is defined. Insertion of the first trocar with the open technique is faster compared with that of the Veress needle (grade A). The RCTs comparing closed (Veress/trocar) versus open approaches have sample sizes that are not sufficient to show any difference in major complications. In large-outcome studies there were fewer complications in the closed group (grade B). The committee analysing the RCTs found the open approach faster and it was associated with a lower incidence of minor complications (grade A). The committee could not favour the use of either access technique. However, the use of either technique may have advantages in specific patient subgroups (grade B).

Update 2006: Meta-analysis of nonrandomised studies comparing open versus closed (Veress/trocar) access concluded a trend towards a reduced risk of major complications, access-site herniation and minor complications in nonobese patients during open access (grade B). Data regarding different closed techniques; direct trocar insertion, Veress/trocar and Veress/radially expanding access (REA) has been added. Major complications in studies of direct trocar versus Veress/trocar were inconclusive (grade B). Minor complications in RCTs were fewer with direct trocar insertion compared with Veress/trocar (grade A). REA versus conventional cutting-tip trocar (second trocar) in a RCT causes less postoperative pain, better patient satisfaction and fewer local wound events (grade A). There is no RTC large enough to address serious complications.

There are four basic techniques used to create pneumoperitoneum: open access technique, blind Veress followed by either a conventional cutting-tip trocar or a REA device, direct trocar insertion with elevation of the rectus sheet and optical trocar insertion.

The true incidence of visceral and vascular injuries of the aforementioned techniques is still unknown but is believed to be less then 1%. Differences that occur by chance would be difficult to discern without exceptionally large sample sizes.

Five randomised clinical trials of different access techniques are described in Table 3.1. Two of these studies included more then 500 patients and both compare direct trocar insertion to Veress/trocar access. It is concluded that the Veress/trocar causes an unacceptably high number of complications, but mostly are minor. The direct trocar insertion is easy and effective (grade A) [1, 8]. The use of the open balloon blunt-tip trocar is described as simple

Table 3.1. Randomised clinical trials of different access techniques

References/ years	No. of patients, and operations	Treatments	Methods	Results	Conclusion
Gunenc et al. [8]/ 2005	578 Randomised method not described, gynaecologic surgery	277–DTI 301–VN[a]	Emphysema, entry failure and other complications	Emphysema: 0–DTI, 11–VN ($p < 0.05$) Entry failure: 2–DTI, 14–VN ($p < 0.05$) Other complications: 2–DTI, 8–VN (NS)	DTI is easy and effective
Agresta et al. [1]/ 2004	598 Single-blind general surgery	275–DTI 323–VN[a]	Feasibility, complications in nonobese patients	Feasibility same Minor complications: 0–DTI, 18–VN ($p < 0.01$) Major complications: 0–DTI, 5–VN (NS)	VN unacceptable; high number of complications (7.4%)
Yim et al. [23]/2001	34 Double-masked[b] adnexal surgery	34–REA 34–CCTT	Severity (VAS) and duration of pain, scar length, patient satisfaction and complications	Reduction in severity and duration of pain, shorter wound length, higher patient satisfaction in REA 4–epigastric bleeding in CCTT	REA had less postoperative pain and better patient satisfaction
Bernik et al. [3]/2001	180 Randomised method not described, chole-cystectomy	118–open BBTT 34–open Hasson 28–VN[a]	Access time and gas leakage	BBTT faster; gas leakage inconclusive	BBTT simple and rapid
Bhoyrul et al. [4]/ 2000	244 Double-blind general surgery	119–REA 125–VN[a]	Complications, pain (VAS) and incisional hernias	Fewer port site complications in REA. Pain similar. No hernias	REA results in fewer local wound events

BBTT balloon blunt-tip trocar, *CCTT* conventional cutting tip trocar, *DTI* direct trocar insertion, *NS* not significant, *REA* radially expanding access, *VAS* visual analogue scale, *VN* Veress needle.
a) Veress needle followed by conventional cutting-tip trocar.
b) Self-controlled study not including primary trocar entrance

and rapid (grade A) [3]. The REA is compared with Veress/trocar in two randomised studies and both conclude that the use of REA is associated with fewer local wound events, better patient satisfaction and less pain (gradeA) [4, 23].

Inclusion criteria were met in 40 studies in a meta-analysis that summarised complications according to open access, Veress/trocar and direct trocar insertion. Fifty-six percent of all major complications were visceral injuries. It was concluded in prospective nonrandomised studies comparing open and closed (Veress/trocar) access that there is a trend in open access towards a reduced risk of major complications, access site herniation and in nonobese patients a reduced risk of minor complications. In prospective nonrandomised studies comparing direct trocar and Veress/trocar access major complications were inconclusive. There were fewer minor complications with direct trocar insertion, predominantly owing to a reduction in extraperitoneal insufflation. Three access-related deaths have been reported (grade B) [10].

Another meta-analysis, including 61 studies, described the overall frequency of bowel injuries of 0.7/1,000 and major vascular injuries in 0.4/1,000 patients. The overall incidence of major injuries at the time of entry was 1.1/1,000. Direct trocar insertion is associated with a significantly reduced major injury incidence of 0.5/1,000, when compared with both open and Veress/trocar entry. In older studies the open entry was often used in high-risk patients, which might be the explanation for the increased incidence of bowel injuries in this group. Open entry appears to minimise vascular injury at the time of entry (grade B) [13].

In a large database study including 14,000 patients, different access techniques were used and the incidence of visceral injuries was 0.13%, major vascular injuries 0.007% and mortality 0.007% (grade B) [19]. In a database analysis of 4,600 patients comparing open versus Veress/trocar access in two different consecutive time cohorts, no cases of major vascular injuries were seen in either group. Visceral injuries were seen in 0.17% of patients in the Veress group and in 0.05% of patients in the open group (not significant) (grade B) [12]. In a consecutive series comparing direct trocar insertion versus Veress/trocar there was a significantly higher overall complication rate in the Veress/trocar group, 14 versus 0.9% ($p < 0.01$). Two major complications, one visceral and one vascular, were seen in the Veress group (grade B) [22]. The REA device is compared to an ordinary cutting-tip trocar used as the secondary port regarding abdominal wall events. REA is free of abdominal wall complications in 99.8% of cases. Cutting-tip trocars have demonstrated increased complication rates for the abdominal wall in terms of bleeding and larger fascia defects that would potentially increase the risk of port site hernias (grade B) [7]. Optical trocar insertion was reported in one retrospective study including 650 patients. The time for entrance was short and a total of 0.3% of bowel injuries were described and no major vascular injuries were reported (grade B) [20].

Insufflation Pressure

Consensus 2002: *The committee recommends use of the lowest intraabdominal pressure (IAP) allowing adequate exposure of the operative field rather than using a routine pressure (grade B). An IAP lower than 14 mmHg is considered safe in a healthy patient (grade A).*

Update 2006: The previous recommendations are still valid and are further supported by less pain and higher quality of life postoperatively using a low insufflation pressure (grade A).

In this update another three RCTs, including a total of 288 patients, were analysed (grade A) [2, 11, 17]. All three studies focussed on postoperative discomfort regarding pain, shoulder-tip pain, analgesia consumption or quality of life (Table 3.2). All three compare low-pressure versus high-pressure pneumoperitoneum. The definition of normal and low laparoscopic insufflation pressure was previously defined in the EAES guidelines as 12–15 and 5–7 mmHg, respectively. These definitions are not in accordance with the definitions used in two of the studies [11, 17]. The largest study of 148 cases used the recommended pressure levels of the two groups mentioned before and demonstrated significantly less pain postoperatively for the first 5 days, less analgesia consumption for the first 4 days and better quality of life concerning physical activity 7 days postoperatively [2]. There was less frequency and intensity of shoulder-tip pain together with less analgesia consumption in another study comparing 9 versus 13 mmHg [17]. The last study compared 10 versus 15 mmHg and does not show any difference between the groups concerning pain or quality of life [11].

The results from these studies further support low-pressure pneumoperitoneum being defined as 7 mmHg or lower. The ASA classification was not addressed separately in these studies. No systematic review or large individual cohort study addressing low-pressure versus high-pressure pneumoperitoneum has been identified.

Warming and Humidifying of Insufflation Gas

Consensus 2002: Warming and humidifying insufflation gas is intended to decrease heat loss; however, compared with external heating devices, the clinical effects of warmed, humidified insufflation gas are minor (grade B). Data on its influence on postoperative pain are contradictory (grade A).

Update 2006: Warming and humidifying insufflation gas compared with standard CO_2 is not associated with any clinically relevant increase in body temperature, especially when an external warming blanket is used in parallel (grade A). There is no clinically relevant effect on postoperative pain for the

Table 3.2. Randomised clinical trials comparing low- and high-pressure pneumoperitoneum. All studies were cholecystectomies

References/ years	No. of patients, operations and ASA classification	CO_2 pressures compared	Method	Results	Conclusion
Koc et al. [11]/2005	50 Double-blind ASA I–III	10 vs 15 mmHg	Pain (VAS), analgesic consumption and QoL	No difference between the groups	Low-pressure PP does not reduce postoperative pain
Barczynski et al. [2]/ 2003	148 Single-blind ASA I–II	7 vs 12 mmHg	Pain (VAS), analgesic consumption and QoL	Less pain, analgesic consumption and better QoL (physical) for low pressure	Recommends low pressure PP if adequate exposure is obtained
Sarli et al. [17]/2000	90 Double-blind ASA I–II	9 vs 13 mmHg	Shoulder-tip pain (VAS) and analgesic consumption	Lower frequency and intensity of shoulder-tip pain and less analgesic consumption in low-pressure group	Low-pressure PP reduces the frequency and intensity of shoulder-tip pain

PP pneumoperitoneum, *QoL* quality of life

two methods (grade A). Warming and humidifying insufflation failed to reduce fogging (grade A).

A total of six RCTs included 279 patients (Table 3.3). A significant increase in body temperature was demonstrated using warmed and humidified CO_2 (grade A) [6, 9, 18, 21] and no differences were found in two studies [5, 15]. Pain, analgesic consumption, recovery and hospital stay failed to demonstrate any difference in four studies [5, 6, 15, 18]. Reduced analgesic consumption was demonstrated in one study [9] and increased pain was demonstrated in another study [21] in the warmed, humidified group. Failure to reduce fogging using warmed and humidified CO_2 was demonstrated in three studies [6, 9, 15].

No systematic review or large individual cohort study has been identified addressing the method of warming and humidifying the insufflation gas.

The application of an external warming device before and during anaesthesia is included as routine in most laparoscopic settings and the possible small effect of humidified and warmed insufflation gas is not justified. Spe-

Table 3.3. Pneumoperitoneum and hypothermia; randomised clinical trials

References/ years	No. of patients, and operations	Treatments and no. in groups	Temperature and measurement	Results	Conclusion
Davis et al. [5]/ 2006	44 Single-blind 4 groups Roux-en-Y	11–standard 11–heated (insufflator tube set) 11–humidified (Insuflow) 11–heated and humidified	Urine bladder	No difference in intra-abdominal humidity or temperature. Pain (VAS), recovery and hospital stay similar	Heating or humidifying of CO_2 not justified
Savel et al. [18]/ 2005	30 Double-blind 2 groups Roux-en-Y	15–standard 15–warmed and humidified (Insuflow)	Oesophageal probe	Temperature increased in warmed/ humidified group. Pain (VAS) and analgesic consumption similar	Warmed and humidified CO_2 was not associated with any significant benefit with regards to postoperative pain
Hamza et al. [9]/ 2005	44 Double-blind 2 groups Roux-en-Y	21–standard 23–warmed and humidified (Insuflow)	Oesophageal probe Tympanic thermometer	Temperature increased and less analgesic consumption in warmed/ humidified group	Insuflow modestly reduced heat loss and analgesic consumption. It failed to reduce fogging of lens
Farley et al. [6]/ 2004	101 Double-blind 2 groups CCE	52–standard 49–warmed and humidified (Insuflow)	Oesophageal probe	Temperature increased in warmed/ humidified group. Pain, recovery and hospital stay similar	No major clinically relevant difference between the groups. Failed to reduce fogging
Nguyen et al. [15]/ 2002	20 Single-blind 2 groups Fundoplication	10–standard 10–heated (warming blanket and Insuflow)	Oesophageal probe Tympanic thermometer	No difference in temperature, pain (VAS), analgesic consumption, hemodynamics and lens fogging	Heated and humidified CO_2 with additional external warming did not influence temperature or pain

Table 3.3 (continued)

References/ years	No. of patients, and operations	Treatments and no. in groups	Temperature and measurement	Results	Conclusion
Wills et al. [21]/2001	40 Double-blind 2 groups Fundoplication	21–standard 19–heated		Increased temperature, pain (VAS) and analgesic consumption in heated group	Heated CO_2 provides no benefit but may be associated with increased early pain

CCE cholecystectomy

cial precautions to minimise gas leakage are essential in laparoscopic surgery for the purpose of reducing the risk of hypothermia.

References

1. Agresta F, DeSimone P, Ciardo LF, Bedin N (2004) Direct trocar insertion vs Veress needle in nonobese patients undergoing laparoscopic procedures. Surg Endosc 18:1778–1781
2. Barczynski M, Herman RM (2003) A prospective randomised trial on comparison of low-pressure (LP) and standard-pressure (SP) pneumoperitoneum for laparoscopic cholecystectomy. Surg Endosc 17:533–538
3. Bernik JR, Trocciola Susan M, Mayer David A, Patane J, Czura CJ, Wallack MK (2001) Balloon blunt-tip trocar for laparoscopic cholecystectomy: improvement over the traditional Hasson and Veress needle methods. J Laparoendosc Adv Surg Tech 11:73–78
4. Bhoyrul S, Payne J, Steffes B, Swanstrom L, Way LW (2000) A randomised prospective study of radially expanding trocars in laparoscopic surgery. J Gastrointest Surg 4:392–397
5. Davis SS, Mikami DJ, Newlin M, Needleman BJ, Barrett MS, Fries R, Larson T, Dundon J, Goldblatt MI, Melvin WS (2006) Heating and humidifying of carbon dioxide during pneumoperitoneum is not indicated. Surg Endosc 20:153–158
6. Farley DR, Grenlee SM, Larson DR, Harrington JR (2004) Double-blind, prospective, randomized study of warmed, humidified carbon dioxide insufflation vs standard carbon dioxide for patients undergoing laparoscopic cholecystectomy. Arch Surg 139:739–744
7. Galen DI (2001) Radially expanding access device for laparoscopic surgery: efficacy and safety in comparison with sharp laparoscopic cannulae. Minim Invasive Ther Allied Technol 10:51–54
8. Günenc MZ, Yesildaglar N, Bingöl B, Önalan G, Tabak S, Gökmen B (2005) The safety and efficacy of direct trocar insertion with elevation of the rectus sheath instead of the skin for pneumoperitoneum. Surg Laparosc Endosc Percutan Tech 15:80–81
9. Hamza MA, Schneider BE, White PF, Recart A, Villegas L, Ogunnaike B, Provost D, Jones D (2005) Heated and humidified insufflation during laparoscopic gastric bypass surgery: effect on temperature, postoperative pain and recovery outcomes. J Laparoendosc Adv Surg Tech 15:6–12
10. Koc M, Ertan T, Tez M, Kocpinar MA, Kilic M, Gocmen E, Kessaf AA (2005) Randomized, prospective comparison of postoperative pain in low- versus high-pressure pneumoperitoneum. ANZ J Surg 75:693–696

11. Merlin TL, Hiller JE, Maddern GJ, Jamieson GG, Brown AR, Kolbe A (2003) Systematic review of the safety and effectiveness of methods used to establish pneumoperitoneum in laparoscopic surgery. Br J Surg 90:668–679
12. Moberg A-C, Montgomery A (2005) Primary access-related complications with laparoscopy. Surg Endosc 19:1196–1199
13. Molloy D, Kaloo PD, Cooper M, Nguyen TV (2002) Laparoscopic entry: a literature review and analysis of techniques and complications of primary port entry. Aust N Z J Obstet Gynaecol 42:246
14. Neudecker J, Sauerland S, Neugebauer E, Bergamaschi R, Bonjer J, Cuschieri A, Fuchs KH, Jacobi CH, Jansen FW, Kovusalo AM, Lacy A, McMahon MJ, Millat B, Schwenk W (2002) The European Association for Endoscopic Surgery clinical practice guideline on the pneumoperitoneum for laparoscopic surgery. Surg Endosc 16:1121–1143
15. Nguyen NT, Furdui G, Fleming NW, Lee SJ, Goldman CD, Singh A, Wolfe BM (2002) Effect of heated and humidified carbon dioxide gas on core temperature and postoperative pain. Surg Endosc 16:1050–1054
16. Sackett DL, Straus SE, Richardson WS, Rosenberg W, Haynes RB (2000) Evidence-based medicine: how to practice and teach EBM, 2nd edn. Churchill Livingston, London
17. Sarli L, Sansebastiano G, Trivelli M, Roncoroni L (2000) Prospective randomized trial of low-pressure pneumoperitoneum for reduction of shoulder-tip pain following laparoscopy. Br J Surg 87:1161–1165
18. Savel RH, Balasubramanya S, Lasheen S, Gaprindashvili T, Arabov E, Fazylov RM, Lazzaro RS, Macura JM (2005) Beneficial effects of humidified, warmed carbon dioxide insufflation during laparoscopic bariatric surgery: a randomized clinical trial. Obes Surg 15:64–69
19. Schäfer M, Lauper M, Krähenbühl L (2001) Trocar and Veress needle injuries during laparoscopy. Surg Endosc 15:275–280
20. String A, Berber E, Foroutani A, Macho JR, Peal JM, Siperstein AE (2001) Use of the optical access trocar for safe and rapid entry in various laparoscopic procedures. Surg Endosc 15:570–573
21. Wills VL, Hunt DR, Armstrong A (2001) A randomised controlled trial assessing the effect of heated carbon dioxide for insufflation on pain and recovery after laparoscopic surgery. Surg Endosc 15:166–170
22. Yerdel MA, Karayalcin K, Koyuncy A, Akin B, Kokoy C, Turkcapar AG, Erverdi N, Alacayir I, Bumin C, Nusret A (1999) Direct trocar insertation versus Veress needle insertion in laparoscopic cholecystectomy. Am J Surg 177:247–249
23. Yim SJF, Yuen PM (2001) Randomised double-masked comparison of radially expanding access device and conventional cutting tip trocar in laparoscopy. Obstet Gynecol 97:435–438

The EAES Clinical Practice Guidelines on Laparoscopic Antireflux Surgery for Gastroesophagel Reflux Disease (1997)

Ernst Eypasch, Edmund A. M. Neugebauer, F. Fischer, Hans Troidl, A. L. Blum, D. Collet, A. Cuschieri, B. Dallemagne, H. Feussner, K.-H. Fuchs, H. Glise, C. K. Kum, T. Lerut, L. Lundell, H. E. Myrvold, A. Peracchia, H. Petersen, J. J. B. van Lanschot

Introduction

In the last 2 years, growing experience and enormous technical developments have made it possible for almost any abdominal operation to be performed via endoscopic surgery. Laparoscopic cholecystectomy, appendectomy, and hernia repair have been going through the characteristic life cycle of technological innovations, and cholecystectomy, at least, seems to have proven a definitive success. To evaluate this life cycle, consensus conferences on these topics have been organized and performed by the EAES [76b].

Currently, the interest of endoscopic abdominal surgery is focusing on antireflux operation. This is documented by an increasing number of operations and publications in the literature. The international societies such as the European Association for Endoscopic Surgery (EAES) have the responsibility to provide a forum for discussion of new developments and to provide guidelines on best practice based on the current state of knowledge. Therefore, a consensus development conference on laparoscopic antireflux surgery for gastroesophageal reflux disease (GERD) was held, which included discussion of some pathophysiological aspects of the disease. Based on the experience of previous consensus conferences (Madrid 1994), the process of the consensus development conference was slightly modified. The development process was concentrated on one subject – reflux disease – and during the 4th International Meeting of the EAES, a long public discussion, including all aspects of the consensus document, was incorporated into the process.

The methods and the results of this consensus conference are presented in this comprehensive article.

Methods

At the Annual Meeting in Luxemburg in 1995, the joint session of the Scientific and Educational Committee of the EAES decided to hold a Consensus Development Conference (CDC) on laparoscopic antireflux surgery for gastroesophageal reflux disease. The 4th International Congress of the EAES in June 1996 in Trondheim should be the forum for the public discussion and finalization of the Consensus Development Conference.

The Cologne group (E. Neugebauer, E. Eypasch, F. Fischer, H. Troidl) was authorized to organize the CDC according to general guidelines. The procedure chosen was the following: A small group of 13 internationally known experts was nominated by the Scientific Committee of the EAES The criteria for selection were:

1. Clinical expertise in the field of endoscopic surgery
2. Academic activity
3. Community influence
4. Geographical location.

Internationally well-known gastroenterologists were asked to participate in the conference in the interest of a balanced discussion between internists and surgeons.

Prior to the conference, each panelist received a document containing guidelines on how to estimate the strength of evidence in the literature for specific endoscopical procedures and a document containing descriptions of the levels of technology assessment (TA) according to Mosteller and Troidl [190 a]. Each panelist was asked to indicate what level of development, in his opinion, laparoscopic antireflux surgery has attained generally, and he was given a form containing specific TA parameters relevant to the endoscopic procedure under assessment. In this form, the panelist was asked to indicate the status of the endoscopic procedure in comparison with conventional open procedures and also to make a comparison between surgical and medical treatment of gastroesophageal reflux disease. The panelist's view must have been supported by evidence in the literature, and a reference list was mandatory for each item. Each panelist was given a list of relevant specific questions pertaining to each procedure (indication, technical aspects, training, postoperative evaluation, etc.). The panelists were asked to provide brief answers with references. Guidelines for response were given and the panelists were asked to send their initial evaluation back to the conference organizers 3 months prior to the conference.

In Cologne, the congress organization team analyzed the individual answers and compiled a preconsensus provisional document.

In particular, the input and comments of gastroenterologists were incorporated to modify the preconsensus document.

The preconsensus documents were posted to each panelist prior to the Trondheim meeting. During the Trondheim conference, in a 3-h session, the preconsensus document was scrutinized word by word and a version to be presented in the public session was prepared. The following day, a 2-h public session took place, during which the text and the tables of the consensus document were read and discussed in great detail. A further 2-h postconference session of the panelists incorporated all suggestions made during the public session. The final postconsensus document was mailed to all expert participants, checked for mistakes and necessary corrections and finalized in September 1996. The full text of the statements is given below.

Consensus Statements on Gastroesophageal Reflux Disease

1. What Are the Epidemiologic Facts in GERD?

In western countries, gastroesophageal reflux has a high prevalence. In the USA and Europe, up to 44% of the adult population describe symptoms characteristic of GERD [124, 127, 242]. Troublesome symptoms characteristic of GERD occur in 10–15% with equal frequency in men and women. Men, however, seem to develop reflux esophagitis and complications of esophagitis more frequently than women [23].

Data from the literature indicate that 10–50% of these subjects will need long-term treatment of some kind for their symptoms and/or esophagitis [34, 195, 225, 242].

The panelists agreed that the natural history of the disease varies widely from very benign and harmless reflux to a disabling stage of the disease with severe symptoms and morphological alterations. There are no good long-term data indicating how the natural history of the disease changes from one stage to the other and when and how complications (esophagitis, stricture, etc.) develop.

Topics which were the subject of considerable debate but which could not be resolved during this conference are listed here [8, 11, 23, 28, 68]:

- The cause of the increasing prevalence of esophagitis
- The cause of the increasing prevalence of Barrett's esophagus and adenocarcinoma
- The discrepancy between clinically and anatomically determined prevalence of Barrett's esophagus
- The problem of ultrashort Barrett's esophagus and its meaning
- The relationship between *Helicobacter pylori* infection and reflux esophagitis
- Gastroesophageal reflux without esophagitis and abnormal sensitivity of the esophagus to acid
- The role of so-called alkaline reflux, which is currently difficult to measure objectively.

2. What Is the Current Pathophysiological Concept of GERD?

GERD is a multifactorial process in which esophageal and gastric changes are involved [27, 65, 98, 251, 283].

Major causes involved in the pathophysiology are incompetence of the lower esophageal sphincter expressed as low sphincter length and pressure, frequent transient lower esophageal sphincter relaxations, insufficient esophageal peristalsis, altered esophageal mucosal resistance, delayed gastric emptying, and antroduodenal motility disorders with pathologic duodenogastroesophageal reflux [27, 65, 92, 95, 134, 251, 283].

Several factors can play an aggravating role: stress, posture, obesity, pregnancy, dietary factors (e.g., fat, chocolate, caffeine, fruit juice, peppermint, alcohol, spicy food), and drugs (e.g., calcium antagonists, anticholinergics, theophylline, (β-blockers, dihydropyridine). All these factors might influence the pressure gradient from the abdomen to the chest either by decreasing the lower esophageal sphincter or by increasing abdominal pressure.

Other parts of the physiological mosaic that might contribute to gastroesophageal reflux include the circadian rhythm of sphincter pressure, gastric and salivary secretion, esophageal clearance mechanisms, as well as hiatal hemia and *H. pylori* infection.

3. What Is a Useful Definition of the Disease?

A universally agreed upon scientific classification of GERD is not yet available. The current model of gastroesophageal reflux disease sees it as an excessive exposure of the mucosa to gastric contents (amount and composition) causing symptoms accompanied and/or caused by different pathophysiological phenomena (sphincter pressure, peristalsis) leading to morphological changes (esophagitis, cell infiltration) [65, 98].

This implies an abnormal exposure to acid and/or other gastric contents like bile and duodenal and pancreatic juice in cases of a combined duodenogastroesophageal reflux.

GERD is frequently classified as a synonym for esophagitis, even though there is considerable evidence that only 60% of patients with reflux disease sustain damage of their mucosa [8, 91, 150, 200, 231, 243]. The MUSE and Savary esophagitis classifications are currently used to stage damage, but they are poor for staging the disease [8].

The modified AFP Score (Anatomy-Function-Pathology) is an attempt to incorporate the presence of hiatus hemia, reflux, and macroscopic and morphologic damage into a classification [83]. However, this classification lacks symptomatology and should be linked to a scoring system for symptoms or quality of life; both scoring systems are extremely important for staging of the disease and for the indication for treatment [195 a, b].

4. What Establishes the Diagnosis of the Disease?

A large variety of different symptoms are described in the context of gastroesophageal reflux disease, such as dysphagia, pharyngeal pain, hoarseness, nausea, belching, epigastric pain, retrostemal pain, acid and food regurgitation, retrostemal burning, heartburn, retrostemal pressure, and coughing. The characteristic symptoms are heartburn (retrosternal buming), regurgitation, pain, and respiratory symptoms [150, 204]. Symptoms are usually related to posture and eating habits.

In addition, typical reflux patients may have symptoms which are not located in the region of the esophagus. Patients with heartbum may or may not have pathological reflux. They may have reflux-type "nonulcer dyspepsia" or other functional disorders.

The diagnostic tests that are needed must follow a certain algorithm. After the history and physical examination of the patients, an upper gastrointestinal endoscopy is performed. A biopsy is taken if any abnormalities (stenosis, strictures, Barrett's, etc.) are found [8].

If no morphologic evidence can be detected, only functional studies, e.g., measuring the acid exposure in the esophageal lumen by 24-h esophageal pH monitoring, are helpful and indicated to detect excessive reflux [65]. It is of vital importance that the pH electrode be accurately positioned in relation to the lower esophageal sphincter (LES). Manometry is the only objective way to assess the location of the LES.

Ordinary esophageal radiologic studies (barium swallow) are considered another mandatory basic imaging study [105 a].

At the next level of investigation there are a number of tests that look for the cause of pathologic reflux using esophageal manometry as a basic investigative tool for this purpose to assess lower esophageal sphincter and esophageal body function [27, 65, 91, 134, 283]. Video esophagography or esophageal emptying scintigraphy may also be helpful.

Optional gastric function studies are 24-h gastric pH monitoring, photooptic bilirubin assessment to assess duodenogastroesophageal reflux, gastric emptying scintigraphy, and antroduodenal manometry [81, 93, 95, 118, 146, 234].

Currently these gastric function studies are of scientific interest but they do not yet play a role in overall clinical patient management, apart from selected patients. The diagnostic test ranking order is displayed in Table 4.1.

Table 4.1. Diagnostic test ranking order for gastroesophageal reflux disease

Basic diagnostic tests	Physiologic/pathologic criteria	References
Endoscopy+ histology	Savary–Miller classification I, II, II, IV, V MUSE classification (M) metaplasia (U) ulcer (S) stricture (E) erosions	Savary and Miller [231], Armstrong et al. [8]
Radiology	Barium swallow	Gelfand [105a]
24-h esophageal pH monitoring	Percentage time below pH 4 DeMeester score	DeMeester et al. [65]
Stationary esophageal manometry [a]	LES: Overall length Intraabdominal length Pressure	DeMeester et al. [65] Dent et al. [69a]
	(Transient LES relaxations) esophageal body disorders weak peristalsis	Eypasch et al. [78]
Optional tests	Persistent gastric acidity	Barlow et al. [14b]
24-h gastric pH monitoring	Excessive duodenogastric reflux	Fuchs et al. [93, 95] Schwizer et al. [234]
Gastric emptying scintigraphy	Delayed gastric emptying	Clark et al. [40]
Photo-optic bilirubin assessment	Esophageal bile exposure	Kauer et al. [146]
	Gastric bile exposure	Fein et al. [81]

[a] The concise numerical values for sphincter length, pressure, and relaxation depend on the respective manometric recording system used in the esophagealfunction lab

5. What Is the Indication for Treatment?

Pivotal criteria for the indication to medical treatment in gastroesophageal reflux disease are the patient's symptoms, reduced quality of life, and the general condition of the patient. When symptoms persist or recur after medication, endoscopy is strongly indicated.

Mucosal damage (esophagitis) indicates a strong need for medical treatment. If the symptoms persist, partially persist, or recur after stopping medication, there is a good indication for doing functional studies. Gastrointestinal endoscopy, already mentioned as the basic imaging examination in GERD, should be performed in context with the functional studies.

Indication for surgery is again centrally based on the patient's symptoms, the duration of the symptoms, and the damage that is present.

Even after successful medical acid suppression the patient can have persistent or recurrent symptoms of epigastric pain and retrosternal pressure as well as food regurgitation due to the incompetent cardia, insufficient peristalsis, and/or a large hiatal hemia.

With respect to indication, one important factor in the patient's general condition is age. On the one hand, age plays a role in the risks stratification when the individual risk of an operation is estimated together with the comorbidity of the patient. On the other hand, age is an economic factor with respect to the break-even point between medical and surgical treatment [21 b].

Concerning the indication for surgery, a differentiation in the symptoms between heartburn and regurgitation is considered important. (Medical treatment appears to be more effective for heartburn than for regurgitation.)

Therefore the indication for surgery is based on the following facts:

- Noncompliance of the patient with ongoing effective medical treatment. Reasons for noncompliance are preference, refusal, reduced quality of life, or drug dependency and drug side effects.
- Persistent or recurrent esophagitis in spite of currently optimal medical treatment and in association with symptoms.
- Complications of the disease (stenoses, ulcers, and Barrett's esophagus [11, 68]) have a minor influence on the indication. Neither medical nor surgical treatment has been shown to alter the extent of Barrett's epithelium.

Therefore mainly symptoms and their relation to ongoing medical treatment play the major role in the indication for surgery. However, antireflux surgery may reduce the need for subsequent endoscopic dilatations [21a]. The participants pointed out that patients with symptoms completely resistant to antisecretory treatment with H_2-blockers or proton-pump inhibitors are bad candidates for surgery. In these individuals other diseases have to be investigated carefully. On the contrary, good candidates for surgery should have a good response to antisecretory drugs. Thus, compliance and preference determine which treatment is chosen (conservative or operative).

6. What Are the Essentials of Laparoscopic Surgical Treatment?

The goal of surgical treatment for GERD is to relieve the symptoms and prevent progression and complications of the disease creating a new anatomical high-pressure zone. This must be achieved without dysphagia, which can occur when the outflow resistance of the reconstructed GE junction exceeds the peristaltic power of the body of the esophagus. Achievement of this goal requires an understanding of the natural history of GERD, the status of the patient's esophageal function, and a selection of the appropriate antireflux procedure.

Since the newly created structure is only a substitute for the lower esophageal sphincter, it is a matter of discussion to what extent it can show physiological reactions (normal resting pressure, reaction to pharmacological stimuli, appropriate relaxations during deglutition, etc.). There is no agreement on how surgical procedures work and restore the gastroesophageal reflux barrier.

With respect to the details of the laparoscopic surgical procedures, the following degree of consensus was attained by the panel (11 present participants) (yes/no):

1. Is there a need for mobilization of the gastric fundus by dividing the short gastric vessels? (7/4)
2. Is there a need for dissection of the crura? (11/0)
3. Is there a need for identification of the vagal trunks? (7/4)
4. Is there a need for removal of the esophageal fat pad? (2/9)
5. Is there a need for closure of the crura posteriorly? (11/0)
6. Should nonabsorbable sutures be used (crura, wrap)? (11/0) [1]
7. Should a large bougie (40–60 French) be used for calibration? (5/6)
8. Should objective assessment be performed (e.g., calibration by a bougie, others) for
   Tightness of the hiatus? (9/0)
   Tightness of the wrap? (9/2)
9. If there is normal peristalsis should one
   routinely use a 360° short floppy fundoplication wrap? (8)
   routinely use a partial fundoplication wrap? (2)
   Use a short wrap equal to or shorter than 2.5 cm? (1)
10. In cases of weak peristalsis, should there be a "tailored approach" (total or partial wrap)? (5/6)[1]

7. Which Are the Important End Points of Treatment Whether Medical or Surgical?

The important end points for the success of conservative/ medical as well as surgical therapy must be a mosaic of different criteria, since neither clinical symptoms, functional criteria, nor the daily activity and quality-of-life assessment can be used *solely* to assess the therapeutic result in this multifactorial disease process.

Patients show great variety in demonstrating and expressing the severity of clinical symptoms and, therefore, they alone are not a reliable guide. Functional criteria can be assessed objectively, but may not be used in the decisionmaking process without looking at the stage of mucosal damage or morphological abnormalities (hiatus hemia, slipped wrap; AFP Score).

---

[1] During the public discussion, Professor Montori (Rome) mentioned the Angelchick prosthesis as a rare alternative – however, this was not discussed in the consensus group

Complete evaluation includes assessment of symptoms, daily activity, and quality of life–ideally, in every single patient.

Instruments: The examples of instruments are listed in [80a, 195a, b].

The earliest point at which one ought to collect functional data after the operation is 6 months. The reasonable time of assessment in the postsurgical follow-up phase is probably 1 year followed by 2-year intervals.

Economic assessment is considered to be a significant end point and is dealt with in a later section.

There is no evidence that laparoscopic surgery should be any better than conventional surgery. If laparoscopic surgery is correctly performed, apart from the problems of abdominal wall complications like hernia, infection, and wound rupture, there should be no difference in outcome as compared to the standard obtained in open surgery.

Laparoscopic surgery, however, has the potential to reduce postoperative pain and limitations of daily activity.

8. What is Failure of Treatment?

In gastroesophageal reflux disease, lifelong medication is needed in many patients, because the disease persists but the acid reduction can take away the symptoms during the time the medication is taken. The disease is treated by reducing the acid and not by treating or correcting the causes of the disease. This latter argument can be used by surgeons, since they mechanically restore the sphincter area and, therefore, correct the most frequent defect associated with the disease.

In surgery, failure of a treatment is defined as the persistence or recurrence of symptoms and/or objective pathologic findings once the treatment phase is finished. In GERD, a definite failure is present when symptoms which are severe enough to require at least intermittent therapy (heartburn, regurgitation) recur after treatment or when other serious problems ("slipped Nissen", severe gas bloat syndrome, dumping syndrome, etc.) arise and when functional studies document that symptoms are due to this problem. Recurrence can occur with or without esophageal damage (esophagitis). Professor Blum (Lausanne) suggested that further long-term outcome studies of medical and surgical treatment are needed.

Quality-of-life measurements are able to differentiate whether and to what extent recurrent symptoms are really impairing the patient's quality of life.

It was agreed upon that a distinction is necessary between the two types of failures of the operation: "the unhappy 5–10%" (i.e. slipped Nissen, etc.) and the 10–40% of individuals who only become aware of their dyspeptic symptoms postoperatively while the reflux-related symptoms are treated. Dyspeptic symptoms occur in the normal population in 20–40% [174b].

Some of the "postfundoplication symptoms" are present already before the operation and are due to the dyspeptic symptomatology associated with GERD.

Patients with failures should be worked up with the available diagnostic tests to detect the underlying cause of the failure. If there is mild recurrent reflux, it usually can be treated by medication as long as the patient is satisfied with this solution and his/her quality of life is good. In the case of severe symptomatic recurrent reflux or other complications, and if endoscopy shows visible esophagitis, the indication for refundoplication after a thorough diagnostic workup must be established. Surgeons very experienced in pathophysiology, diagnosis, and the surgical technique of the disease should perform these redo operations. Expert management of patients undergoing redo surgery for a benign condition is of extreme importance.

9. What Are the Issues in an Economic Evaluation?

With respect to a complete economic evaluation the panelists refer to the available literature [14a, 76a].

Cost, cost minimization, and cost-effectiveness analyses of gastroesophageal reflux disease must take into account the following issues (list incomplete):

1. Costs of medications
2. Costs of office visits
3. Costs of routine endoscopies
4. Frequency of sick leaves at work
5. Frequency of restricted family or hobby activity at home
6. Assessment of job performance and restrictions due to the disease
7. Costs of diagnostic workup including functional studies and specialized investigations
8. Costs of surgical intervention
9. Costs for treatment of surgical complications
10. Costs of treatment of complications of maintenance medical therapy, such as emergency hospital admissions, e.g., swallowing discomfort, bolus entrapment in peptic stenoses
11. Perspective of the analysis (patient, hospital, society)
12. Health care system (socialized, private).

A special issue is the so-called break-even point between medical and surgical treatment (duration and cost of medical treatment vs laparoscopic antireflux treatment) [21b].

Ultimately, the results of medical or surgical treatment, especially with respect to age of the patient, should be translated into quality-adjusted life-years (QALYs) to differentiate which treatment is better for what age, comorbidity, and stage of disease.

Literature List with Ratings of References

All literature submitted by the panelists as supportive evidence for their evaluation was compiled and rated. The ratings of the references are based on the panelists' evaluation. The number of references is incomplete for the case series without controls and anecdotal reports. The result of the panelists' evaluation is given in Table 4.2 for the endoscopic antireflux operations and in Table 4.3 for medical treatments (all options). The consensus statements are based on these published results. A complete list of all references mentioned in Tables 4.2 and 4.3 is included.

Question 1. What Stage of Technological Development is Endoscopic Antireflux Operations at (in June 1996)?

The definitions for the stages in technological development follow the recommendations of the Committee for Evaluating Medical Technologies in Clinical Use [190 a] (Mosteller F, 1985) extended by criteria introduced by Troidl (1995). The panel's evaluation as to the attainment of each technological stage by endoscopic antireflux surgery, together with the strength of evidence in the literature, is presented in Table 4.4.

Technical performance and applicability were demonstrated by several authors as early as 1992/1993. The results on safety, complications, morbidity, and mortality data depend on the leaming phase (more than 50 cases) of the operations. The complication, reoperation, and conversion rates are higher in the first 20 cases of an individual surgeon. It is strongly advocated that experienced supervision be sought by surgeons beginning laparoscopic fund-

Table 4.2. Ratings of published literature on antireflux operations and medical treatment: strength of evidence in the literature-antireflux operations

Study type	Strength of evidence	References
Clinical randomized controlled studies with power and relevant clinical end points	III	[202, 203, 246, 274]
Cohort studies with controls prospective, parallel controls prospective, historical controls	II	[32, 37, 49, 80 87, 110 130 147, 163, 188, 217, 221, 272, 274, 281]
Case-control studies Cohort studies with literature controls Analysis of databases Reports of expert committees	I	[3, 4, 12, 19, 22, 36, 44, 47, 49, 55, 60 61, 63, 72, 73, 95, 89, 107, 113, 126, 132, 159, 162, 163, 177, 184, 187, 190 192, 208, 212, 213, 216, 219, 237, 255, 267]
Case series without controls Anecdotal reports Belief	0	Numerous

Table 4.3. Ratings of published literature on antireflux operations and medical treatment strength of evidence in the literature-medical treatment

Study type	Strength of evidence	References
Clinical randomized controlled studies with power and relevant clinical end points	III	[10 17, 24, 26, 39, 56, 70 112, 115, 116, 120 121, 139, 151, 161, 168, 171, 180 189, 202, 223, 224, 227, 228, 240 244, 246, 263, 265, 268, 270 274, 282, 284]
Cohort studies with controls: ■ Prospective, parallel controls ■ Prospective, historical controls	II	[3, 6, 23, 29, 38, 85, 101, 130 135, 139]
Case-control studies Cohort studies with literature controls Analysis of databases Reports of expert committees	I	[16, 23, 50, 72, 117, 123, 135, 152, 157, 172, 174, 200 229, 241, 260, 264]
Case series without controls Anecdotal reports Belief	0	Numerous

Table 4.4. Evaluation of the status of endoscopic antireflux surgery 1996: level attained and strength of evidence

Stages in technology assessment[a]	Level attained/ strength of evidence[b]	Consensus (%)[c]
1. Feasibility Technical performance, applicability, safety, complications, morbidity, mortality	II	64 (7/11)
2. Efficacy ■ Benefit for the *patient* demonstrated in centers of excellence	II	64 (7/11)
■ Benefit for the *surgeon* (shorter operating time, easier technique)	0–I	67 (6/9)
3. Effectiveness Benefit for the patient under normal clinical conditions, i.e., good results reproducible with widespread application	II	60 (6/10)
4. Costs Benefit in terms of cost-effectiveness	I–II	70 (7/10)
5. Ethics Issues of concern may be long operation times, frequency of thrombo-embolization, incidence of reoperations, altered indication for surgery, etc.[c]	0	57 (4/7)
6. Recommendation	Yes	100 (11/11)

[a] Mosteller [190a] and Troidl [265a]
[b] Level attained to the definitions of the different grades
[c] Percentage of consensus was calculated by dividing the number of panelists who voted 0, I, II or III by total number of panelists who submitted their evaluation forms

oplication during their first 20 procedures [278a, b]. Data on *efficacy* (benefit for the patient) demonstrated in centers of excellence were based on type II studies. The benefit for the surgeon in terms of elegance, ease, and speed of the procedure is not yet clear cut. The operation time is the same or longer, and the technique is harder initially – however, the view of the operating field is better. The effectiveness data are still insufficient, long-term results are missing, and the results reported come mainly from interested centers and multicenter studies. It is important to audit continually the results of antireflux operations, especially because different techniques are used. The economic evaluation of laparoscopic antireflux surgery is still premature (few data from small studies only). Future studies are recommended in different health care systems, assessing the relative economic advantages of laparoscopic antireflux surgery in comparison to the available and paid medical treatment.

A major issue of ethical concern is the altered indication for surgery. A change of indication might produce more cost and harm in inappropriately selected patients. Laparoscopic antireflux surgery should be recommended in centers with sufficient experience and an adequate number of individuals with the disease. Randomized controlled studies are recommended to compare medical vs laparoscopic surgical treatment and partial vs total fundoplication wraps.

Question 2. What is the Current Status of Laparoscopic Antireflux Surgery vs Open Conventional Procedures in Terms of Feasibility and Efficacy parameters?

Tables with specific parameters relevant to open and laparoscopic antireflux procedures summarize the current status (Tables 4.5, 4.6). The evaluation is mainly based on type I and type II studies (see list of references).

The results show that safety is comparable and rather favorable compared to the open technique. The incidence for complications, morbidity, and mortality is similar to the open technique once the learning phase has been surpassed. For specific intraoperative and postoperative adverse events see Tables 4.5 and 4.6.

In terms of *efficacy*, significant advantages of the endoscopic antireflux operations are: less postoperative pain, shorter hospital stay, and earlier return to normal activities and work.

In general, laparoscopic antireflux surgery has advantages over open conventional procedures if performed by trained surgeons.

Laparoscopic antireflux surgery has the potential to improve reflux treatment provided that appropriate diagnostic facilities for functional esophageal studies and adequately trained and dedicated surgeons are available.

Table 4.5. Antireflux surgery vs open conventional procedures: evaluation of feasibility parameters by all panelists at CDC in Trondheim

Stages of technology assessment	Assessment based on evidence in the literature					Consensus[b]	Strength of evidence 0–III[c]
	Definitely better[a]	Probably better	Similar	Probably worse	Definitely worse		
Safety/intraop. adverse events	1		6	4		55% (6/11) similar	I–II
Gastric or esophageal leaks/perforations							
Hiatal entrapments of gastric warp with necrosis	1		9	1		82% (9/11) similar	I–II
Vascular injury, bleeding, splenic injury	2	4	5			55% (6/11) better	I–II
Emphysema	1		3	4	2	60% (6/10) worse	II
Operation time			3	5	1	67% (6/9) worse	II
Postoperative adverse events	1	2	8			73% (8/11) similar	I–II
Bleeding							
Wound infection	3	6	2			82% (9/11) better	I–II
Reoperation		2	6	3		55% (6/11) similar	I–II
Warp disorders		1	8	2		73% (8/11) similar	I–II
Hemias of abdominal wall	3	6	2			82% (9/11) better	I–II
Thrombosis/pulmonary embolism	1	3	6	1		55% (6/11) similar	I
Mortality		3	7			70% (7/10) similar	I–II

a) Comparison: laparoscopic fundoplication techniques vs open conventional procedure
b) Percentage of consensus was calculated by dividing the number of panelists who voted better (probably and definitely), similar, or worse (probably and definitely) by the total number of panelist's who submitted their evaluation forms
c) Refer to Table 4.1

Table 4.6. Antireflux surgery vs open conventional procedures: evaluation of efficacy parameters by all panelists prior to CDC in Trondheim

Stages of technology assessment	Assessment based on evidence in the literature					Consensus[b]	Strength of evidence 0–III[c]
	Definitely better[a]	Probably better	Similar	Probably worse	Definitely worse		
Postoperative pain	6	4				100% (10/10) better	I–II
Postoperative disorders			9	1		90% (9/10) similar	I–II
Bloating							
Flatulence			10	1		91% (10/11) similar	I–II
Dysphagia			9	2		82% (9/11) similar	I–II
Recurrent reflux			10			100% (10/10) similar	I–II
Hospital stay	4	7				100% (10/10) better	I–II
Return to normal activities and work	7	3				91% (10/11) better	I–II
Cosmesis	7	2	2			82% (9/11) better	I–II
Effectiveness (overall assessment)	1	5	4			60% (6/10)	I–II

a) Comparison: laparoscopic fundoplication techniques vs open conventional procedure
b) Percentage of consensus was calculated by dividing the number of panelists who voted better (probably and definitely), similar, or worse (probably and definitely) by the total number of panelists who submitted their evaluation forms
c) Refer to Table 4.1

References

1. Ackermann C, Margreth L, Müller C, Harder F (1988) Das Langzeitresultat nach Fundoplication. Schweiz Med Wochenschr 118:774
2. Allison PR (1951) Reflux oesophagitis, sliding hemia and the anatomy of repair. Surg Gynecol Obstet 92:419–431
3. Anvari N, Allen C (1996) Incidence of dysphagia following laparoscopic Nissen fundoplication without division of short gastrics. Surg Endosc 10:199
4. Anvari M, Allen C, Born A (1995) Laparoscopic Nissen fundoplication is a satisfactory alternative to long-term omeprazole therapy. Br J Surg 82:938–942
5. Apelgren K (1996) Hospital charges for Nissen fundoplication and other laparoscopic procedures. Surg Endosc 10:359–360
6. Armstrong D, Blum AL (1989) Full-dose H2-receptor antagonist prophylaxis does not prevent relapse of reflux oesophagitis. Gut 30:A1494
7. Armstrong D, Monnier P, Nicolet M, Blum AC, Savary M (1991) Endoscopic assessment of esophagitis. Gullet 1:63–67
8. Armstrong D, Blum AL, Savary M (1992) Reflux disease and Barrett's esophagus. Endoscopy 24:9–17
9. Armstrong D, Nicolet M, Monnier P, Chapuis G, Savary M, Blum AL (1992) Maintenance therapy: is there still a place for antireflux surgery? [Review]. World J Surg 16:300–307
10. Arvanitakis C, Nikopoulos A, Theoharidis A (1993) Cisapride and ranitidine in the treatment of gastro-oesophageal reflux disease – a comparative randomized double-blind trial. Aliment Phannacol Ther 7:635–641
11. Attwood SEA, Barlow AP, Norris TL, Watson A (1992) Barrett's oesophagus: effect of antireflux surgery on symptom control and development of complications. Br J Surg 79:1060–1063
12. Aye RW, Hill LD, Kraemer SJ, Snopkowski P (1994) Early results with the laparoscopic Hill repair. Am J Surg 167:542–546
13. Bagnato VJ (1992) Laparoscopic Nissen fundoplication. Surg Laparosc Endosc 2:188–190
14. Ball CS, Norris T, Watson A (1988) Acid sensitivity in reflux oesophagitis with and without complications. Gut 29:799
14a. Barnes BA (1982) Cost benefit and cost effectiveness analysis in surgery. Surg Clin North Am 62:737–748
14b. Barlow AP, DeMeester TR, Boll CS, Eypasch EP (1989) The significance of gastric hypersecretion in gastroesophageal reflux disease. Arch Surg 124:937–940
15. Bechi P, Pucciani F, Baldini F (1993) Long-term ambulatory enterogastric reflux monitoring. Validation of a new fiber optic technique. Dig Dis Sci 38:1297–1306
16. Beck IT, Connon J, Lemire S, Thomson ABR (1992) Canadian consensus conference on the treatment of gastroesophageal reflux disease. Can J Gastroenterol 6:277–289
17. Behar J, Sheahan DG, Biancani B, Spiro HM, Storer EH (1975) Medical and surgical management of reflux esophagitis: a 38-month report on a prospective clinical trial. N Engl J Med 293:263–268
18. Bell NJV, Burget B, Howden CW (1992) Appropriate acid suppression for the management of gastro-oesophageal reflux disease. Digestion 51:59–67
19. Bell RCW, Hanna P, Treibling A (1996) Experience with 1202 laparoscopic Toupet fundoplications. Surg Endosc 10:198
20. Belsey R (1977) Mark IV repair of hiatal hernia by the transthoracic approach. World J Surg 1:475–483
21. Berguer R, Stiegmann GV, Yamamoto M, Kim J, Mansour A, Denton J, Norton LW, Angelchik JP (1991) Minimal access surgery for gastroesophageal reflux: laparoscopic placement of the Angelchik prosthesis in pigs. Surg Endosc 5:123–126
21a. Bonavina L, Bardini R, Baessato M, Peracchia A (1993) Surgical treatment of reflux stricture of the esophagus. Br J Surg 80:317

21b. Boom VDG, Go PMMYH, Hameeteman W, Dallemagne B (1996) Costeffectiveness of medical versus surgical treatment in patients with severe or refractory gastroesophageal reflux in The Netherlands. Scand J Gastroenterol 31:1–9

22. Bittner HB, Meyers WC, Brazer SR, Pappas TN (1944) Laparoscopic Nissen fundoplication operative results and short-term follow-up. Am J Surg 167:193–200

23. Blum AL (1990) Treatment of acid-related disorders with gastric acid inhibitors: the state of the art. Digestion 47:3–10

24. Blum AL (1990) Cisapride prevents the relapse of reflux esophagitis. Gastroenterology 98:A22

25. Blum AL, The EUROCIS-trialists (1990) Cisapride reduces the relapse rate on reflux esophagitis. World Congress of Gastroenterology, Sydney, Australia

26. Blum AL, Adami B, Bouzo MH (1991) Effect of cisapride on relapse of esophagitis. A multinational placebo-controlled trial in patients healed with an antisecretory drug. Dig Dis Sci 38:551–560

27. Bonavina L, Evander A, DeMeester TR, Walther B, Cheng SC, Palazzo L, Concannon JL (1986) Length of the distal esophageal sphincter and competency of the cardia. Am J Surg 151:25–34

28. Brossard E, Monnier PH, Olhyo JB (1991) Serious complications – stenosis, ulcer and Barrett's epithelium – develop in 21.6% of adults with erosive reflux esophagitis. Gastroenterology 100:A36

29. Brunner G, Creutzfeldt W (1989) Omeprazole in the long-term management of patients with acid-related diseases resistant to ranitidine. Scand J Gastroenterol 24:101–105

30. Cadiere GB, Houben JJ, Bruyns J, Himpens J, Panzer JM, Gelin M (1994) Laparoscopic Nissen fundoplication technique and preliminary results. Br J Surg 81:400–403

31. Cadiere GB, Himpens J, Bruyns J (1995) How to avoid esophageal perforation while performing laparoscopic dissection of the hiatus. Surg Endosc 9:450–452

32. Cadiere GB, Bruyns J, Himpens J, Vertuyen M (1996) Intrathoracic migration of the wrap after laparoscopic Nissen fundoplication. Surg Endosc 10:187

33. Castell DO (1985) Introduction to pathophysiology of gastroesophageal reflux. In: Castell DO, Wu WC, Ott DJ (eds) Gastrooesophageal reflux disease: pathogenesis, diagnosis, therapy. Future, New York, pp 3–9

34. Castell DO (1994) Management of gastro-esophageal reflux disease 1995. Maintenance medical therapy of gastro-esophageal reflux – which drugs and how long? Dis Esophagus 7:230–233

35. Cederberg C, Andersson T, Skanberg I (1989) Omeprazole: pharmacokinetics and metabolism in man. Scand J Gastroenterol 24:33–40

36. Champault G (1994) Gastroesophageal reflux. Treatment by laparoscopy. 940 cases – French experience. Ann Chir 48:159–164

37. Champion JK, Mc Keman JB (1995) Technical aspects for laparoscopic Nissen fundoplication. Surg Technol Int IV:103–106

38. Chiban N, Wilkinson J, Hurst RH (1943) Symptom relief in erosive GERD, a meta-analysis. Am J Gastroenterol 88 9

39. Chopra BK, Kazal HL, Mittal PK, Sibia SS (1992) A comparison of the clinical efficacy of ranitidine and sucralfate in reflux oesophagitis. J Assoc Physicians India 40:162–163

40. Clark GWB, Jamieson JR, Hinder RA, Polishuk PV, DeMeester TR, Gupta N, Cheng SC (1993) The relationship of gastric pH and the emptying of solid, semisold and liquid meals. J Gastrointest Mot 5:273–279

41. Cloud ML, Offen WW, Robinson M (1994) Nizatidine versus placebo in gastro-oesophageal reflux disease: a 12-week, multicentre, randomised, double-blind study. Br J Clin Pract 76:3–10

42. Cloyd DW (1994) Laparoscopic repair of incarcerated paraesophageal hemias. Surg Endosc 8:893–897

43. Coley CR, Bang MJ, Spechler SJ, Williford WO, Mulley AG (1993) Initial medical vs surgical therapy for complicated or chronic gastroesophageal reflux disease. A cost effectiveness analysis. Gastroenterology 104:AS

44. Collard JM, de Gheldere CA, De Keck M, Otte JB, Kestens PJ (1994) Laparoscopic anti-reflux surgery. What is real progress? Ann Surg 220:146–154
45. Collard JM, Romagnoli R, Kestens PJ (1996) Reoperation for unsatisfactory outcome alter laparoscopic antireflux surgery. Dis Esophagus 9:56–62
46. Collen MJ, Strong RM (1992) Comparison of omeprazole and ranitidine in treatment of refractory gastroesophageal reflux disease in patients with gastric acid hypersecretion. Dig Dis Sci 37:897–903
47. Collet D, Cadiere GB, the Formation for the Development of Laparoscopic Surgery for Gastroesophageal Reflux Disease Group (1995) Conversions and complications of laparoscopic treatment of gastroesophageal reflux disease. Am J Surg 169:622–626
48. Congrave DP (1992) Brief clinical report. Laparoscopic paraesophageal hemia repair. J Laparoendosc Surg 2:45–48
49. Coster DD, Bower WH, Wilson VT, Butler DA, Locker SC, Brebrick RT (1995) Laparoscopic Nissen fundoplication a curative, safe, and cost-effective procedure for complicated gastroesophageal reflux disease. Surg Laparosc Endosc 5:111–117
50. Creutzfeldt W (1994) Risk-benefit assessment of omeprazole in the treatment of gastrointestinal disorders. Drug Saf 10:66–82
51. Crist DW, Gradaez TR (1993) Complications of laparoscopic surgery. Surg Clin North Am 73:265–289
52. Csendes A, Braghetto I, Korn 0, Cortes C (1989) Late subjective and objective evaluations of antireflux surgery in patients with reflux esophagitis: analysis of 215 patients. Surgery 105:374–82
53. Cuschieri A (1993) Laparoscopic antireflux surgery and repair of hiatal hemia. World J Surg 17:40–45
54. Cuschieri A, Shimi S, Nathansson LK (1992) Laparoscopic reduction – crural repair and fundoplication of large hiatal hernia. Am J Surg 163:425–430
55. Cuschieri A, Hunter J, Wolfe B, Swanstrom LL, Hutson W (1993) Multicenter prospective evaluation of laparoscopic antireflux surgery. Preliminary report. Surg Endosc 7:505–510
56. Dahhach M, Scott GB (1994) Comparing the efficacy of cisapride and ranitidine in esophagitis: a double-blind, parallel group study in general practice. Br J Clin Pract 48:10–14
57. Dallemagne B, Weerts JM, Jehaes C, Markiewicz S, Lombard R (1991) Laparoscopic Nissen fundoplication preliminary report. Surg Laparosc Endosc 1:138–143
58. Dallemagne B, Weerts JM, Jehaes C, Markiewicz S, Lombard R (1992) Laparoscopic Nissen fundoplication preliminary report. Surg Laparosc Endosc 2:188–190
59. Dallemagne B, Weerts JM, Jehaes C, Markiewicz S, Lombard R (1993) Techniques and results of endoscopic fundoplication. Endosc Surg Allied Technol 1:72–75
60. Dallemagne B, Taziaux P, Weerts J, Jehaes C, Markiewicz S(1995) Laparoscopic surgery of gastroesophageal reflux. Ann Chir 49:30–36
61. Dallemagne B, Weerts JM, Jehaes C, Markiewicz S(1996) Causes of failures of laparoscopic antireflux operations. Surg Endosc 10:305–310
62. DeMeester TR (1989) Prolonged esophageal pH monitoring? In Read NW (ed) Gastrointestinal motility: which tests? Wrightson Biomedical, Petersfield, UK, pp 41–51
63. DeMeester TR (1994) Antireflux surgery. J Am Coll Surg 179:385–393
64. DeMeester TR, Johnson LF, Kent AH (1974) Evaluations of current operations for the prevention of gastroesophageal reflux. Ann Surg 180:511–523
65. DeMeester TR, Johnson LS, Joseph GJ, Toscano MS, Hall AW, Skinner DB (1976) Patterns of gastroesophageal reflux in health and disease. Ann Surg 184:459–470
66. DeMeester TR, Bonavina L, Albertucci N (1986) Nissen fundoplication for gastroesophageal disease: evaluation of primary repair in 100 consecutive patients. Ann Surg 204:9–20
67. DeMeester TR, Fuchs KK, Ball CS (1987) Experimental and clinical results with proximal end-to-end duodenojejunostomy for pathologic duodenogastric reflux. Ann Surg 206:414–426

68. DeMeester TR, Attwood SEA, Smyrk TC, Therkildsen DH, Hinder RA (1990) Surgical therapy in Barrett's esophagus. Ann Surg 212:528–542
69. Demmy TL, Caron NR, Curtis JJ (1994) Severe dysphagia from an Angelchik prothesis: utility of routine esophageal testing. Ann Thorac Surg 57:1660–1661
69a. Dent JA, Dodds WJ, Friedman RH, Sekeguchi P, Hogen WJ, Arndorfer EC, Petrie DJ (1980) Mechanisms of gastroesophageal reflux in recumbent human subjects. J Clin Invest 65:256–267
70. Dent J, Yeomans ND, Mackinnon M, Reed W, Narielvala FM, Hetzel DJ, Solcia E, Sheannan DJC (1994) Omeprazole vs ranitidine for prevention of relapse in reflux oesophagitia. A controlled double blind trial of their efficacy and safety. Gut 35:590–598
71. DePaula AL, Hashiba K, Bafutto M, Machado CA (1995) Laparoscopic reoperations after failed and complicated antireflux operations. Surg Endosc 9:681–686
72. DeVault KR (1994) Current diagnosis and treatment of gastroesophageal reflux disease. Mayo Clin Proc 69:867–876
73. Deveney K, Swanstrom L, Shepard B, Deneney C (1996) A statewide registry for outcome of open and laparoscopic anti-reflux procedures. Surg Endosc 10:197
74. Dimenäs E (1993) Methodological aspect of evaluation of quality of life in upper gastrointestinal diseases. Scand J Gastroenterol 28:18–21
75. Donahue PE, Samelson S, Nyhus LM, Bombeck T (1985) The floppy Nissen fundoplication. Effective long-term control of pathological reflux. Arch Surg 120:663–668
76. Dor J, Humbert P, Dor V (1962) L'interet de la technique de Nissen modifie dans la prevention du reflux apres cardiomyotomie extramuqueuse de Heller. Mem Acad Chir Paris 27:877
76a. Drummond MF, Stoddart GL, Torrance GW (1987) Methods for the economic evaluation of health care programmes. Oxford University Press, Oxford
76b. Educational Committee of the European Association for Endoscopic Surgery and other interventional techniques (E.A.E.S.) Conference Organizers: Neugebauer E, Troidl H, Kum CK, Eypasch E, Miserez M, Paul A (1995) The E.A.E.S. Consensus Development Conferences on Laparoscopic Cholecystectomy, Appendectomy, and Hernia Repair. Consensus Statements. Surg Endosc 9:550–563
77. Eller R, Olsen D, Sharp K, Richards W (1996) Is division of the short gastric vessels necessary? Surg Endosc 10:199
78. Eypasch EP, Stein H, DeMeester TR, Johansson K-E, Barlow AP, Schneider GT (1990) A new technique to define and clarify esophageal motor disorders. Am J Surg 159:144
79. Eypasch E, Spangenberger W, Neugebauer E, Troidl H (1992) Frühe postoperative Verbesserung der Lebensqualität nach laparoskopischer Cholezystektomie. In: Häring R (ed) Diagnostik und Therapie des Gallensteinleidens. Blackwell, Berlin
80. Eypasch R, Holthausen U, Wellens E, Troidl H (1994) Laparoscopic Nissen fundoplication: potential benefits and burdens. Update in gastric surgery. In: Röher HD (ed) Grenzland Symposium, Düsseldorf. Thieme, Stuttgart
80a. Eypasch E, Williams JI, Wood-Dauphinée S, Ure BM, Schmülling C, Neugebauer E, Troidl H (1995) The Gastrointestinal Quality of Life Index (GIQLI): development and validation of a new instrument. Br J Surg 82:216–222
81. Fein M, Fuchs K-H, Bohrer T, Freys S, Thiede A (1996) Fiberoptic technique for 24 hour bile reflux monitoring – standards and normal values for gastric monitoring. Dig Dis Sci 41:216–225
82. Feussner H, Stein HJ (1994) Minimally invasive esophageal surgery. Laparoscopic antireflux surgery and cardiomyotomy. Dis Esophagus 7:17–23
83. Feussner H, Petri A, Walker S, Bollschweiler E, Siewert JR (1991) The modified AFP score: an attempt to make the results of anti-reflux surgery comparable. Br J Surg 78:942–946
84. Filipi CJ, Hinder RA, DePaula AL, Hunter JG, Swanstrom LL, Stalter KD (1996) Mechanisms and avoidance of esophageal perforation by bougie and nasogastric intubation. Surg Endosc 10:198

85. Fiorucci ST, Santucci L, Morelli A (1990) Effects of omeprazole and high doses of ranitidine on gastric acidity and GOR in patients with moderate-severe oesophagitis. Am J Gastroenterol 85:1485–1462
86. Fontaumard E, Espalieu P, Boulez J (1995) Laparoscopic Nissen-Rosetti fundoplication. Surg Endosc 9:869–873
87. Frantzides CT, Carlson MA (1992) Laparoscopic vs conventional fundoplication. J Laparoendosc Surg 5:137–143
88. Freston JW, Malagelada JR. Petersen H, McClay RF (1995) Critical issues in the management of gastroesophageal reflux disease. Eur J Gastroenterol Hepatol 7:577–586
89. Fuchs KH (1993) Operative procedures in antireflux surgery. Endosc Laparosc Surg 1:65–71
90. Fuchs KH, DeMeester TR (1987) Cost benefit aspects in the management of gastroesophageal reflux disease. In: Siewert JR, Hoelscher AH (eds) Diseases of the esophagus. Springer, Berlin Heidelberg New York, pp 857–861
91. Fuchs KH, DeMeester TR, Albertucci M (1987) Specificity and sensitivity of objective diagnosis of gastroesophageal reflux disease. Surgery 102:575–580
92. Fuchs KH, DeMeester TR, Albertucci M, Schwizer W (1987) Quantification of the duodenogastric reflux in gastroesophageal reflux disease. In: Siewerter JR (ed) Diseases of the esophagus. Springer, Berlin Heidelberg New York, pp 831–835
93. Fuchs KH, DeMeester TR, Hinder RA, Stein HJ, Barlow AP, Gupta NC (1991) Computerized identification of pathological duodenogastric reflux using 24-hour gastric pH monitoring. Ann Surg 213:13–20
94. Fuchs KH, Freys SM, Heimbucher J (1992) Indications and technique of laparoscopic antireflux operations. In: Nabeya K, Hanaoka T, Nogami H (eds) Recent advances in diseases of the esophagus. Springer, Berlin Heidelberg New York, pp 43–50
95. Fuchs KH, Selch A, Freys SM, DeMeester TR (1992) Gastric acid secretion and gastric pH measurement in peptic ulcer disease. Prob Gen Surg 9:138–151
96. Fuchs KH, Freys SM, Heimbucher J (1993) Erfahrungen mit der laparoskopischen Technik in der Antirefluxchirurgie. Chirurg 64:317–323
97. Fuchs KH, Heimbucher J, Freys SM, Thiede A (1994) Management of gastro-esophageal reflux disease 1995. Tailored concept of antireflux operations. Dis Esophagus 7:250–254
98. Fuchs KH, Freys SM, Heimbucher J, Fein M, Thiede A (1995) Pathophysiologic spectrum in patients with gastroesophageal reflux disease in a surgical GI function laboratory. Dis Esophagus 8:211–217
99. Funch-Jens P (1995) Is this a reflux patient or is it a patient with functional dyspepsia with additional reflux symptoms? Scand J Gastroenterol 30:29–31
100. Gallup Ltd. (1989) Gallup poll – UK attitudes to heartburn and reflux. Gallup, New Maldeu
101. Galmiche JP, Brandstötter G, Evreex M (1988) Combined therapy with cisapride and cometidine in treatment of reflux esophagitis. Dig Dis Sci 35:675–681
102. Galmiche JP, Bruley des Varannes S(1994) Symptoms and disease severity in gastroesophageal reflux disease. Scand J Gastroenterol 29:62–68
103. Gamett WR (1993) Efficacy, safety, and cost issues in managing patients with gastroesophageal reflux disease. Am J Hosp Pharm 50:11–18
104. Geagea T (1991) Laparoscopic Nissen's fundoplication: preliminary report on ten cases. Surg Endosc 5:170–173
105. Geagea T (1994) Laparoscopic Nissen-Rossetti fundoplication. Surg Endosc 8:1080–1084
105a. Gelfand DW (1988) Radiologic evaluation of the pharynx and esophagus. In: Gelfand DW, Richter JE (eds) Dysphagia – diagnosis and treatment. Ikagu-Shoiq, New York, pp 45–83
106. Glise H (1989) Healing relapse rate and prophylaxis of reflux esophagitis. Scand J Gastroenterol 24:57–64
107. Glise H, Hallerbäck B (1996) Principles of operative treatment for GR and critical review of results of such operations. SAGES postgraduate course: problem solving in endoscopic surgery. SAGES, Santa Monica

108. Glise H, Hallerbäck B, Johansson B (1995) Quality of life assessments in evaluation of laparoscopic Rosetti fundoplication. Surg Endosc 9:183–189
109. Glise H, Johansson B, Rosseland AR, Hallerbäck B, Hultén S, Carling L, Knapstad LJ (2006) Gastroesophageal reflux symptoms – clinical findings and effect of ranitidine treatment (submitted)
110. Gooszen HG, Weidema WF, Ringers J, Horbach JM, Maschee AA, Lamers CB (1993) Initial experience with laparoscopic fundoplication in The Netherlands and comparison with an established technique (Belsey Mark IV). Scand J Gastroenterol 200:24–27
111. Grande L, Toledo-Pimentel V, Manterola C, Lacima G, Ros E, Garcia-Valdecasas JC, Fuster J, Visa J, Pera C (1994) Value of Nissen fundoplication in patients with gastro-oesophageal reflux judged by long-term symptom control. Br J Surg 81:548–550
112. HallerbäckB, Unge P, Carling L, Edwin B, Glise H, Haw N, Lyrenäs E, Lundberg K (1994) Omeprazole or ranitidine in long term treatment of reflux oesophagitis. Gastroenterology 107:1305–1311
113. Hallerbäck B, Glise H, Johansson B, Rödmark T(1994) Laparoscopic Rossetti fundoplication. Surg Endosc 8:1417–1422
114. Hamelin B, Amould B, Barbier JP (1994) Cost-effectiveness comparison between omeprazole and ranitidine for treatment of reflux. Gastroenterology 106:88
115. Hatlebakk JG, Berstad A, Carling L, Svedberg LE, Unge P, Ekstrom P, Halvorsen L, Stallemo A, Hovdenak N, Trondstad R (1993) Lansoprazole versus omeprazole in short-term treatment of reflux oesophagitis. Results of a Scandinavian multicentre trial. Scand J Gastroenterol 28:224–228
116. Havelund T, Laurenssen LS, Skoubo-Kristensen R (1988) Omeprazole and ranitidine in the treatment of reflux esophagitis: double blind comparative trial. Br Med J 296:89–92
117. Heading RC (1995) Long-term management of gastroesophageal reflux disease. Scand J Gastroenterol 30:25–30
118. Heimbucher J, Kauer WKH, Peters JH (1994) Physiologic basis of peptic ulcer therapy. In: Peter JH, DeMeester TR (eds) Minimally invasive surgery of the foregut. Quality Medical, St Louis, pp 199–214
119. Hendel L, Hage E, Hendel J, Stentoft P (1992) Omeprazole in the longterm treatment of severe gastro-oesophageal reflux disease in patients with systemic sclerosis. Aliment Phannacol Ther 6:565–577
120. Hetzel DJ (1992) Controlled clinical trials of omeprazole in the longterm management of reflux disease. Digestion 51:35–42
121. Hetzel DJ, Dent J, Reed W (1988) Healing and relapse of severe peptic esophagitis after treatment with Omeprazole. Gastroenterology 95:903–912
122. Hill AD, Walsh TN, Bolger CM, Byrne PJ, Hennessy TP (1994) Randomized controlled trial comparing Nisson fundoplication and the Angelchik prosthesis. Br J Surg 81:72–74
123. Hillman AL (1994) Economic analysis of alternative treatments for persistent gastroesophageal reflux disease. Scand J Gastroenterol 29:98–102
124. Hillman AL, Bloom BS, Fendrick AM, Schwartr JS (1992) Cost and quality effects of alternative treatments for persistent gastroesophageal reflux disease. Arch Int Med 152:1467–1472
125. Hinder RA, Filipi CJ (1992) The technique of laparoscopic Nissen fundoplication (Review). Surgical Laparosc Endosc 2:265–272
126. Hinder RA, Filipi CJ, Weltscher G, Neary P, DeMeester TR, Perdikis G (1994) Laparoscopic Nissen fundoplication is an effective treatment of gastroesophageal reflux disease. Ann Surg 220:481–483
127. Howard J, Heading RC (1992) Epidemiology of gastro-esophageal reflux disease. World J Surg 16:288–293
128. Howden DW, Castell DO, Cohen S, Frestn IW, Orlando RC, Robinson M(1995) The rationale for continuous maintenance treatment of reflux esophagitis. Arch Int Med 155:1465–1471

129. Hunt RH (1995) The relationship between the control of pH and healing and symptom relief in gastro-oesophageal reflux disease. Aliment Phannacol Ther 9:3–7
130. Incarbone R, Peters JH, Heimbucher J, Dvorak D, DeMeester CG, Bremner TR (1995) A contemporaneous comparison of hospital charges for laparoscopic and open Nissen fundoplication. Surg Endosc 9:151–154
131. Isal JB, Zeitun B, Barbier B (1990) Comparison of two dosage regimens of omeprazole – 10 mg once daily and 20 mg week-ends – as prophylaxis against recurrence of reflux esophagitis. Gastroenterology 98:A63
132. Jamieson GG, Watson DI, Britten-Jones R, Mitchell PC, Anvari M (1992) Laparoscopic Nissen fundoplication on esophageal motor function. Arch Surg 127:788–791
133. Jamieson CG, Watson DI, Britten-Jones R, Mitchell PC, Anvari M (1994) Laparoscopic Nissen fundoplication. Ann Surg 220:137–145
134. Joelsson BE, DeMeester TR, Skinner DB (1982) The role of the esophageal body in the antireflux mechanism. Surgery 92:417–424
135. Joelsson S, Joelson IB, Lundberg PP, Wolan A, Wallander MA (1992) Safety experience from long-term treatment with omeprazole. Digestion 51:93–101
136. Jönsson B, Stålhammer NO (1993) The cost-effectiveness of omeprazole and ranitidine in intemittent and maintenance treatment of reflux esophagititis cases of Sweden. Br J Med Econ 6:111–126
137. Johansson B, Glise H, Hallerback B (1995) Thoracic herniation and intrathoracic gastric perforation after laparoscopic fundoplication. Surg Endosc 9:917–918
138. Johansson J, Johnsson F, Joelsson B, Floren CH, Walther B (1993) Outcome 5 years after 360 degree fundoplication for gastrooesophageal reflux disease. Br J Surg 80:46–49
139. Johansson KE, Tibbling L (1986) Maintenance treatmentwith Ranitidine compared with fundoplication in gastro-oesophageal reflux disease. Scand J Gastroenterol 21:779–788
140. Johnsen R, Bernersen B, Straume B, Forde OH, Bostad L, Burhol PG (1991) Prevalences of endoscopic and histological findings in subjects with and without dyspepsia. Br Med J 302:749–752
141. Johnsson F, Joelsson B, Gudmundson K, Greif L (1987) Symptoms and endoscopic findings in diagnosis of gastro-oesophageal reflux disease. Scand J Gastroenterol 22:714–718
142. Jones R (1995) Gastro-oesophageal reflux disease in general practice. Scand J Gastroenterol 30:35–38
143. Jones R, Lydeard S(1989) Prevalence of dyspepsia in the community. Br Med J 298:30–32
144. Jones RH, Lydeard SE, Hobbs FRD (1990) Dyspepsia in England and Scotland. Gut 31:401–405
145. Katada N, Hinder RA, Raiser F, McBride P, Filipi CJ (1995) Laparoscopic Nissen fundoplicatioa Gastroenterologist 3:95-104
146. Kauer W, Peters JH, DeMeester TR, Ireland AP, Bremner CG, Hagen JA (1995) Mixed reflux of gastric and duodenal juices is more harmful to the esophagus than gastric-juice alone. Ann Surg 222:525–533
147. Kauer WK, Peters JH, DeMeester TR, Heimbucher J, Ireland AP, Bremner CG (1995) A tailored approach to antireflux surgery. J Thorac Cardiovasc Surg 110:141–146
148. Kimmig JM (1995) Treatment and prevention of relapse of mild oesophagitiswith omeprazole and cisapride: comparison of two strategies. Aliment Pharmacol Ther 9:281–286
149. Kiviluto T, Luukkonen P, Salo J (1994) Laparoscopic gastro-oesophageal antireflux surgery. Ann Chir Gynaecol 83:101–106
150. Klauser AG, Schindlbeck NE, Müller-Lissner SA (1990) Symptoms in gastro-oesophageal reflux disease. Lancet 335:205–208
151. Klinkenberg-Knol EC (1992) The role of omeprazole in healing and prevention of reflux disease. Hepatogastroenterology 39:27–30

152. Klinkenberg-Knol EC, Meuwissen SGM (1992) Medical therapy of patients with reflux oesophagitis poorly responsive to H2-receptor antagonist therapy. Digestion 51:44–48
153. Klinkenberg-Knol EC, Jansen JMBJ, Festen HPM, Meuwissen SGM, Lamers CBHW (1987) Double-blind multicentre comparison of omeprazole and ranitidine in the treatment of reflux oesophagitis. Lancet 1:349–351
154. Klinkenberg-Knol EC, Jansen JBM, Lamers CBHW (1989) Use of omeprazole in the management of reflux oesophagitis resistant to H2-receptor antagonists. Scand J Gastroenterol 24:88–93
155. Klinkenberg-Knol EC, Festen HPM, Janesen JBM (1994) Longterm treatment with omeprazole for refractory esophagitis: efficacy and safety. Ann Intern Med 121:161–167
156. Klinkenberg-Knol EC, Festen HP, Meuwissen SG (1995) Pharmacological management of gastro-oesophageal reflux disease. Drugs 49:695–710
157. Koelz HR (1989) Treatment of reflux esophagitis with H2-blockers, antacids and prokinetic drugs: an analysis of randomized clinical trials. Scand J Gastroenterol 24:25–36
158. Koop H, Arnold R(1991) Long-term maintenance treatment of reflux esophagitis with omeprazole. Prospective study with H2-blocker-resistant esophagitis. Dig Dis Sci 36:552
159. Kraemer SJ, Aye R, Kozarek RA, Hill LD (1994) Laparoscopic Hill repair. Gastrointest Endosc 40:155–159
160. Kuster SGR, Gilroy S(1993) Laparoscopic repair of paraesophageal hiatal hemia. Surg Endosc 7:362–363
161. Laursen LS, Bondesen S, Hansen J (1992) Omeprazol 10 mg or 20 mg daily for the prevention of relapse in gastroesophageal reflux disease? A double-blind comparative study. Gastroenterology 102:A109
162. Laycock WS, Mauren S, Waring JP, Trus T, Branum G, Hunter JG (1995) Improvement in quality of life measures following laparoscopic antireflux surgery. Gastroenterology 108:A1128
163. Laycock WS, Oddsdottir M, Franco A, Mansour K, Hunter JG (1995) Laparoscopic Nissen fundoplication is less expensive than open Belsey Mark IV. Surg Endosc 9:426–429
164. Laycock WS, Trus TL, Hunter GE (1996) New technology for the division of short gastric vessels during laparoscopic Nissen fundoplication. Surg Endosc 10:71–73
165. Lernt T, Coosemans W, Christiaeus R, Gmwez JA (1990) The Belsey Mark IV antireflux, procedure: indications and long-term results. In: Little AG, Ferguson MK, Skinner DP (eds) Diseases of the esophagus, vol II: Benign diseases. Futura, Mount Kisco, pp 181–188
166. Liebermann DA (1987) Medical therapy for chronic reflux esophagitis: long-term follow-up. Arch Intem Med 147:1717–1720
167. Low DG, Hill LD (1989) Fifteen to 20-year results following the Hill antireflux operation. Thorac Cardiovasc Surg 98:444–450
168. Lundell L, Backman L, Ekström P (1990) Omeprazole or high-dose ranitidine in the treatment of patients with reflux esophagitis not responding to standard doses of H2-receptor antagonists. Aliment Phannacol Ther 4:145–155
169. Lundell L, Backman L, Ekström P (1990) Prevention of relapse of esophagitis after endoscopic healing: the efficacy of omeprazole compared with ranitidine. Gastroenterology 98:A82
170. Lundell L (1992) Acid suppression in the long-term treatment of peptic stricture and Barrett's oesophagus. Digestion 51:49–58
171. Lundell L (1994) The knife or the pill in the long-term treatment of gastroesophageal reflux disease? Yale J Biol Med 67:233–246
172. Lundell L (1994) Long-term treatment of gastro-oesophageal reflux disease with omeprazole. Scand J Gastroenterol 29:74–78
173. Lundell L, Abrahamsson H, Ruth N, Sandberg N, Olbe LC (1991) Lower esophageal sphincter characteristics and esophageal acid exposure following partial 360° fundoplication results of a prospective randomized clinical study. World J Surg 15:115–121

174. Lundell L, Backman L, Enström D (1991) Prevention of relapse of reflux esophagitis after endoscopic healing. The efficacity and safety of omeprazole compared with ranitidine. Scand J Gastroenterol 26:248–256

174a. Lundell L, Abrahamson H, Ruth M, Rydberg C et al. (1996) Long-term results of a prospective randomized comparison of total fundic wrap (Nissen-Rossetti) vs semifundoplication (Toupet) for gastro-esophageal reflux. Br J Surg 83:830–835

174b. Jones RH, Lydeard SE, Hobes FDR, Kenkre JE, Williams EI, Jones, SJ, Repper JA, Caldow JL, Dunwoodie WMB, Bottomley JM (1990) Dyspepsia in England and Scotland. Gut 31:402–405

175. Luostarinen R (1993) Nissen fundoplication for reflux esophagitis. Long-term clinical and endoscopic results in 109 of 127 consecutive patients. Ann Surg 217:329–337

176. Luostarinen M (1995) Nissen fundoplication for gastro-oesophageal reflux disease: long-term results. Ann Chir Gynaecol 84:115–120

177. Luostarinen M, Isolauri J, Laitinen J (1993) Fate of Nissen fundoplication after 20 years: a clinical, endoscopical and functional analysis. Gut 34:1015–1020

178. Luostarinen M, Koskinen M, Reinikainen P, Karvonen J, Isolauri J (1995) Two antireflux operations: floppy vs standard Nissen fundoplicatioa Ann Med 27:199–205

179. Mangar D, Kirchhoff GT, Leal JJ, Laborde R, Fu E (1994) Pneumothorax during laparoscopic Nissen fundoplication. Can J Aneasth 41:854–856

180. Marks R, Richter J, Rizzo J (1994) Omeprazole vs H2-receptor antagonists in treating patients with peptic stricture and esophagitis. Gastroenterology 106:907–915

181. Marrero JM, de Caestecker JS, Maxwell JD (1994) Effect of famotidine on oesophageal sensitivity in gastro-oesophageal reflux disease. Gut 35:447–450

182. Matthews HR (1996) A proposed classification for hiatal hemia and gastroesophageal reflux. Dis Esophagus 9:1–3

183. McAnena OJ, Willson PD, Evans DF, Kadirkamanathan SS, Mannur KR, Wingte DL (1995) Physiological and symptomatic outcome after laparoscopic fundoplication. Br J Surg 82: 795–797

184. McKernan JB (1994) Laparoscopic antireflux surgery. Int Surg 79:342–345

185. McKernan JB (1994) Laparoscopic repair of gastroesophageal reflux disease. Toupet partial fundoplication vs Nissen fundoplication. Surg Endosc 8:851–856

186. McKernan JB, Laws HL (1994) Laparoscopic Nissen fundoplication for the treatment of gastroesophageal reflux disease. Am Surg 60:87–93

187. McKernan JB, Champion JK (1995) Laparoscopic antireflux surgery. Am Surg 61:530–536

188. Meyer C, de Manzini N, Rohr S, Thiry CL, Perraud V (1994–1995) Laparoscopic treatment of gastroesophageal reflux Cardiopexia with the round ligament versus Nissen's type fundoplication. Chirurgie 120:107–112

189. Mössner J, Hölscher AH, Herz R, Schneider A (1995) A double-blind study of pantoprazole and omeprazole in the treatment of reflux oesophagitis: a multicenter trial. Aliment Pharmacol Ther 9:321–326

190. Mosnier H, Leport J, Aubert A, Kianmanesh R, Sbai Idrissi MS, Guivarch M (1995) A 270 degree laparoscopic posterior fundoplasty in the treatment of gastroesophageal reflux. J Am Coll Surg 181:220–224

190a. Mosteller F (1985) Assessing Medical Technologies. National Academic Press, Washington, DC

191. Mouiel J, Katkhouda N (1995) Laparoscopic Rossetti fundoplication. Surg Technol Int III:207–213

192. Mouiel J, Katkhouda N, Jugenheim J (1993) Reflux gastrooesophagie: experience laparoscopique. In: Mouiel J (ed) Actualite digestives medico-chirurgicals. 14e serie. Massoq Paris, pp 26–33

193. Myrvold HE (1995) Laparoscopic reflux surgery; the merits and the problems. Ann Med 27:29–33

194. Nathanson LK, Shimi S, Cushieri A (1991) Laparoscopic ligamentum teres (round ligament) cardiopexy. Br J Surg 78 947–951

195. Nebel OT, Fornes MF, Castsell DO (1976) Symptomatic gastroesophageal reflux incidence and precipitating factors. Am J Dig Dis 21953–956
195a. Neugebauer E, Troidl H, Wood-Dauphinee S, Bullinger M, Eypasch E (1991) Meran Consensus Conference Quality-of-Life-Assessment in Surgery, 3–8 October 1990. Part I and Part II. Theor Surg 6:121–165, 195–220
195b. Neugebauer E, Troidl H, Wood-Dauphinee S, Bullinger M, Eypasch E (1992) Meran Consensus Conference Quality-of-Life-Assessment in Surgery, 3–8 October 1990. Part III. Theor Surg 7:14–38
196. Neunheim KS, Baue AE (1994) Paraesophageal hiatal hernia. In: Shield TW (ed) General thoracic surgery. Williams & Wilkins, Philadelphia, pp 644–651
197. Nissen R (1956) Eine einfache Operation zur Beeinflussung der Reflux Esophagitis. Schweiz Med Wochenschr 86:590–592
198. Nowzaradan Y, Bames P (1993) Laparoscopic Nissen fundoplication. J Laparoendosc Surg 3:429–438
199. Oddsdotti M, Franco AL, Laycock WS, Warring JP, Hunter JE (1995) Laparoscopic repair of paraesophageal hernia. New access, old technique. Surg Endosc 9:164–168
200. Ollyo JB, Monnier P, Fontalliet C (1993) The natural history and incidence of reflux esophagitis. Gullet 3:3–10
201. O'Reilly MJ, Mullins SG (1993) Laparoscopic Nissen fundoplication report of first 15 cases. J Laparoendosc Surg 3:317–324
202. Ortiz A, Martinez de Haro LF, Parilla P, Morales G, Molina J, Bertnejo J, Liron R, Aguilar J (1996) Conservative treatment versus antireflux surgery in Barrett's oesophagus: long-term results of a prospective study. Br J Surg 83:274–278
203. Ovaska J, Rantala A, Laine S, Gullichsen R (1996) Laparoscopic vs conventional Nissen fundoplication a prospective randomized study. Surg Endosc 10:178
204. Palmer ED (1958) Hiatus hemia in the adult: clinical manifestations. Am J Dig Dis 3:45–58
205. Paluch TA (1996) Ambulatory laparoscopic Nissen fundoplication a preliminary report. Surg Endosc 10:198
206. Paluch TA, Hilford MA, Feitelbert SP (1996) Laparoscopic fundoplication and managed care: cost effective in the treatment of gastroesophageal reflux. Surg Endosc 10:187
207. Paritek D, Tam PKH (1991) Results of fundoplication in a UK Paediatric centre. Br J Surg 78:346–348
208. Patti MG, Arcerito M, Pellegrini CA, Mulvihill SJ, Tong J, Way LW (1995) Minimally invasive surgery for gastroesophageal reflux disease. Am J Surg 170:614–618
209. Peillon C, Manouvrier JL, Labreche J, Kaeffer N, Denis P, Testart J (1994) Should the vagus nerves be isolated from the fundoplication wrap? A prospective study. Arch Surg 129:814–818
210. Pellegrini CA (1994) The role of minimal-access surgery in esophageal disease. Curr Opin Gen Surg 117–119
211. Pellegrini CA (1995) Therapy for gastroesophageal reflux disease: the new kid on the block. Editorial. J Am Coll Surg 180:485–487
212. Peracchia A, Bancewicz J, Bonavina L (1995) Fundoplication is an effective treatment for gastroesophageal reflux disease. Gastroenterol Intem 8:1–7
213. Perissat J, Collet D (1995) Laparoscopic treatment of gastroesophageal reflux disease. Surg Technol Int III:201–205
214. Perissat J, Collet D, Edye M (1992) Therapeutic laparoscopy. Endoscopy 24:138–143
215. Peters JH, DeMeester TR (1995) Indications, principles of procedure selection end technique of laparoscopic Nissen fundoplication. Semin Laparosc Surg 2:27–44
216. Peters JK, DeMeester TR (1995) Early experience with laparoscopic Nissen fundoplication. Surg Technol Int IV: 109–113
217. Peters JH, Heimbucher J, Kauer WKH, Incarbone R, Bremner CG, DeMeester TR (1995) Clinical and physiologic comparison of laparoscopic and open Nissen fundoplication. J Am Coll Surg 180:385–393

218. Peterson H (1995) The prevalence of gastro-esophageal reflux disease. Scand J Gastroenterol 30:5–6
219. Pitcher DE, Curet MJ, Martin DT (1994) Successful management of severe gastroesophageal reflux disease with laparoscopic Nissen fundoplication. Am J Surg 168:547–554
220. Raiser F, Hinder RA, McBride PJ, Katada N, Filipi CJ (1995) The technique of laparoscopic Nissen fundoplication. Chest Surg Clin North Am 5:437–448
221. Rattner DW, Brooks DC (1995) Patient satisfaction following laparoscopic and open antireflux surgery. Arch Surg 130:289–294
222. Richter JE, Long JF (1995) Cisapride for gastroesophageal reflux disease: a placebo-controlled, double-blind study. Am J Gastroenterol 90:423–430
223. Robertson CS, Evans DF, Ledingham SJ, Atkinson M (1993) Cisapride in the treatment of gastro-oesophageal reflux disease. Aliment Phannacol Ther 7:181–190
224. Robinson M, Decktor DL, Maton PN, Sabesin S, Roufail W, Kogut D, Roberts W, McCullough A, Pardoll P, Saco L (1993) Omeprazole is superior to ranitidine plus metoclopramide in the short-term treatment of erosive oesophagitis. Aliment Phannacol Ther 7:67–73
225. Rösch W (1987) Erosion of the upper gastrointestinal tract. Clin Gastroenterol 7:623
226. Rosetti N, Hell K (1977) Fundoplication for treatment of gastroesophageal reflux in hiatal hemia. World J Surg 1:439-444
227. Rush DR. Stelmach WJ, Young TL, Kirchdoerfer LJ, Scott-Lennox J, Holverson HE, Sabesin SM, Nicholas TA (1995) Clinical effectiveness and quality of life with ranitidine vs placebo in gastroesophageal reflux disease patients: a clinical experience network (CEN) study. J Fam Pract 41:126–136
228. Sandmark S, Carlson R, Fauser 0, Lundell L (1988) Omeprazole or ranitidine in the treatment of reflux esophagitis. Results of a double-blind randomized Scandinavian multi-center study. Scand J Gastroenterol 23:625–632
229. Santag SJ (1990) The medical management of reflux oesophagitis. Gastroenterol Clin North Am 19:683–709
230. Sato TL, Wu WC, Castell DO (1992) Randomized, double-blind, placebo-controlled crossover trial of pirenzepine in patients with gastroesophageal reflux. Dig Dis Sci 37:297–302
231. Savary N, Miller G (1978) The esophagus: handbook and atlas of endoscopy. In: Fassman AG (ed) Solothertn, Switzerland, p 135
232. Schauer PR, Meyers WC, Eubanks S (1996) Mechanism of gastric and esophageal perforations during laparoscopic Nissen fundoplication. Ann Surg 223:43–52
233. Schindlbeck NE, Klauser AG, Berghammer G, Londong W, Muller-Lissner SAL (1992) Three year follow up of patients with gastrooesophageal reflux disease. Gut 33:1016–1019
234. Schwizer W, Hinder RA, DeMeester TR (1989) Does delayed gastric emptying contribute to gastroesophageal reflux disease? Am J Surg 157:74–81
235. Siewert JR, Feussner H (1987) Early and long-term results of antireflux surgery. A critical look. Bailliere clinical gastroenterology. Saunders, Oxford, pp 821–842
236. Siewert JR, Isolauri J, Feussner H (1989) Reoperation following failed fundoplication. World J Surg 13: 791
237. Siewert JR, Stein HJ, Feussner H (1995) Reoperations after failed antireflux procedures. Ann Chir Gynaecol 84:122–128
238. Sito E, Thor PJ, Maczka M, Lorens K, Konturek SJ, Maj A (1993) Double-blind cross-over study of ranitidine and ebrotidine in gastroesophageal reflux disease. J Physiol Phannacol 44:259–272
239. Skinner DB, Belsey R (1967) Surgical management of esophageal reflux and hiatus hemia: long-term results with 1030 patients. J Thorac Cardiovasc Surg 53:33–54
240. Smith PM, Kerr GD, Cockel R, Ross BA, Bate CM, Brown P, Dronfield MW, Green JRB, Hislop WS, Theodossi A, McFarland RJ, Watts DA, Taylor MD, Richardson PDI, The Restore Investigator Group (1994) A comparison of omeprazole and ranitidine in the prevention or recurrence of benign esophageal stricture. Gastroenterology 107:1312–1318
241. Sölvell L (1989) The clinical safety of omeprazole. Scand J Gastroenterol 24:106–110

242. Sonntag SJ (1993) Rolling review: gastroesophageal reflux disease. Aliment Phannacol Ther 7:293–312
243. Sonntag SJ, Schnell TG, Miller TQ (1991) The importance of hiatal hernia in reflux esophagitis comapred with lower esophageal sphincter pressure or smoking. J Clin Gastroenterol 13:628–643
244. Sonntag S, Robinson M, Roufail W (1992) Daily dose of omeprazole (OME) is needed to maintain healing an erosive esophagitis (BE). Am J Gastroenterol 87:1258
245. Soper NJ, Brunt LM, Kerbl K (1994) Laparoscopic general surgery. N Engl J Med 330:409–419
246. Spechler SJP, Veterans Affairs Gastroesophageal Reflux Disease Study Group (1992) Comparison of medical and surgical therapy for complicated gastroesophageal reflux disease. N Engl J Med 326:786–792
247. Spechler SJ, Gordon DW, Cohen J, Williford WO, Krol W (1995) The effects of antireflux therapy on pulmonary function in patients with severe gastroesophageal reflux disease. Am J Gastroenterol 90:915–918
248. Staerk-Laursen L, Havelund T, Bondsen S(1995) Omeprazole in the long-term treatment of gastroesophageal reflux disease. Scand J Gastroenterol 30:839–846
249. Stein HJ, DeMeester TR (1992) Who benefits from antireflux study? World J Surg 16:312
250. Stein HJ, Feussner H, Siewert JR (1992) Minimally invasive antireflux procedures. World J Surg 16:347–348
251. Stein HJ, Barlow AP, DeMeester TR, Hinder RA (1992) Complications of gastroesophageal reflux disease: role of the lower esophageal sphincter, esophageal acid/alkaline exposure, and duodenogastric reflux. Ann Surg 216:35–43
252. Stein HJ, Feussner H, Siewert JR (1996) Failure of antireflux surgery: causes and management strategies. Am J Surg 171:36–40
253. Stewart KC, Urschel JD, Hallgren RA (1994) Reoperation for complications of the Angelchik antireflux prothesis (see comments). Source Thorac Surg 57:1557–1558
254. Stipa S, Fegiz G, Iascone C, Paolini A, Moraldi A, De Marchi C, Chieco PA (1989) Belsey and Nissen operations for gastroesophageal reflux. Ann Surg 210:583–589
255. Swanström L, Wayne R (1994) Spectrum of gastrointestinal symptoms after laparoscopic fundoplication. Am J Surg 167:538–541
256. Swanstrom L, Pennings J (1995) Safe laparoscopic dissection of the gastroesophageal junction. Am J Surg 169:507–511
257. Tack J, Coremans G, Janssens J (1995) A risk-benefit assessment of Cisaprise in the treatment of gastro-intestinal disorders. Drug Safe 12:384–392
258. Than KBA, Silaner T (1989) A long term randomized prospective trial of the Nissen procedure versus a modified Toupet technique. Ann Surg 210:719–724
259. Thibault C, Marceau P, Biron S, Borque RA, Beland L, Potvin M (1994) The Angelchik antireflux prosthesis: long-term clinical end technical follow-up. Can J Surg 37:12–17
260. Thomson ABR (1992) Medical treatment of gastro-esophageal reflux disease: options and priorities. Hepetogastroenterology 39:14–23
261. Timmer R, Breumelhof R, Nadorp JHSM, Smout AJPM (1993) Recent advances in the pathophysiology of gastroesophageal reflux disease. Fur J Gastroenterol Hepatol 5:485–491
262. Toupet A (1963) Technique d'oesophago-gastroplastie avec phrenogastropexie appliqué dans la eure radicale des hernies hiatales et comme complétement de l'opération d'Heller dans les cardiospasmes. Mem Acad Chir 89:384
263. Toussaint J, Gussuin A, Deruuttre M (1991) Healing and prevention of a relapse esophagitis by cisapride. Gut 32:1280–1285
264. Tytgat NJ, Nuo CY, Schotborgh RY (1990) Reflux esophagitis. Scand J Gastroenterol 25:1–12
265. Tytgat GNJ, Anker-Hansen OJ, Carling L (1992) Effect of cisapride on relapse of reflux esophagitis, healed with an antisecretory drug. Scand J Gastroenterol 27:175–183
265a. Troidl H (1995) Endoscopic Surgery – a Fascinating Idea Requires Responsibility in Evaluation and Handling. Minimal Access Surgery, Surg Tech Int III:111–117

266. Urschel JD (1993) Complications of antireflux surgery. Am J Surg 166:68–70
267. Van den Boom G, Go PMM, Hamelteman W, Dallemagne B, Ament AJHA (1996) Cost effectiveness of medical versus surgical treatment in patients with severe or refractory gastroesophageal reflux disease in The Netherlands. Scand J Gastroenterol 31:1–9
268. Van Trappen G, Rutgeer TSL, Schurmans P, Coenegrachts JL (1988) Omeprazole (40 mg) is superior to ranitidine in the short-term treatment of ulcerative reflux esophagitis. Dig Dis Sci 33:523
269. Verlinden M (1990) Healing and prevention of relapse of reflux oesophagitis by cisapride. Gastroenterol 98:A144
270. Vigneri S, Tertnini R, Leandro G (1995) A comparison of five maintenance therapies for reflux esophagitis. N Engl J Med 333:1106–1110
271. Waterfall WE, Craven MA, Allen CJ (1986) Gastroesophageal reflux: clinical presentations, diagnosis and management. Can Med Assoc J 135:1101–1109
272. Watson A, Spychal RT, Brown MG, Peck N, Callander N (1995) Laparoscopic physiological antireflux procedure: preliminary results of a prospective symptomatic and objective study. Br J Surg 82:651–656
273. Watson DI, Reed MWR, Johnson AG (1994) Laparoscopic fundoplication for gastroesophageal reflux. Ann R Coll Surg Engl 76:264–268
274. Watson DI, Gourlay R, Globe J, Reed MWR, Johnson AG, Stoddart CJ (1994) Prospective randomized trial of laparoscopic (LNF) versus open (ONF) Nissen fundoplication. Gut 35:S15
275. Watson DI, Jamieson GG, Devitt PG, Matthew G, Britten-Jones RE, Garne PA, Williams RS (1995) Changing strategies in the performance of laparoscopic Nissen fundoplication as a result of experience with 230 operations. Surg Endosc 9:961–966
276. Watson DI, Jamieson GG, Mitchell PC, Devitt PG, Britten-Jones R (1995) Stenosis of the esophageal hiatus following laparoscopic fundoplication. Arch Surg 130:1014–1016
277. Watson DI, Jamieson GG, Devitt OG, Mitchell PC, Garne PA (1995) Paraesophageal hiatus hernia: an important complication of laparoscopic Nissen fundoplication. Br J Surg 82:521–523
278. Watson DI, Jamieson GG, Nyers JC, Tews JP (1996) The effect of 12 weeks Cisapride on esophageal and gastric function in patients with gastroesophageal reflux disease. Dis Esophagus 9:48–52
278a. Watson DI, Baigrie RJ, Jamieson GG (1996) A leaming curve for laparoscopic fundoplication definable, avoidable, or a waste of time? Ann Surg 224:198–203
278b. Watson DI, Jamieson GG, Baigrie RJ, Mathew G, Devitt PG, Garne PA, Britten-Jones R (1996) Laparoscopic surgery for gastroesophageal reflux: beyond the leaming curve. Br J Surg 83:1284–1287
279. Weerts JM, Dallemagne B, Hamoir E, Demarche M, Markiewicz S, Jehaes C, Lombard R, Demoulin JC, Etienne M, Ferron PE (1993) Laparoscopic Nissen fundoplication detailed analysis of 132 patients. Surg Laparosc Endosc 3:359–364
280. Weerts JM, Dallemagne B, Jehaes C, Markiewicz S (1996) Laparoscopic management after failed reflux operations. Surg Endosc 10:198
281. Wu JS, Dunnegan DL, Luttman DR, Soper NJ (1996) The influence of surgical technique on early clinical outcome of laparoscopic Nissen Fundoplication. Surg Endosc 10:187
282. Zaitown P, Rampol P, Barbier P (1989) Omeprazole (20 mg om) versus ranitidine (150 mg diad) in reflux esophagitis. Results of a double-blind randomized trial. Gastroenterol Clin Biol 13:457–462
283. Zaninotto G, DeMeester TR, Schwites W (1988) The lower esophageal sphincter in health and disease. Am J Surg 155:104–111
284. Zeitoun P (1989) Comparison of omeprazole with ranitidine in the treatment of reflux oesophagitis. Scand J Gastroenterol 24:83–87

Gastroesophageal Reflux Disease – Update 2006

Karl-Hermann Fuchs, Ernst Eypasch

Introduction

Gastroesophageal reflux disease (GERD) is one of the most frequent benign functional disorders in humans concerning the gastrointestinal tract. It is a multifactorial process although the majority of patients develop this disease from a failure of the gastroesophageal junction to hold gastric contents in the stomach [20, 23, 36]. The disease presents typically with symptoms such as heartburn and/or regurgitation, but can present with dysphagia, extraesophageal symptoms such as epigastric pain, respiratory symptoms and others. Gastroenterologists and surgeons are the major medical subspecialties that are involved in the diagnosis, treatment and research of this disease. In addition, many other disciplines, such as pulmonologists, ENT physicians, radiologists, pathologists and others must be involved in the management of the disease because of its multifactorial background and its multifactorial problems.

The European Association for Endoscopic Surgery (EAES) has established consensus conferences regarding special medical problems involving minimally invasive surgery and endoscopy. Ten years ago a first consensus development conference was organized, focusing on GERD and the results were subsequently published in *Surgical Endoscopy* [28]. The purpose of this chapter is a critical overview of questions and consensus statements published at the time and a current analysis of important literature and randomized trials on GERD in 2006.

Consensus Subjects in Management of GERD

Epidemiologic Background in GERD

GERD is mainly established and develops predominantly in modern industrial societies such as Europe and the USA [23]. There is a high prevalence of the disease in these societies in 20–40% of the adult population. It was agreed that the natural history of the disease varies in a wide spectrum between a very mild form of the disease with occasional symptoms, and an advanced stage of GERD with severe symptoms and endoscopic alterations. Many special topics were discussed and could not be resolved within the conference, such as the cause of increasing prevalence, special aspects of Barrett's esophagus and its development to adenocarcinoma, the meaning of ultrashort Barrett's esophagus and the relationship of GERD to *Helicobacter pylori* as well as GERD without the presence of esophagitis, abnormal sensitivity of the esophagus, and the acid and the so-called alkaline reflux.

Currently, the prevalence of GERD including all forms of manifestations can be determined as high as 10–20% in Western societies [5]. An increasing incidence of GERD is highly probable. Epidemiologic studies show a prevalence for at least one episode of heartburn per week in 11–18% of the population [5, 46, 55, 56].

The Pathophysiologic Background of GERD

GERD is a multifactorial process, in which esophageal and gastric changes are involved. The major pathophysiologic causes are the incompetence of the lower esophageal sphincter, transient sphincter relaxations, insufficient esophageal peristaltisis, altered esophageal mucosal resistance, delayed gastric emptying and antroduodenal motility disorders with pathologic duodeno-gastro-esophageal reflux [20, 23, 30, 36, 75, 81]. Several factors, such as stress, obesity, pregnancy and dietary factors as well as drugs, play an aggravating role in this process.

Currently no spectacular new insights into the pathophysiology of GERD have emerged. It is a multifactorial determined disease, in which without any doubt the gastroesophageal junction with its special anatomical and functional components are important. Since there is some evidence that different stages of severity of GERD might have a different background, this leaves us with more questions than evidence-based facts [48, 51, 74].

The Useful Definition of the Disease

A universally agreed scientific definition of GERD was not available at the time; therefore, a model of GERD as increased exposure of the mucosa to gastric contents causing symptoms and morphologic changes was used. This implied an abnormal exposure to acid and/or other gastric contents, like bile, duodenal and pancreatic juice in cases of combined duodeno-gastro-esophageal reflux.

In the past 5–10 years several attempts have been made by both gastroenterologists and surgeons to establish a definition that can be used by both subspecialties to fulfill requirements for research projects and the clinical management of the disease. Often these definitions are characterized by the individual view of the predominant organizing bodies of these consensus projects such as the GENVAL workshop, the impedance workshop and, for example, the German Society of Gastroenterology workshop guidelines project [26, 35, 51].

In summary, the definition can be established as follows: GERD is present when there is a risk for organic complications by increased gastroesophageal reflux and/or a significant limitation of health-related well-being such as quality of life due to reflux symptoms.

This definition resulting from the GENVAL workshop in 1999 is generally enough to cover all problems [26]; however, in daily clinical practice a more precise definition must be used based on diagnostic findings to determine whether the individual patient has the disease or not. Therefore, it is important to realize that morphologic complications of reflux can develop in the esophagus, such as esophagitis, stricture and Barrett's esophagus as well as extraesophageal symptoms. The presence of GERD is highly probable, when reflux symptoms occur once or twice per week accompanied by the limitation in quality of life [74].

Currently, GERD is differentiated in nonerosive reflux disease (NERD), erosive reflux disease with esophagitis (ERD) and Barrett's esophagus as well as extraesophageal manifestations [48, 74].

The natural course of GERD has not been studied extensively. The initial stages of NERD and ERD are usually not progressive in most patients; therefore, a repetitive endoscopic evaluation to verify the change from one stage into the next is not necessary. On the other hand, the spontaneous disappearance of reflux disease after a long period of time occurs rather seldom. In a minority of patients with GERD, severe forms of the disease can progress over the years; however, this observation is not well documented and evidence is minimal, since these patients are constantly treated by medication and are usually seen in surgical centers after some time.

The Diagnostic Workup of GERD

A large variety of different symptoms were described in the context of GERD, such as dysphagia, odynophagia, hoarseness, nausea, belching, epigastric pain, retrosternal pain, acid and food regurgitation, retrosternal burning, heartburn, retrosternal pressure, coughing and epigastric pressure [7, 16, 49]. The most typical symptoms are heartburn, retrosternal burning, and food and acid regurgitation [48, 49]. Symptoms are usually related to posture and eating habits. If typical symptoms are present, there is already a high probability of the presence of the disease; however, symptoms are not a reliable guide to document the presence of GERD [16]. Therefore, morphologic and functional evaluation is important. Morphologic tests are endoscopy and radiography. If no morphologic evidence can be found, functional studies such as 24-h esophageal pH monitoring and esophageal manometry are required. In the 1996 consensus conference a certain diagnostic test ranking order for GERD was established: endoscopy, radiology, 24-h esophageal pH monitoring and esophageal manometry as basic diagnostic tests and 24-h gastric pH monitoring and gastric emptying scintigraphy as well as bilirubin monitoring as optional tests [28].

Today, in 2006, true heartburn is considered a very important chief complain in GERD [9, 48]. When this symptom is present, there is a probability of more than 75% that the individual patient suffers from reflux disease [63]. With all other symptoms, this probability is much less and other diseases, especially functional dyspepsia, can be the cause.

Endoscopy is especially important in exclusion of malignant disease and when alarm symptoms such as dysphagia, retrosternal pain and bleeding are present [49, 53]. With endoscopy, it is possible to establish the diagnosis of GERD and its grade of severity, if reflux esophagitis is present. If esophagitis is excluded, the presence of NERD must be established using other techniques [38].

Twenty-four-hour pH monitoring is considered to be the gold standard investigation for the quantitative evaluation of acid exposure in the distal esophagus [34, 54]. Most gastroenterologists prefer pH monitoring only in the absence of esophagitis. Since esophagitis can also be due to ulcers from medication and since many studies and much of the surgical literature show the value of pH monitoring in the detection of the presence of the disease, preoperative workup should include pH monitoring [9, 69].

For diagnostic workup prior to surgery endoscopy, 24-h pH monitoring and manometry are important for the optimal selection for patients. For the surgically relevant pathophysiologic background it is important to determine either the incompetence of the lower esophageal sphincter by esophageal manometry or the increased incidence of transient sphincter relaxations by sleeve manometry [7, 14, 20, 23, 25, 30, 34, 36, 54, 64, 75, 80]. Manometry prior to surgery is important in order to exclude spastic esophageal motility disorders.

The Indication for Treatment of GERD

The indication for medical treatment of GERD should be established in patients with symptoms and reduced quality of life. When these symptoms persist over weeks the indication for medical treatment is useful. If mucosal damage such as esophagitis is present, medical therapy is necessary.

In 1996, the indication for surgery was based on the patient's symptoms, the duration of the symptoms and the presence of damage [28]. Even after successful medical acid suppression, patients can have persistent or recurrent symptoms of epigastric pain and retrosternal pressure as well as food regurgitation due to an incompetent cardia, insufficient peristaltisis and/or a large hiatal hernia. Concerning the indication for surgery, a differentiation in symptoms between heartburn and regurgitation is important. Medical treatment can resolve heartburn, but usually does not interfere with regurgitation; therefore, the indication for surgery at the time was based on the following facts:

- Noncompliance of the patient with on-going effective medical therapy. The reasons for noncompliance were preference, refusal, reduced quality of life or drug dependency and side effects.
- Persistent or recurrent esophagitis despite adequate medical treatment.
- Complications of the disease such as stenosis, ulcers and Barrett's esophagus have a minor influence on the indication, since neither medical nor surgical treatment has been shown to alter the extent of Barrett's epithelium. At the time the participants pointed out that patients with symptoms completely resistant to antisecretory treatment are bad candidates for surgery. In these individuals other diseases have to be investigated carefully.

Today, in the majority of cases, patients with NERD and ERD need medical therapy with proton pump inhibitors (PPIs). A vast amount of data is available today to show the benefit of PPI therapy in GERD. All patients with acute symptoms of reflux disease should undergo PPI treatment. After stopping this medication, the patient's symptoms will relapse. As a consequence, a long-term maintenance therapy must be established for many patients (ERD and NERD).

The basis for establishing an indication for antireflux surgery is the necessity of long-term treatment with PPI [30, 50]. There is always a controversial discussion between gastroenterologists and surgeons about the precise criteria for surgery and this will continue in the next few years. It is a matter of individual discussion and interpretation of data. Rather unquestionable criteria or indications for surgery are proven PPI side effects in the individual patient, intolerable persisting symptoms despite inadequate PPI dose (usually regurgitation and aspiration and volume reflux). A relative indication is the wish of the patient despite satisfactory quality of life under PPI treatment [26, 28, 33, 37].

Predictive factors for a good postoperative result are a positive response to PPI therapy, a documented pathologic acid exposure of the esophagus by 24-h pH monitoring and the presence of typical reflux symptoms [9].

Technical Essentials of Laparoscopic Antireflux Surgery

In 1996, it was stated, that the goal of surgical treatment for GERD is to relieve the symptoms and to prevent progression and the development of complications of the disease by the creation of a new anatomic high-pressure zone [28]. This must be achieved without dysphagia, which can occur when the outflow resistance of the reconstructed gastroesophageal junction exceeds the peristaltic power of the body of the esophagus. Achievement of this goal requires an understanding of the natural history of GERD, the status of the patient's esophageal function and the selection of the appropriate reflux procedure. Today in 2006, this goal of surgical treatment is still the same; however, the understanding of surgical therapy has changed to some extent.

At the time, 11 participants at the consensus conference discussed in detail the laparoscopic surgical techniques and established a list of ten technical features, which are presented as follows according to the degree of consensus that was attained by the panel (agreement yes/no):

1. Need for mobilization of the gastric fundus (7/4)
2. Need for dissection of the crura (11/0)
3. Need for identification of the vagus truncs (7/4)
4. Need for removal of the esophageal fat pad (2/9)
5. Need for closure of the crura posteriorly (11/0)
6. Use of nonabsorbable sutures for crura and wrap (11/0)
7. Use of large bougie (40–60 French) for calibration (5/6)
8. Objective assessment for tightness of hiatus and tightness of wrap (9/0 or 9/2)
9. Normal peristalsis routinely uses 360° short floppy wrap (8/3)
10. Weak peristalsis tailored approach (total or partial wrap) (5/6)

In the past 10 years a number of randomized trials regarding different techniques have been published. Of special interest are the randomized comparisons between medical and surgical technique, randomized comparison of open versus laparoscopic technique, partial versus total fundoplication and randomized comparisons regarding different technical aspects such as division of short gastric vessels, dissection of the vagus and anterior versus posterior hiatoplasty or crural closure.

It must also be emphasized that there were some controversial aspects regarding the results of randomized trials compared with the results of prospective series from single centers with considerable experience of the disease and its surgical therapy, which should also be kept in mind regarding clinical relevance. Another important issue regarding the value of randomized trials is the selection criteria or definitions that are used for patients to enter these studies in order to reflect the comparability between different randomized trials. In some randomized trials only symptoms were used as the criterion for the presence of the disease, while in others additional results of objective testing, such as esophageal acid exposure or endoscopic findings, were used as criteria [3, 4, 12, 21, 22, 29, 41, 42].

Reviewing the literature of the past 10 years will show that nonfundoplication techniques such as the Angelchik prothesis, the ligamentum teres plasty or the Hill operation have not been the subject of comparisons or reports in large series and therefore their impact can be neglected.

In many publications from experienced centers with a large case load the results for open antireflux surgery after 5 years were reported with a success rate between 28 and 95%, after 5–10 years between 66 and 96% and with a follow-up for more than 10 years between 56 and 85% [22, 24, 33]. With the application of minimal access technique the success rates after 5 years were in the range 85–95% and in the very few studies with a follow-up time longer than 5 years after a laparoscopic procedure they were between 85 and 91%, where nonspecialized centers show clearly worse results [8, 10, 17, 28, 32, 35, 37, 39, 40, 43–45, 47, 59, 60, 71, 73, 81].

Comparison of Medical Versus Operative Therapy

Table 5.1 demonstrates the current overview of very few studies focusing on this comparison between medical and surgical therapy. The classic paper reporting the use of omeprazole as a PPI versus open surgical therapy from Scandinavia shows in a 5-year follow-up no advantage of either management strategy and a similar rate of failure for PPIs and surgical therapy [58]. Although not published as a full paper, there is a report showing an advantage for surgical therapy after 7 years of follow-up, with this difference just reaching a statistical significance. In a second study, early results already show an advantage regarding acid exposure in the esophagus and quality of life criteria after 6 months of follow-up in favor of laparoscopic fundoplica-

Table 5.1. Randomized comparison between medical proton pump inhibitor therapy and antireflux surgery

Author/year	N	Follow-up	Failure rate	Quality of life
Lundell et al. [58]/2001	155 Omeprazole	5 years	75%	
	155 Open ARS	5 years	70%	
Mahon et al. [62]/2005	108 PPI	12 months		Score 136
	104 LARS	12 months		Score 142*
European trial	>500	<3 years		
	PPI versus LARS			

ARS antireflux surgery, *LARS* laparoscopic antireflux surgery, *PPI* proton pump inhibitor
*p<0.003

tion [62]. Currently a large European randomized trial is under way with the recruitment of more than 500 patients; however, follow-up is still too short.

Randomized Comparison of Open Versus Laparoscopic Technique

There are several studies showing an advantage for special parameters such as immunologic factors or respiratory function in favor of the laparoscopic technique compared with the open technique [68, 82] (Table 5.2). The first randomized trial comparing these two techniques was published in 1997 by Laine et al. [52] and shows a longer operation time with laparoscopic technique. Fifty-five patients were compared with 55 patients with a significantly longer hospitalization for the open technique. The functional result was there was no significant different between the two groups.

Another study created a large controversial discussion, since the laparoscopic arm showed after a few months many patients with dysphagia, compared with the conventional technique [4]. Nilsson et al. [66] published the results of their randomized comparison between open and conventional antireflux surgery after 5 years in 2004. This study is of special interest, since owing to the special design, the patients and personal were blind to the choice of technique. In the laparoscopic group, there was significantly less use of analgesia, better postoperative respiratory function and shorter hospitalization. The 5-year follow-up data showed no difference in the functional result regarding the access technique, but a good functional result after 5 years in both groups.

In summary, from the available randomized trials comparing open versus laparoscopic technique it must be emphasized how important the experience of the surgeon is, especially in the laparoscopic group, and that obviously some degree of inexperience can cause excessive dyphagia and other side effects.

Randomized Comparison of Total Versus Partial Fundoplication

The discussion regarding these two procedures has been controversial in the past few years and still is. Several randomized trials have shown that there is no difference in functional outcome regarding reflux persistence or recurrence. In some trials the side effects of the operations are significantly less after partial fundoplication. Table 5.3 demonstrates the overview of this comparison. Even though the randomized trials have not shown any problems in durability after partial fundoplication, several prospective cohort studies from high-volume, very experienced centers have shown the problems with durability after partial fundoplication. The latter fact will cause further controversial discussions within the surgical community, because of its clinical relevance.

Table 5.2. Randomized comparison between open and laparoscopic technique: perioperative data

Author/recruitment	Randomized groups	Morbidity N (%)	Operation time (min)	Hospitalization (days)	Return to work (days)
Laine et al. [52]/1992–1995	Open 55	7 (13)	57	6.4	37
	Laparoscopic 55	3 (8)	88	3.2	15
Heikkinen et al. [42]/1995–1996	Open 20	5 (25)	74	5.5	44
	Laparoscopic 22	3 (14)	98	3.0	21
Bais et al. [4]/1997–1998	Open 46	8 (17)	–	–	–
	Laparoscopic 57	5 (9)			
Luostarinen and Isolauri [61]/1994–1995	Open 15	0	30	5.0	30
	Laparoscopic 13	1 (8)	105	4.0	17
Chrysos et al. [13]/1993–1998	Open 50	38 (76)	83	5.9	–
	Laparoscopic 56	12 (21)	77	2.4	
Nilsson et al. [66]/1995–1997	Open 30	0	109	3.0	32
	Laparoscopic 30	0	148	3.0	27

Table 5.3. Randomized comparison between open and laparoscopic technique: follow-up data

Author/recruitment	Randomized groups	Patients at follow-up	Reflux recurrence N (%)	Dysphagia N (%)	Bloating N (%)	Reoperation N (%)
Laine et al. [52]/1992–1995	Open 55	30 (12 months)	3 (10)	4 (13)	2 (7)	0
	Laparoscopic 55	18 (12 months)	0	0	3 (17)	0
Heikkinen et al. [42]/1995–1996	Open 20	19 (24 months))	2 (11)	11 (58)	10 (53)	0
	Laparoscopic 22	19 (24 months))	0	9 (48)	11 (58)	0
Bais et al. [4]/1997–1998	Open 46	46 (3 months)	1 (2)	0	–	0
	Laparoscopic 57	57 (3 months)	2 (4)	7 (12)$\star$	–	4 (7)
Luostarinen and Isolauri [61]/1994–1995	Open 15	13 (17 months)	0	6 (46)	–	0
	Laparoscopic 13	13 (17 months)	0	4 (31)	–	1 (8)
Chrysos et al. [13]/1993–1998	Open 50	50 (12 months)	1 (2)	2 (4)	3 (6)	0
	Laparoscopic 56	56 (12 months)	2 (4)	2 (4)	0	0
Nilsson et al. [66]/1995–1997	Open 30	23 (60 months)	4 (17)	5 (22)	10 (43)	1 (4)
	Laparoscopic 30	17 (60 months)	2 (12)	7 (41)	8 (47)	2 (12)

$\star p < 0.05$

Comparison of Mobilization of the Gastric Fundus by Division of the Short Gastric Vessels

A few randomized trials were focused on this question and have shown that the results are rather in favor of leaving the fundic attachments intact rather than mobilizing the fundus totally (Table 5.4). Since the way of wrapping the fundus around the lower esophageal sphincter depends on the method of mobilization of the fundus, this question remains open. The symmetric wrap which is favored by some authors is impossible to perform with a non-mobilized fundus. Also the extent of mobilization might have an influence on the results of the comparative groups, which is another criticism of those who favor the mobilization of the fundus. Table 5.5 demonstrates some of the results of the available randomized trials. In summary, it can be stated that on the basis of these data it is not a mistake to leave the fundic attachments towards the spleen intact.

Management of the Vagus Nerve

There is only one study which has investigated the advantage or disadvantage of the dissection of the vagus and has documented an anatomic position of the vagus. Peillon et al. [72] investigated this issue and did not find any significant difference in outcome between those patients in whom they dissected the vagus and clearly defined its localization and in those patients on whom they did not perform this additional step.

The Value of a Hiatoplasty (Crural Closure) and Cardia Calibration

Twenty years ago, there was a remarkable discussion among surgeons regarding the necessity and benefit of crural closure. Interesting enough, for the participants of the consensus conference of 1996 there wes only one issue that was without controversial discussion [28]. This was the total agreement of the necessity of performing a precise crural dissection and a crural closure. There is one trial showing that anterior closure is as good as posterior closure [78]. The importance of the crural closure has gained even more clinical relevance in patients with large hiatal hernias or redo cases, where the weakness of the hiatal and crural material leads to migration of the wrap. In these cases, there is some new evidence that the use of a mesh in onlay technique will reduce the failures substantially. Two randomized trials have confirmed this view [31, 41].

Another randomized trial focused on the value of the cardia calibration by using a large bougie. Patterson et al. [70] showed an advantage of patients with a cardia calibration by using a bougie during the suture of the fundoplication since those patients with no calibration during the operation had significantly more severe side effects.

Important End Points of Treatment (Medical and Surgical)

In 1996 it was stated that the important end point of the success of conservative medical as well as surgical therapy must be a mosaic of different criteria. Today many gastroenterologists are convinced that symptoms and quality of life are the crucial end points in the treatment of GERD and that it is of less importance whether there is still some degree of esophagitis after treatment. For years in many surgical studies the postoperative presence of esophagitis was still considered as a sign of failure. This controversy is still being discussed at present and more data are needed. This seems to be a reasonable concept in times of financial restrictions and the problematic possibility of repeating expensive investigations for follow-up patients with GERD.

As a consequence, treatment failure is defined in many newly designed studies as the persistence or recurrence of symptoms during the follow-up time [58]. Measures of quality of life must be included in the evaluation of retreatment and posttreatment status in order to have a quantitative assessment. The statement in the 1996 consensus report therefore is still valid: In GERD a definite failure is present when symptoms which are severe enough to require at least intermittent therapy (heartburn and regurgitation) recur after treatment or when other serious problems (like severe gas bloat, dumping syndrome, etc.) arise and when functional studies document that symptoms are due to this problem. Recurrence can occur with or without esophageal damage.

The Issue of an Economic Evaluation

At the time, the judgment over a complete economic evaluation was referred by the panelists to the available literature [28]. It was recognized that these issues have considerable importance. However, today it must also be emphasized that economic considerations depend very heavily on the economic and financial situation as well as the structure of the health insurance system in the individual countries [1, 15, 65]. As a consequence, no general conclusions can be drawn Europe-wide. This question interferes with the establishment of the indication for surgery. Prior to surgery, a long period of adequate PPI treatment is absolutely necessary. The break-even point between the expense of long-term medical treatment (this depends also on the costs of PPIs, which have been decreasing in the past few years) and the expense of one-time surgical therapy are difficult to calculate. One must keep in mind that a failure rate of surgical therapy of 5–10% is a realistic figure and is a very expensive burden that the surgical treatment arm has to carry.

Endoscopic Antireflux Therapy

In the past few years several forms of endoscopic antireflux therapy have been established, such as the Stretta procedure, the Enteryx injection, the gastroplication by Endocinch, the Gate Keeper technique and the Plicator gastroplication [2, 11]. Most of these techniques have been stopped in the last 24 months owing either to their insufficiency and high rate of recurrence and/or severe side effects and complications. Currently, the Stretta procedure still in use is, which is the application of radiofrequency waves in the lower esophageal sphincter in order to cause a scaring and have a mechanical effect on the gastroesophageal junction. It is also speculated that there might be an effect on the number of transient sphincter relaxations. The Plicator technique is currently under clinical investigation and no long-term data are available.

In summary, these endoscopic antireflux therapies, performed by flexible endoscopy, were considered 5 years ago as a tremendous achievement with many possibilities and a great prospect of becoming a third arm of therapy in the management of GERD. After the problems regarding these techniques in the past 24 months it is too early to consider this option of therapy as a major and clinically relevant treatment option at present.

What iss the stage of technological development or endoscopic antireflux operations and what iss the current status of antireflux surgery versus open, conventional procedures in terms of visibility and efficacy parameters?

This issue was basically answered in question 6. Laparoscopic antireflux surgery is a well-established and safe technique 15 years after its first application by Bernard Dallemagne in 1991 [18, 19]. Today, antireflux procedures should be performed laparoscopically because they have a proven advantage and this should be the standard.

Conclusions

GERD is a multifactorial process. In the past 10 years many new insights have been gained owing to the research work and clinical experience with patients with this disease. There is a well-established medical therapy with PPIs for the vast majority of patients. The mainstay of diagnostic workup is endoscopy, 24-h esophageal pH monitoring and esophageal manometry as well as radiography. The minimally invasive technique has become the standard access technique in all specialized centers around the world. The past 10 years has shown a tremendous boom in surgical activity causing a widespread application of this operative technique as well as research activities and randomized trials to establish evidence-based criteria.

Careful selection of patients after adequate PPI therapy for surgery and a precise diagnostic workup with 24-h esophageal pH monitoring, endoscopy as well as esophageal manometry to exclude motility disorders is important. Two major antireflux procedures that have been used worldwide in most cases are the 360° short floppy Nissen fundoplication and the posterior partial Toupet-hemifundoplication. Randomized trials as well as a few long-term follow-up studies have shown good results in 80–90% of patients.

References

1. Arguedas MR, Heudebert GR, Klapow JC, Centor RM, Eloubeidi MA, Wilcox CM, Spechler SJ (2004) Re-examination of the cost-effectiveness of surgical versus medical therapy in patients with gastroesophageal reflux disease: the value of long-term data collection. Am J Gastroenterol 99:1023–1028
2. Arts J, Lerut T, Rutgeerts P, Sifrim D, Janssens J, Tack J (2005) A one-year follow-up study of endoluminal gastroplication (Endocinch) in GERD patients refractory to proton pump inhibitor therapy. Dig Dis Sci 50:351–356
3. Baigrie RJ, Cullis SN, Ndhluni AJ, Cariem A (2005) Randomized double-blind trial of laparoscopic Nissen fundoplication versus anterior partial fundoplication. Br J Surg 92:819–823
4. Bais JE, Bartelsman JF, Bonjer HJ, Cuesta MA, Go PM, Klinkenberg-Knol EC, van Lanschot JJB, Nadorp JH, Smout AJ, van der Graaf Y (The Netherlands Antireflux Surgery Study Group) (2000) Laparoscopic or conventional Nissen fundoplication for gastroesophageal reflux disease: randomized clinical trial. Lancet 355:170–174
5. Bardhan KD, Royston C, Nayyar AK (2000) Reflux rising! A disease in evolution? Gastroenterology 118:A478
6. Blomqvist A, Dalenbäck J, Hagedorn C, Lönroth H, Lundell L (2000) Impact of complete gastric fundus mobilisation on outcome after laparoscopic total fundoplication. J Gastrointest Surg 4:493–500
7. Breumelhof R, Smout AJ (1991) The symptom sensitivity index: a valuable additional parameter in 24-hour esophageal pH recording. Am J Gastroenterol 86:160–164
8. Byrne JP, Smithers BM, Nathanson Lymphknoten, Martin I, Ong HS, Gotley DC (2005) Symptomatic and functional outcome after laparoscopic reoperation for failed antireflux surgery. Br J Surg 92:996–1001
9. Campos GM, Peters JH, DeMeester TR, Oberg S, Crookes PF, Tan S, DeMeester SR, Hagen JA, Bremner CG (1999) Multivariate analysis of factors predicting outcome after laparoscopic Nissen fundoplication. J Gastrointest Surg 3:292–300
10. Catarci M, Gentileschi P, Papi C, Carrara A, Marrese R, Gaspari AL, Grassi GB (2004) Evidence-based appraisal of antireflux fundoplication. Ann Surg 239:325–337
11. Chen YK, Raijman I, Ben-Menachem T, Starpoli AA, Liu J, Pazwash H, Weiland S, Shahrier M, Fortajada E, Saltzmann JR, Carr-Locke DL (2005) Long-term outcomes of endoluminal gastroplication: a US multicenter trial. Gastrointest Endosc 61:659–667
12. Chrysos E, Tzortzinis A, Tsiaoussis J, Athanasakis H, Vassilakis J, Xynos E (2001) Prospective randomized trial comparing Nissen to Nissen-Rossetti technique for laparoscopic fundoplication. Am J Surg 182:215–221
13. Chrysos E, Tsiaoussis J, Athanasakis E, Vassilakis J, Xynos E (2002) Laparoscopic versus open approach for Nissen fundoplication. Surg Endosc 16:1679–1684
14. Cole SJ, van den Bogaerde JB, van der Walt H (2005) Preoperative esophageal manometry does not predict postoperative dysphagia following anti-reflux surgery. Dis Esophagus 18:51–56
15. Cookson R, Flood C, Koo B, Mahon D, Rhodes M (2005) Short-term cost effectiveness and long-term cost analysis comparing laparoscopic Nissen fundoplication with proton-pump inhibitor maintenance for gastro-esophageal reflux disease. Br J Surg 92:700–706
16. Costantini M, Crookes PF, Bremner RM, Hoeft SF, Ehsan A, Peters JH, Bremner CG, DeMeester TR (1993) Value of physiologic assessment of foregut symptoms in a surgical practice. Surgery 114:780–786

17. Cuschieri A, Hunter J, Wolfe B, Swanstrom LL, Hutson W (1993) Multicenter prospective evaluation of laparoscopic antireflux surgery. Surg Endosc 7:505–510
18. Dallemagne B, Weerts JM, Jehaes C (1991) Laparoscopic Nissen fundoplication: preliminary reports. Surg Laparosc Endosc 1:138–143
19. Dallemagne B, Weerts JM, Jehaes C, Markiewicz S (1996) Causes of failures of laparoscopic antireflux operations. Surg Endosc 10:305–310
20. DeMeester TR (1987) Definition, detection and pathophysiology of gastroesophageal reflux disease. In: DeMeester TR, Matthews HR (eds) International trends in general thoracic surgery, vol 3. Benign esophageal disease. Mosby, St Louis, pp 99–127
21. DeMeester TR, Fuchs KH (1988) Comparison of operations for uncomplicated reflux disease. In: Jamieson GG (ed) Surgery of the oesophagus. Churchill Livingstone, London, pp 299–308
22. DeMeester TR, Johnson LF, Kent AH (1974) Evaluation of current operations for the prevention of gastroesophageal reflux. Ann Surg 180:511–525
23. DeMeester TR, Johnson LS, Joseph GJ, Toscano MS, Hall AW, Skinner DB (1976) Patterns of gastroesophageal reflux in health and disease. Ann Surg 184:459–470
24. DeMeester TR, Bonavina L, Abertucci M (1986) Nissen fundoplication for gastroesophageal reflux disease. Evaluation of primary repair in 100 consecutive patients. Ann Surg 204:19
25. Dent J, Holloway RH, Toouli J, Dodds WJ (1988) Mechanisms of lower oesophageal sphincter incompetence in patients with symptomatic gastro-oesophageal reflux. Gut 29:1020–1028
26. Dent J, Brun J, Fendrick AM, Fennerry MB, Janssens J et al (1999) Genval Workshop Group: an evidence-based appraisal of reflux disease management. Gut 44:S1–16
27. Engstrom C, Blomqvist A, Dalenback J, Lonroth H, Ruth M, Lundell L (2004) Mechanical consequences of short gastric vessel division at the time of laparoscopic total fundoplication. J Gastrointest Surg 8:442–447
28. Eypasch E, Neugebauer E, Fischer F, Troidl H (1997) Laparoscopic antireflux surgery for gastroesophageal reflux disease (GERD). Results of a consensus development conference. Surg Endoscopy 11:413–426
29. Eyre-Brook IA, Codling BW, Gear MWL (1993) Results of a prospective randomized trial of the Angelchik prosthesis and of a consecutive series of 119 patients. Br J Surg 80:602–604
30. Fein M, Ireland AP, Ritter MP, Peters JH, Hagen JA, Bremner CG, DeMeester TR (1997) Duodenogastric reflux potentiates the injurious effects of gastroesophageal reflux. J Gastrointest Surg 1:27–33
31. Frantzides CT, Madan AK, Carlson MA, Stavrpoulos GP (2002) A prospective randomized trial of laparoscopic polytetrafluoroethylene (PTFE) patch repair vs simple cruroplasty for large hiatal hernia. Arch Surg 137:649–652
32. Franzen T, Anderberg B, Wiren M, Johansson KE (2005) Long-term outcome is worse after laparoscopic than after conventional Nissen fundoplication. Scand J Gastroenterol 40:1261–1268
33. Fuchs KH (2005) Conventional and minimally invasive surgical methods for gastroesophageal reflux. Chirurg 76:370–378
34. Fuchs KH, DeMeester TR, Albertucci M (1987) Specificity and sensitivity of objective diagnosis of gastroesophageal reflux disease. Surgery 102:575–580
35. Fuchs KH, Heimbucher J, Freys SM, Thiede A (1995) Management of gastro-esophageal reflux disease 1995. Tailored concept of anti-reflux operations. Dis Esophagus 7:250–254
36. Fuchs KH, Freys SM, Heimbucher J, Fein M, Thiede A (1995) Pathophysiologic spectrum in patients with gastroesophageal reflux disease in a surgical GI function laboratory. Dis Esophagus 8:211–217
37. Fuchs KH, Feussner H, Bonavina L, Collard JM, Coosemans W for the European Study Group for Antireflux Surgery (1997) Current status and trends in laparoscopic antireflux surgery: results of a consensus meeting. Endoscopy 29:298–308
38. Galmiche JP, des Varannes SB (2001) Endoscopy-negative reflux disease. Curr Gastroenterol Rep 3:206–214

39. Gotley DC, Smithers BM, Rhodes M, Menzies B, Branicki FJ, Nathanson (1996) Laparoscopic Nissen fundoplication – 200 consecutive cases. Gut 38:487–491
40. Grande L, Toledo-Pimentel V, Manterola C, Lacima G, Ros E, Garcia-Valdecasas JC, Fuster J, Visa J, Pera C (1994) Value of Nissen fundoplication in patients with gastro-oesophageal reflux judged by long-term symptom control. Br J Surg 81:548
41. Granderath FA, Schweiger UM, Kamolz T, Asche KU, Pointner R (2005) Laparoscopic Nissen fundoplication with prosthetic hiatal closure reduces postoperative intrathoracic wrap herniation: preliminary results of a prospective randomized functional and clinical study. Arch Surg 140:40–48
42. Heikkinen TJ, Hakipuro K, Bringman S (2000) Comparison of laparoscopic and open Nissen fundoplication 2 years after operation. A prospective randomized trial. Surg Endosc 355:170–174
43. Hinder RA, Filipi CJ, Wetscher G, Neary P, DeMeester TR, Perdikis G (1994) Laparoscopic Nissen fundoplication is an effective treatment for gastroesophageal reflux disease. Ann Surg 220:472–483
44. Horvath KD, Jobe BA, Herron DM, Swanström LL (1999) Laparoscopic Toupet fundoplication is an inadequate procedure for patients with severe reflux disease. J Gastrointest Surg 3:583–591
45. Hunter JG, Smith CD, Branum GD et al (1999) Laparoscopic fundoplication failures. Ann Surg 230:595–606
46. Isolauri J, Laippala P (1995) Prevalence of symptoms suggestive of gastroesophageal reflux disease in an adult population. Ann Med 27:67–70
47. Jobe BA, Wallace J, Hansen PD, Swanström LL (1997) Evaluation of laparoscopic Toupet fundoplication as a primary repair for all patients with medically resistant gastroesophageal reflux. Surg Endosc 11:1080–1083
48. Kennedy T, Jones R (2000) The prevalence of gastroesophageal reflux symptoms in a UK population and the consultation behaviour of patients with these symptoms. Aliment Pharmacol Ther 14:1589–1594
49. Klauser AG, Schindlbeck NE, Müller-Lissner SA (1990) Symptoms in gastroesophageal reflux disease. Lancet 335:205–208
50. Klinkenberg-Knol EC, Nelis F, Dent J et al (2000) Long-term omeprazole treatment in resistant gastroesophageal reflux disease: efficacy, safety, and influence on gastric mucosa. Gastroenterology 118:661–669
51. Koop H, Shepp S, Müller-Lissner S, Madisch A, Micklefield G, Messmann H, Fuchs KH, Hotz J (2005) GERD, results of an evidence based consensus conference of the German Society of Gastroenterology. Z Gastroenterol 43:163–164
52. Laine S, Rantala A, Gullichsen R, Ovaska J (1997) Laparoscopic vs conventional Nissen fundoplication. A prospective randomized study. Surg Endosc 11:441–444
53. Laws HL, Clements RH, Swillie CM (1997) A randomized, prospective comparison of the Nissen fundoplication versus the Toupet fundoplication for gastroesophageal reflux disease. Ann Surg 225:647–653; discussion 654
54. Locke GR, Talley NJ (1993) 24-hour monitoring for gastroesophageal reflux disease. Lancet 342:1246–1247
55. Locke GR, Talley NJ, Fett SL et al (1997) Prevalence and clinical spectrum of gastroesophageal reflux: a population-based study in Olsted county, Minnesota. Gastroenterology 112:1448–1456
56. Louis E, DeLooze D, Deprez P et al (2002) Heartburn in Belgium: prevalence, impact on daily life, and utilization of medical resources. Eur J Gastroenterol Hepatol 14:279–284
57. Lundell L, Abrahamsson H, Ruth M, Rydberg L, Lonroth H, Olbe L (1996) Long-term results of a prospective randomized comparison of total fundic wrap (Nissen-Rossetti) or semifundoplication (Toupet) for gastro-oesophageal reflux. Br J Surg 83:830–835
58. Lundell L, Miettinen P, Myrvold HE, Pedersen SA, Liedman B, Hatlebakk JG, Julkonen R, Levander K, Carlsson J, Lamm M, Wiklund I (2001) Continued (5-year) followup of a randomized clinical study comparing antireflux surgery and omeprazole in gastroesophageal reflux disease. J Am Coll Surg 192:172–179; discussion 179–181

59. Luostarinen M (1993) Nissen fundoplication for reflux esophagitis. Long-term clinical and endoscopic results in 109 of 127 consecutive patients. Ann Surg 217:329
60. Luostarinen ME, Isolauri JO (1999) Surgical experience improves the long-term results of Nissen fundoplication. Scand J Gastroenterol 34:117–120
61. Luostarinen MES, Isolauri JO (1999) Randomized trial to study the effect of fundic mobiization on long-term results of Nissen fundoplication. Br J Surg 86:614–618
62. Mahon D, Rhodes M, Decadt B, Hindmarsh A, Lowndes R, Beckingham I, Koo B, Newcombe RG (2005) Randomized clinical trial of laparoscopic Nissen fundoplication compared with proton-pump inhibitors for treatment of chronic gastroesophageal reflux. Br J Surg 92:695–699
63. Martinez-Serna T, Tercero FJ, Filipi CJ et al (1999) Symptom priority ranking in the care of gastroesophageal reflux: a review of 1,850 cases. Dig Dis 17:219–224
64. Mittal RK, Holloway RH, Penagini R, Blackshaw A, Dent J (1995) Transient lower esophageal sphincter relaxations. Gastroenterology 109:601–610
65. Myrvold HE, Lundell L et al and the Nordic GERD Study Group (2001) The cost of long-term therapy for GERD: a randomized trial comparing omeprazole and open antireflux surgery. Gut 49:488–494
66. Nilsson G, Wenner J, Larsson S, Johnsson F (2004) Randomized clinical trial of laparoscopic versus open fundoplication for gastro-oesophageal reflux. Br J Surg 91:552–559
67. O'Boyle CJ, Watson DI, Jamieson GG, Myers JC, Game PA, Devitt PG (2002) Division of short gastric vessels at laparoscopic Nissen fundoplication: a prospective double-blind randomized trial with 5-year follow-up. Ann Surg 235:165–170
68. Olsen MF, Josefson K, Dalenback J, Lundell L, Lonroth H (1997) Respiratory function after laparoscopic and open fundoplication. Eur J Surg 163:667–672
69. Pandolfino JE, Richter JE, Ours T, Guardino JM, Chapman J, Kahrilas PJ (2003) Ambulatory esophageal pH monitoring using a wireless system. Am J Surg 98:740–749
70. Patterson EJ, Herron DM, Hansen PD, Ramzi N, Standage BA, Swanstrom LL (2000) Effect of an esophageal bougie on the incidence of dysphagia following nissen fundoplication; a prospectiv, blinded, randomized clinical trial. Arch Surg 135:1055–1061; discussion 1061–1062
71. Patti MG, Robinson T, Galvani C, Gorodner MV, Fisichella PM, Way LW (2004) Total fundoplication is superior to partial fundoplication even when esophageal peristalsis is weak. J Am Coll Surg 198:863–869; discussion 869–870
72. Peillon C, Manouvrier JL, Labreche J, Kaeffer N, Denis P (1994) Testart. Should vagus nerves be isolated from the fundoplication wrap? A prospective study. Arch Surg 129:814–818
73. Perdikis G, Hinder RA, Lund RJ, Raiser F, Katada N (1997) Laparoscopic Nissen fundoplication: where do we stand? Surg Laparosc Endosc 7:117–121
74. Schepp W, Allescher HD, Frieling T, Katschinski M, Malfertheiner P, Pehl C, Peitz U, Rösch W, Hotz J (2005) GERD: definitions, epidemiology and natural course. Z Gastroenterol 43:165–168
75. Tack J, Koek G, Demedts I, Sifrim D, Janssens J (2004) Gastroesophageal reflux disease poorly responsive to single-dose proton pump inhibitors in patients without Barrett's esophagus: acid reflux, bile reflux, or both? Am J Gastroenterol 99:981–988
76. Thor KBA, Silander T (1989) A long-term randomized prospective trial of the Nissen procedure versus a modified Toupet technique. Ann Surg 210:719
77. Walker SJ, Holt S, Sanderson CJ, Stoddard CJ (1992) Comparison of Nissen total and Lind partial transabdominal fundoplication in the treatment of gastro-oesophageal reflux. Br J Surg 79:410
78. Watson DI, Jamieson GG, Devitt PG, Kennedy JA, Ellis T, Ackroyd R, Lafullarde T, Game PA (2001) A prospective randomized trial of laparoscopic Nissen fundoplication anterior vs posterior hiatal repair. Arch Surg 136:745–751
79. Watson DI, Jamieson GG, Ludemann R, Game PA, Devitt PG (2004) Laparoscopic total versus anterior 180 degree fundoplication – five year follow-up of a prospective randomised trial. Dis Esophagus 17(Suppl 1):A81–88

80. Zaninotto G, DeMeester TR, Schwizer W, Johansson KE, Cheng SC (1988) The lower esophageal sphincter in health and disease. Am J Surg 155:104–111
81. Zaninotto G, Molena D, Ancona E, and the Study Group for the Laparoscopic Treatment of Gastroesophageal Reflux Disease of the Italian Society of Endoscopic Surgery (2000) A prospective multicenter study on laparoscopic treatment of gastroesophageal reflux disease in Italy. Surg Endosc 14:282–288
82. Zieren J, Jacobi CA, Wenger FA, Volk HD, Muller JM (2000) Fundoplication: a model for immunologic aspects of laparoscopic and conventional surgery. J Laparoendosc Adv Surg Tech A 10:35–40
83. Zornig C, Strate U, Fibbe C, Emmermann A, Layer P (2002) Nissen vs Toupet laparoscopic fundoplication. Surg Endosc 16:758–766

The EAES Clinical Practice Guidelines on the Diagnosis and Treatment of Diverticular Disease (1999)

Lothar Köhler, Stefan Sauerland, Edmund A.M. Neugebauer, R. Caprilli, A. Fingerhut, N.Y. Haboubi, L. Hultén, C.G.S. Hüscher, A. Jansen, H.-U. Kauczor, M.R.B. Keighley, F. Köckerling, W. Kruis, A. Lacy, K. Lauterbach, J. Leroy, J.M. Müller, H.E. Myrvold, P. Spinelli

Introduction

Colonic diverticulosis is an increasingly common condition. About a third of the population is affected by the sixth decade and a half by the ninth decade. The estimated incidence of diverticulitis is approximately ten patients/100,000/year [3, 8]. In the USA, approximately 200,000 admissions to hospital annually are due to diverticular disease. Over the preceding century, the sex predilection has changed from a male to a female predominance. It is well documented that the disease is more common in Western societies than in developing countries [55, 61]; this prevalence can be explained by the etiology of the disease [4]. In East Asia, right-side colonic diverticula or bilateral disease has been found to be more common [54, 58].

Owing to the worldwide importance of the disease and the newly emerging possibilities and controversies in diagnosis and therapy, the European Association for Endoscopic Surgery (EAES) decided to hold a consensus development conference (CDC) during the Sixth International Congress of the EAES, held in Rome, Italy, in 1998.

Methods

With the authorization of the EAES, the planning committee together with the Scientific Committee of the EAES nominated 16 experts as panel members. As with previous conferences [69], the criteria for selection were clinical and scientific expertise in the field of diverticular disease, along with geographical location. In addition, all medical specialties involved in diverticular disease were represented on the panel, so that recommendations would derive from a more complete perspective of the disease.

Prior to the conference, all panelists were asked to search the literature, list all relevant articles, and estimate the strength of evidence for every article cited (see footnote to Table 6.1 for categories of evidence) [1]. They were asked to answer 12 questions on subjects ranging from natural history and diagnosis to aspects of therapy. When assessing laparoscopic sigmoid resection, the levels of technology according to Mosteller [60] and Troidl [83] had to be ranked.

Table 6.1. Laparoscopic surgery for diverticular disease

Stages in technology assessment	Definitely better	Probably better	Similar	Probably worse	Definitely worse	Strength of evidence[a]	References
Feasibility							
Safety/ intraoperative adverse events			X			III	[15, 21, 27, 35, 43, 48, 49, 53, 78, 82, 89, 92]
Operation time				X		III	[15, 21, 27, 35, 43, 48, 49, 53, 78, 82, 89, 92]
Postoperative adverse events	X	X				III	[15, 21, 27, 35, 43, 48, 49, 53, 78, 82, 89, 92]
Mortality			X			III	[15, 21, 27, 35, 43, 48, 49, 53, 78, 82, 89, 92]
Efficacy							
Postoperative pain and other disorders		X				III	[21, 49, 53, 82, 89]
Hospital stay		X				III	[15, 21, 35, 43, 49, 53, 78, 82, 89]
Return to normal activities and work		X				IV	No data
Cosmesis	X					IV	82
Effectiveness (overall assessment)		X				III	

Ia evidence from metaanalysis of randomized controlled trials;
Ib evidence from at least one randomized controlled trial;
IIa evidence from at least one controlled study without randomization;
IIb evidence from at least one other type of quasi-experimental study;
III evidence from descriptive studies, such as comparative studies, correlation studies, and case-control studies;
IV evidence from expert committee reports or opinions or clinical experience of respected authorities, or both
[a] Categories of evidence (as defined by AHCPR [1])

All answers received from the panel members were analyzed and subsequently combined into a provisional preconsensus statement. Each member was then informed about the identity of the other members, which had not been disclosed thus far.

In Rome, all panel members met for a first meeting on June 4, 1998. At this time, the provisional statement was scrutinized, word by word, in a 5-h session. The following day, the modified statement was presented to the audience for public discussion (1.5-h session). During a postconsensus meeting on the same day, all suggestions from the audience were discussed again by the panelists, and the statement was further modified. The final statement was mailed to all panelists for a final Delphi process.

Consensus Statements on Diverticular Disease

1. Definition

In the literature, there is as yet no uniform definition of diverticular disease [30, 36, 80]. Consensus on the following terminology was achieved: Colonic diverticular disease is a condition seen mostly in the sigmoid region. It is characterized structurally by mucosal herniation through the colonic wall, generally accompanied by muscular thickening, elastosis of the taenia coli, and mucosal folding [40, 90]. This condition may be asymptomatic (*diverticulosis*) or associated with "symptoms," termed *diverticular disease*, which may be complicated or uncomplicated. The term *diverticulitis* is used to indicate superadded inflammation involving the bowel wall. Other pathologic complications include perforation, fistula, obstruction, and bleeding.

2. Natural History

The *natural history* of this condition has not been very well investigated within prospective studies [8, 29, 68, 79]. No good indicators are available to distinguish patients who will become symptomatic from those who will not.

3. Etiology

The etiology of diverticular disease is generally accepted as being associated with a lifelong *deficiency of dietary fiber* [19, 22]. It is believed that such a diet results in a small stool, the propulsion of which requires a high intracolonic pressure (equivalent to 150 mmHg or more) [84]. At the vulnerable regions where blood vessels enter the colonic wall, herniation is found. Muscular thickening and elastosis of the taenia coli have also been documented.

A high-roughage diet, such as that consumed by vegetarians, protects against diverticular disease [38]. This type of diet offers an opportunity for primary disease prevention. In Western countries, however, the decline of dietary fiber intake, mainly from cereal grains, has resulted in a high prevalence of disease, in sharp contrast to the data from developing countries.

Aging is associated with decreased tensile strength of both the collagen and the muscle fibers of the colon. In diverticulosis, similar changes occur, but they exceed the effect ascribed to aging alone [87, 88]. Nevertheless, with increasing age, the prevalence of diverticular disease rises steadily. Moderate and vigorous *physical activity* stimulates bowel activity and therefore may have a protective effect, at least in men [2]. Because *obesity* correlates with low physical activity levels and low fiber intake, it is associated with diverticular disease [74], but it plays no causal role.

Some *hereditary diseases*, such as polycystic kidney disease, Marfan's and Ehlers–Danlos syndrome, are associated with an increased incidence of disease, since, these diseases impair the strength of the submucosa.

Smoking may modestly increase the risk of developing diverticular disease. *Alcohol* and *caffeine* consumption do not play major roles in the etiology [3].

Immunosuppressed patients (mainly transplant recipients) have an increased susceptibility to diverticular disease [25].

Acute attacks of diverticulitis may be associated with hard feces becoming trapped in a diverticulum, causing mucosal ulceration and bacterial migration into the surrounding pericolic fat.

4. Classification

Diverticular disease can be classified with regard to the following aspects of the disease: localization, distribution, clinical symptoms and presentation, and pathology [58]. Two classifications are of importance – the *clinical classification and the Hinchey classification*.

Clinical classification: Subjective disease is difficult to grade, but we consider crampy pain, fever, and subjective patient evaluations to be symptomatic. Disease is classified as follows:
- Symptomatic uncomplicated disease
- Recurrent symptomatic disease
- Complicated disease (hemorrhage, abscess, phlegmon, perforation, purulent and fecal peritonitis, stricture, fistula, small-bowel obstruction due to postinflammatory adhesions)

Hinchey classification: The modified *Hinchey classification* [44, 78] should be used to describe the clinical stages of *perforated diverticular disease:*
- Stage I: pericolic abscess
- Stage IIa: distant abscess amenable to percutaneous drainage
- Stage IIb: complex abscess associated with/without fistula

- Stage III: generalized purulent peritonitis
- Stage IV: fecal peritonitis

However, neither classification is validated according to established criteria [72].

5. Diagnosis

The choice of diagnostic procedure depends on the clinical presentation. Differential diagnosis in coexisting intestinal disease has to be considered. The first step in making the diagnosis is to establish patient history with respect to type, severity, and course of the symptoms. The second step may require barium enema, colonoscopy, laboratory tests, CT, sonography, or radiograph [18]. The order of the procedures depends on the clinical decision and the availability of the methods.

In *uncomplicated cases*, a colonoscopy with biopsy and/or a barium enema [39, 71] is necessary to rule out adenoma, carcinoma, colitis, and Crohn's disease [64]. There is no consensus on which method should be used first, or whether biopsy is mandatory or recommended.

Patients with *recurrent symptomatic disease* who are eligible for surgery, especially if an endoscopic procedure is planned, should undergo CT and/or barium enema to provide information on location of the disease process, extraluminal changes, and coexisting abdominal abnormalities [10].

In *complicated diverticular disease* (except bleeding) cross-sectional imaging such as computed tomography (CT) should be used in addition to radiography [12, 41, 45, 57, 81]. CT has been reported to have more than 90% sensitivity and specificity [6, 23]. Ultrasonography may serve as another good diagnostic tool [77, 86], but its usefulness depends on the experience of the examiner [75, 91]. If CT is unavailable or does not yield a conclusive diagnosis, a low-pressure, water-soluble contrast enema can be considered. Flexible endoscopy is not recommended in suspected perforation or abscess formation, since it may perforate the colonic wall. The value of magnetic resonance imaging (MRI) has not yet been studied in acute diverticular disease and therefore be evaluated by water-soluble contrast enema to confirm the should be considered experimental.

Cases of *acute obstructive diverticular disease* should obstruction. If the patient has a chronic obstructive situation, colonoscopy with biopsy should be performed.

In cases presenting with *massive bleeding*, a number of different approaches have been used successfully, including selective arteriography, endoscopy, and radionuclide scans [24, 67]. However, there is no consensus on which of these diagnostic tools is preferable as a first choice.

6. Criteria for Making the Treatment Decision

There is general consensus that *disease-dependent criteria* for the treatment decision include number of previous attacks, fever, anemia, leukocytosis, intraluminal narrowing, obstruction, fistulas, abscess formation, free air, intraabdominal fluid, and thickening of the wall verified by CT scan [10, 26].

Patient-dependent criteria include age and concomitant disease, functional and emotional status, degree of disability, cognitive function, and subjective well-being of the patient. However, these criteria have not been thoroughly studied in previous trials.

The number of diverticula, their distribution, and manometry data should have no influence on decision making.

7. Indications for Conservative Treatment

There is a consensus that conservative treatment is indicated in cases with a first attack of uncomplicated diverticulitis [51]. The rationale is that approximately 50–70% of patients treated for a first episode of acute diverticulitis will recover and have no further problems. Only approximately 20% of patients with a first attack develop any complications. Those with recurrent attacks are at 60% risk to develop complications [29]. The members agreed that a detailed description of conservative treatment was outside the scope of the consensus conference, and stated that conservative treatment strategies should be followed as suggested in a recent review article [30]. Appropriate conservative therapy in mild cases consists of oral hydration, oral antibiotics (i.e., ciprofloxacin and metronidazol [66]) and antispasmodics. In moderate or severe cases, oral feeding should be stopped to allow bowel rest [11]. Hydration and antibiotics should be given intravenously. Analgesics can be given as required, including narcotics, but morphine should be avoided because of its potential to cause colonic spasm and hypersegmentation [65].

Patients with diverticular disease who are not suffering from an acute attack should be instructed to maintain a diet high in fiber [19]. Patients who continued to experience discomfort (such as mild cramps, meteorism, or stool irregularities) may benefit from the addition of bulking agents (i.e., plantago) or antispasmodics.

8. Indications for Operative Treatment

There is a consensus that prophylactic sigmoid colectomy is not justified in asymptomatic patients who have no history of inflammatory attacks. There is also agreement that prophylactic sigmoid colectomy should not be performed for symptomatic diverticular disease in the belief that complications would be prevented thereby. Patients should be considered for elective surgery if they have had at least two attacks of symptomatic diverticular disease [7]. There are no available data on symptoms or signs that might predict the occurrence or severity of an attack. The decision should be made by the treating doctor. At the same time, the benefits of resection for recurrent symptoms must be weighed against the risks of surgery in old, fragile patients and those with concurrent disease. This situation must be fully explained to patients (consensus). Surgery may also be indicated after the first attack in patients who require chronic immunosuppression. Chronic complications such as colovesicular or colovaginal fistulas, stenoses, and bleeding are further indications for operation. If a concomitant carcinoma cannot be excluded, surgery is also recommended.

9. Type of Operation

For *symptomatic, uncomplicated disease*, there is a consensus that the diseased segment – usually the sigmoid colon – should be resected. Sigmoid myotomy is nowadays an outmoded procedure. It is not necessary to remove all diverticula [93]. The distal resection line should be just below the level of the rectosigmoid junction, and anastomosis is performed with the proximal rectum to prevent recurrent disease [37]. The extent to which the colon is resected in the oral direction is controversial. Many surgeons claim that the colon should be divided when the bowel is soft, even in the presence of diverticula; whereas others suggest complete proximal resection of macroscopically involved bowel to achieve normal wall thickness without diverticula at the line of resection. There are insufficient data to resolve this issue [14, 93]. The left ureter should always be identified before resection is performed. During resection, the presacral nerves should be identified and preserved from damage.

Hinchey I (abscess confined to mesentery) should first be treated by percutaneous drainage where possible, followed by sigmoid colectomy and primary anastomosis in fit patients (consensus).

Hinchey II (pelvic abscess, whatever the localization) should also be treated by percutaneous drainage, and followed later by sigmoid resection in most cases, but the risk in patients with comorbidity must be considered in the final decision (consensus) [9].

Hinchey III (purulent peritonitis) is a problematical situation: There are no valid data regarding its best treatment. Options include Hartmann resection, or resection with primary anastomosis with or without a covering stoma [28, 42, 50]. There is a need for randomized trials here (consensus).

Hinchey IV (fecal peritonitis) should be treated by the Hartmann procedure after intense preoperative resuscitation measures [13]. Drainage alone by open operation is not viable for Hinchey III and IV (consensus).

Patients should be informed that the chance of restoring intestinal continuity is only 60% at best after a Hartmann procedure [62]. Open surgery to restore continuity after a Hartmann operation is a major undertaking, and it is associated with a high potential for complications (consensus).

If continuous and severe *bleeding* is caused by diverticular disease, the involved segment should be resected [17, 31, 56, 67]. On-table lavage and endoscopy should be considered to localize the bleeding [5]. However, exact localization is often impossible [32]. In these cases, subtotal colectomy with ileorectal anastomosis is indicated. Selective intraarterial infusion of vasopressin and endoscopic injection hemostasis have been shown to be effective [47, 70], but elective surgery should be considered to prevent recurrence in the long term [20].

10. Place of Laparoscopic Procedures

There is a consensus that elective laparoscopic sigmoid resection (for procedures, see Appendix) may be an acceptable alternative to conventional sigmoid resection in patients with recurrent diverticular disease or stenosis [21, 27, 33, 34, 48, 49, 53, 78] (Table 6.1).

In Hinchey I and II patients, the laparoscopic approach is not the first choice, but it may be justified if no gross abnormalities are found during diagnostic laparoscopy [43]. In some patients, peritoneal lavage or drainage of a localized abscess can be undertaken by laparoscopy [52].

There is no place today for laparoscopic resections in Hinchey III (diverticulitis with purulent peritonitis) and Hinchey IV (diverticulitis with fecal peritonitis) patients [35, 46, 59, 63, 76, 85]. Laparoscopic hookup after a Hartmann resection may reduce morbidity [62], but there may be a high conversion rate.

All surgeons engaged in laparoscopic-assisted sigmoid colectomy must have a low threshold for converting to an open operation if difficulties are encountered or if the anatomy of the abdomen and pelvis cannot be clearly defined [92]. The procedures should be restricted to surgeons experienced in laparoscopic techniques.

11. Laparoscopic Technique

The aim of laparoscopic surgery is to minimize surgical trauma. The same principles as those used in conventional surgery must be applied to the laparoscopic technique.

12. Avoiding Recurrent Disease

In uncomplicated nonoperated cases, recurrent attacks can be prevented by bulking agents, such as plantago. During the operation, the proper height of the proximal resection of the diseased bowel is still a controversial topic [16]. The distal resection should be performed to the level of the rectum, where the taenia disappears [14]. A specimen of 20 cm or more should be resected [16].

13. Long-Term Results and Sequelae of Therapeutic Interventions

In *uncomplicated disease*, the data indicate that a high-fiber diet provides symptomatic relief and protects from complications (below 1% per patient year follow-up) [42].

In *complicated disease*, after successful conservative treatment, the risk of further episodes of complications is approximately 2% per patient year [42, 73]. Resection was required in 3% or less of patients in collected series.

Only a few studies have focused on the outcome for the patients. Quality-of-life measurements are missing. Functional data concerning stool frequency, bowel habits, and continence after the operation are scarce. The persistence of intermitted pain in the lower abdomen after sigmoid resection is surprisingly high (1–27%) [93].

14. Economics

Extensive literature reviews have turned up very little in the way of economic data on the treatment of diverticular disease, especially data that would allow a comparison of treatment options. We recommend that choice of treatment not be based on economic data currently, because costs may vary from one locale to another. Further studies in this area are indicated.

Appendix:
Operative Technique for Laparoscopic Sigmoidectomy

The patient is positioned in a modified Trendelenburg position. The pneumoperitoneum should not exceed a pressure of more than 12 mmHg.

Usually four trocars are used, but more trocars can be used in cases of difficulties. The optic trocar is inserted above the umbilicus in the midline. Another 5- or 10-mm trocar is positioned in the left lower quadrant, and two further trocars (10 and 12 mm) are placed in the lower right quadrant.

The dissection begins in the basis of the mesosigmoid, where the vessels are located and divided after identification of the left ureter. Some surgeons prefer the primary mobilization of the sigmoid colon after identification of the left ureter; others prefer to ligate the superior rectal artery or dissect even closer to the bowel. The mesenteric attachments are freed widely. The parietal peritoneum is divided up to the splenic flexure. Mobilizing the splenic flexure may be useful in creating a tension-free suture. After presacral nerves are identified, the rectosigmoid junction is divided by stapler. A mini-laparotomy is performed in the left lower quadrant, or in the right lower quadrant, or a Pfannenstiel incision is done.

The bowel is extracted through the mini-laparotomy, and proximal resection is completed. Some surgeons use a bag to remove the specimen. The anvil of the stapling device is placed after performing a purse-string suture. After reestablishing the pneumoperitoneum, the stapler is introduced peranally, and the anastomosis is completed. The completeness of the resection ring has to be examined. Integrity of the anastomosis is checked either by endoscope, by air, or by methylene blue-colored water. Drainage of the pelvis is facultative.

References

1. AHCPR (United States Agency for Health Care Policy and Research) (1992) Acute pain management. Operative or medical procedures and trauma. Rockville, MD
2. Aldoori WH, Giovannucci EL, Rimm EB, Ascherio A, Stampfer MJ, Colditz GA, Wing AL, Trichopoulos DV, Willett WC (1995) Prospective study of physical activity and the risk of symptomatic diverticular disease in men. Gut 36:276–282
3. Aldoori WH, Giovannucci EL, Rimm EB, Wing AL, Trichopoulos DV, Willett WC (1995) A prospective study of alcohol, smoking, caffeine, and the risk of symptomatic diverticular disease in men. Ann Epidemiol 5:221–228
4. Almy TP, Howell DA (1980) Diverticular disease of the colon. N Engl J Med 302:324–331
5. Allen Mersh TG (1993) Should primary anastomosis and on-table colonic lavage be standard treatment for left colon emergencies? Ann R Coll Surg Engl 75:195–198
6. Ambrosetti P, Grossholz M, Becker C, Terrier F, Morel P (1997) Computed tomography in acute left colonic diverticulitis. Br J Surg 84:532–534
7. Ambrosetti P, Robert JH, Witzig JA, Mirescu D, Mathey P, Borst F, Rohner A (1994) Acute left colonic diverticulitis in young patients. J Am Coll Surg 179:156–160
8. Ambrosetti P, Robert JH, Witzig JA, Mirescu D, Mathey P, Borst F, Rohner A (1994) Acute left colonic diverticulitis: a prospective analysis of 226 consecutive cases. Surgery 115:546–550
9. Ambrosetti P, Robert J, Witzig JA, Mirescu D, de Gautard R, Borst F, Rohner A (1992) Incidence, outcome, and proposed management of isolated abscesses complicating acute left-sided colonic diverticulitis. A prospective study of 140 patients. Dis Colon Rectum 35:1072–1076
10. Ambrosetti P, Robert J, Witzig JA, Mirescu D, de Gautard R, Borst F, Meyer P, Rohner A (1992) Prognostic factors from computed tomography in acute left colonic diverticulitis. Br J Surg 79:117–119
11. Arfwidsson S (1984) Pathogenesis of multiple diverticula of the sigmoid colon in diverticular disease. Acta Chir Scand [Suppl] 342:1–68
12. Balthazar EJ, Megibow A, Schinella RA, Gordon R (1990) Limitations in the CT diagnosis of acute diverticulitis: comparison of CT, contrast enema, and pathologic findings in 16 patients. Am J Roentgenol 154:281–285

13. Belmonte C, Klas JV, Perez JJ, Wong WD, Rothenberger DA, Goldberg SM, Madoff RD (1996) The Hartmann procedure. First choice or last resort in diverticular disease? Arch Surg 131:616–617

14. Benn PL, Wolff BG, Ilstrup DM (1986) Level of anastomosis and recurrent colonic diverticulitis. Am J Surg 151:269–271

15. Bergamaschi R, Arnaud J (1997) Immediately recognizable benefits and drawbacks after laparoscopic colon resection for benign disease. Surg Endosc 11:802–804

16. Bergamaschi R, Arnaud J (1998) Anastomosis level and specimen length in surgery for uncomplicated diverticulitis of the sigmoid. Surg Endosc 12:1149–1151

17. Bokhari M, Vernava AM, Ure T, Longo WE (1996) Diverticular hemorrhage in the elderly – is it well tolerated? Dis Colon Rectum 39:191–195

18. Brewster NT, Grieve DC, Saunders JH (1994) Double-contrast barium enema and flexible sigmoidoscopy for routine colonic investigation. Br J Surg 81:445–447

19. Brodribb AJM, Humphreys DM (1976) Diverticular disease: three studies. Br Med J 1:424–430

20. Browder W, Cerise EJ, Litwin MS (1986) Impact of emergency angiography in massive lower gastrointestinal bleeding. Ann Surg 204:530–536

21. Bruce CJ, Coller JA, Murray JJ, Schoetz DJ, Roberts PL, Rusin LC(1996) Laparoscopic resection for diverticular disease. Dis Colon Rectum 39:S1–S6

22. Burkitt DP, Walker ARP, Painter NS (1974) Dietary fiber and disease. JAMA 229:1068–1074

23. Cho KC, Morehouse HT, Alterman DD, Thornhill BA (1990) Sigmoid diverticulitis: diagnostic role of CT. Comparison with barium enema studies. Radiology 176:111–115

24. Colombo PL, Todde A, Belisomo M, Bianchi C, Sciutto AM, Tinozzi S (1986) L'emorragia massiva da diverticolosi colica. Ann Ital Chir 65:89–97

25. Detry O, Defraigne JO, Meurisse M, Bertrand O, Demoulin JC, Honore P, Jacquet N, Limet R (1996) Acute diverticulitis in heart transplant recipients. Transpl Int 9:376–379

26. Detry R, Jamez J, Kartheuser A, Zech F, Vanheuverzwijn R, Hoang P, Kestens PJ (1992) Acute localized diverticulitis: optimum management requires accurate staging. Int J Colorectal Dis 7:38–42

27. Eijsbouts QA, Cuesta MA, de Brauw LM, Sietses C (1997) Elective laparoscopic-assisted sigmoid resection for diverticular disease. Surg Endosc 11:750–753

28. Elliott TB, Yego S, Irvin TT (1997) Five-year audit of the acute complications of diverticular disease. Br J Surg 84:535–539

29. Farmakis N, Tudor RG, Keighley MR (1994) The 5-year natural history of complicated diverticular disease. Br J Surg 81:733–735

30. Ferzoco LB, Raptopoulos V, Silen W (1998) Acute diverticulitis. N Engl J Med 338:1521–1526

31. Foutch PG (1995) Diverticular bleeding: are nonsteroidal anti-inflammatory drugs risk factors for hemorrhage and can colonoscopy predict outcome for patients? Am J Gastroenterol 90:1779–1784

32. Forde KA (1981) Colonoscopy in acute rectal bleeding. Gastrointest Endosc 27:219–220

33. Fowler DL, White SA, Anderson CA (1995) Laparoscopic colon resection: 60 cases. Surg Laparosc Endosc 5:468–471

34. Franklin ME (1995) Laparoscopic management of colorectal disease. The United States experience. Dig Surg 12:284–287

35. Franklin ME, Dorman JP, Jacobs M, Plasencia G (1997) Is laparoscopic surgery applicable to complicated colonic diverticular disease? Surg Endosc 11:1021–1025

36. Freeman SR, McNally PR (1993) Diverticulitis. Med Clin North Am 77:1149–1167

37. Frizelle FA, Dominguez JM, Santoro GA (1997) Management of post-operative recurrent diverticulitis: a review of the literature. J R Coll Surg Edinb 42:186–188

38. Gear JSS, Ware A, Fursdon P, Mann JI, Nolan DJ, Brodribb AJM, Vessey MP (1979) Symptomless diverticular disease and intake of dietary fiber. Lancet i:511–514

39. Goldstein NS, Ahmad E (1997) Histology of the mucosa in sigmoid colon specimens with diverticular disease: observations for the interpretation of sigmoid colonoscopic biopsy specimens. Am J Clin Pathol 107:438–444
40. Graser E (1899) Über multiple falsche Darmdivertikel in der Flexura sigmoidea. Münch Med Wochenschr 22:721–723
41. Hachigian MP, Honickman S, Eisenstat TE, Rubin RJ, Salvati EP (1992) Computed tomography in the initial management of acute left-sided diverticulitis. Dis Colon Rectum 35:1123–1129
42. Haglund U, Hellberg R, Johnsén C, Hultén L (1979) Complicated diverticular disease of the sigmoid colon. An analysis of short and long term outcome in 392 patients. Ann Chir Gynaecol 68:41–46
43. Hewett PJ, Stitz R (1995) The treatment of internal fistulae that complicate diverticular disease of the sigmoid colon by laparoscopically assisted colectomy. Surg Endosc 9:411–413
44. Hinchey EJ, Schaal PGH, Richards GK (1978) Treatment of perforated diverticular disease of the colon. Adv Surg 12:85–109
45. Hulnick DH, Megibow AJ, Balthazar EJ, Naidich DP, Bosniak MA (1984) Computed tomography in the evaluation of diverticulitis. Radiology 152:491–495
46. Khan AL, Ah See AK, Crofts TJ, Heys SD, Eremin O (1995) Surgical management of the septic complications of diverticular disease. Ann R Coll Surg Engl 77:16–20
47. Kim YI, Marcon NE (1993) Injection therapy for colonic diverticular bleeding. A case study. J Clin Gastroenterol 17:46–48
48. Köckerling F, Schneider C, Reymond MA, Scheidbach H, Konradt J, Bärlehner E, Bruch HP, Kuthe A, Troidl H, Hohenberger W, Laparoscopic Colorectal Study Group (1998) Early results of a prospective multicenter study on 500 consecutive cases of laparoscopic colorectal surgery. Surg Endosc 12:37–41
49. Köhler L, Rixen D, Troidl H (1998) Laparoscopic colorectal resection for diverticulitis. Int J Colorect Dis 13:43–47
50. Kronborg O (1993) Treatment of perforated sigmoid diverticulitis: a prospective randomized trial. Br J Surg 80:505–507
51. Larson DM, Masters SM, Spiro HM (1976) Medical and surgical therapy in diverticular disease. A comparative study. Gastroenterology 71:734–737
52. Lee EC, Murray JJ, Coller JA, Roberts PL, Schoetz DJ (1997) Intraoperative colonic lavage in nonelective surgery for diverticular disease. Dis Colon Rectum 40:669–674
53. Liberman MA, Phillips EH, Carroll BJ, Fallas M, Rosenthal R (1996) Laparoscopic colectomy vs traditional colectomy for diverticulitis: outcome and costs. Surg Endosc 10:15–18
54. Lo CY, Chu KW (1996) Acute diverticulitis of the right colon. Am J Surg 171:244–246
55. Manousos O, Day NE, Tzonou A, Papadimitriou C, Kapetanakis A, Polychronopoulou-Trichopoulou A, Trichopoulos D (1985) Diet and other factors in the aetiology of diverticulosis: an epidemiological study in Greece. Gut 26:544–549
56. McGuire HH (1994) Bleeding colonic diverticula. A reappraisal of natural history and management. Ann Surg 220:653–656
57. McKee RF, Diegnan RW, Krukowski ZH (1993) Radiological investigation in acute diverticulitis. Br J Surg 80:560–565
58. Miura S, Kodaira S, Aoki H, Hosoda Y (1996) Bilateral type diverticular disease of the colon. Int J Colorectal Dis 11:71–75
59. Morton DG, Keighley MR (1995) Prospektive nationale Studie zur komplizierten Divertikulitis in Grossbritannien. Chirurg 66:1173–1176
60. Mosteller F (1985) Assessing medical technologies. National Academic Press, Washington, DC
61. Munakata A, Nakaji S, Takami H, Nakajima H, Iwane S, Tuchida S (1993) Epidemiological evaluation of colonic diverticulosis and dietary fiber in Japan. Tohoku J Exp Med 171:145–151

62. Navarra G, Occhionorelli S, Marcello D, Bresadola V, Santini M, Rubbini M (1995) Gasless video-assisted reversal of Hartmann's procedure. Surg Endosc 9:687–689

63. O'Sullivan GC, Murphy D, O'Brien MG, Ireland A (1996) Laparoscopic management of generalized peritonitis due to perforated colonic diverticula. Am J Surg 171:432–434

64. Padidar AM, Jeffrey RB, Mindelzun RE, Dolph JF (1994) Differentiating sigmoid diverticulitis from carcinoma on CT scans: mesenteric inflammation suggests diverticulitis. Am J Roentgenol 163:81–83

65. Painter NA (1968) Diverticular disease of the colon. Br Med J 3:475–479

66. Papi C, Ciaco A, Koch M, Capurso L (1995) Efficacy of rifaximin in the treatment of symptomatic diverticular disease of the colon. A multicenter double-blind placebo-controlled trial. Aliment Pharmacol Ther 9:33–39

67. Parkes BM, Obeid FN, Sorensen VJ, Horst HM, Fath JJ (1993) The management of massive lower gastrointestinal bleeding. Am Surg 59:676–678

68. Parkes TG (1969) Natural history of diverticular disease of the colon. A review of 521 cases. Br Med J 4:639–645

69. Paul A, Millat B, Holthausen U, Sauerland S, Neugebauer E, for the Scientific Committee of the European Association of Endoscopic Surgery (1998) Diagnosis and treatment of common bile duct stones (CBDS): results of a consensus development conference. Surg Endosc 12:856–864

70. Ramirez FC, Johnson DA, Zierer ST, Walker GJ, Sanowski RA (1996) Successful endoscopic hemostasis of bleeding colonic diverticula with epinephrine injection. Gastrointest Endosc 43:167–170

71. Rex DK, Mark D, Clarke B, Lappas JC, Lehman GA (1995) Flexible sigmoidoscopy plus air-contrast barium enema versus colonoscopy for evaluation of symptomatic patients without evidence of bleeding. Gastrointest Endosc 42:132–138

72. Rothman KJ, Greenland S (eds) (1998) Modern epidemiology. 2nd ed. Lippincott-Raven, Philadelphia

73. Sarin S, Boulos PB (1994) Long-term outcome of patients presenting with acute complications of diverticular disease. Ann R Coll Surg Engl 76:117–120

74. Schauer PR, Ramos R, Ghiatas AA, Sirinek KR (1992) Virulent diverticular disease in young obese men. Am J Surg 164:446–448

75. Schiller VL, Schreiber L, Seaton C, Sarti DA (1995) Transvaginal sonographic diagnosis of sigmoid diverticulitis. Abdom Imaging 20:253–255

76. Schulz C, Lemmens HP, Weidemann H, Rivas E, Neuhaus P (1994) Die Resektion mit primärer Anastomose bei der komplizierten Diverticulitis. Eine Risikoanalyse. Chirurg 65:50–53

77. Schwerk WB, Schwarz S, Rothmund M (1992) Sonography in acute colonic diverticulitis. A prospective study. Dis Colon Rectum 35:1077–1084

78. Sher ME, Agachan F, Bortul M, Nogueras JJ, Weiss EG, Wexner SD (1997) Laparoscopic surgery for diverticulitis. Surg Endosc 11:264–267

79. Sheppard AA, Keighley MRB (1986) Audit of complicated diverticular disease. Ann R Coll Surg Engl 68:8–10

80. Standards Task Force, American Society of Colon and Rectal Surgeons (1995) Practice parameters for sigmoid diverticulitis. Dis Colon Rectum 38:125–132

81. Stefansson T, Nyman R, Nilsson S, Ekbom A, Pahlman L (1997) Diverticulitis of the sigmoid colon. A comparison of CT, colonic enema and laparoscopy. Acta Radiol 38:313–319

82. Stevenson AR, Stitz RW, Lumley JW, Fielding GA (1998) Laparoscopically assisted anterior resection for diverticular disease: follow-up of 100 consecutive patients. Ann Surg 227:335–342

83. Troidl H (1994) Endoscopic surgery – a fascinating idea requires responsibility in evaluation and handling. In: Szabó Z, Kerstein MD, Lewis JE (eds) Surgical technology international III. Universal Medical Press, San Francisco, pp 111–117

84. Trotman IF, Misiewicz JJ (1988) Sigmoid motility in diverticular disease and the irritable bowel syndrome. Gut 29:218–222

85. Tucci G, Torquati A, Grande M, Stroppa I, Sianesi M, Farinon AM (1996) Major acute inflammatory complications of diverticular disease of the colon: planning of surgical management. Hepatogastroenterology 43:839–845
86. Verbanck J, Lambrecht S, Rutgeerts L, Ghillebert G, Buyse T, Naesnes M, Tytgat H (1989) Can sonography diagnose acute colonic diverticulitis in patients with acute intestinal inflammation? A prospective study. J Clin Ultrasound 17:661–666
87. Wess L, Eastwood MA, Edwards CA, Busuttil A, Miller A (1996) Collagen alteration in an animal model of colonic diverticulosis. Gut 38:701–706
88. Wess L, Eastwood MA, Wess TJ, Busuttil A, Miller A (1995) Cross linking of collagen is increased in colonic diverticulosis. Gut 37:91–94
89. Wexner SD, Reissman P, Pfeifer J, Bernstein M, Geron N (1996) Laparoscopic colorectal surgery. Surg Endosc 10:133–136
90. Whiteway J, Morson BC (1985) Elastosis in diverticular disease of the sigmoid colon. Gut 26:258–266
91. Wilson SR, Toi A (1990) The value of sonography in the diagnosis of acute diverticulitis of the colon. Am J Roentgenol 154:1199–1202
92. Wishner JD, Baker JW, Hoffman GC, Hubbard GW, Gould RJ, Wohlgemuth SD, Ruffin WK, Melick CF (1995) Laparoscopic-assisted colectomy: the learning curve. Surg Endosc 9:1179–1183
93. Wolff BG, Ready RL, MacCarty RL, Dozois RR, Beart RW (1984) Influence of sigmoid resection on progression of diverticular disease of the colon. Dis Colon Rectum 27:645–647

Diverticular Disease – Update 2006

M. E. Kreis, K. W. Jauch

Definition, Epidemiology and Clinical Course

A commonly accepted uniform definition of diverticular disease is not available. The mere presence of diverticula which are herniations of the mucosal layer through the colonic wall is referred to as diverticulosis. It is debatable whether diverticulosis on its own without further complications causes symptoms and whether this condition should be named diverticular disease. However, problems secondary to diverticulosis such as diverticulitis, perforation, fistula, obstruction and bleeding definitely justify the use of the term diverticular disease, which, then, may also be classified as complicated diverticular disease.

Diagnostics

The diagnostic workup for diverticular disease has been virtually unchanged throughout recent years. With the high-resolution CT scanners that are available nowadays, most clinicians and radiologists prefer the CT scan to diagnose diverticula compared with the more time-consuming barium enema, although the latter is still a useful examination. Furthermore, imaging of diverticular is also elegantly possible with modern MRI scans [1]. It is of note that colonoscopy, which frequently detects diverticula as an irrelevant finding during screening for colorectal cancer, was found to be a useful procedure even for acute diverticulitis in order to diagnose associated pathology [2]. In this study, the rate of perforation was low so that this risk does not really justify renouncing colonoscopy during an acute attack.

Operative Versus Conservative Treatment

There is still consensus that the patients should not undergo sigmoid colectomy after the first attack of uncomplicated diverticulitis. Elective sigmoid colectomy is recommended for patients who have a second attack. This algorithm is now further supported by a recent study reporting data from a large database [3]. In this study, 13.3% of the patients who had an initial episode of acute diverticulitis had a recurrence, while this rate went up to 29.3% in those patients that had not been operated on following two episodes. It is debatable whether younger patients should be operated on earlier, i.e., upon initial presentation with acute diverticulitis. Approximately half of the studies that address this issue argue in favor of this approach [4–7], while the other half argue against it [8–11]. This issue, therefore, remains unsettled.

The historic paper by Farmakis et al. [12] that reported lethal complications in almost 10% of patients during recurrent divertiular was recently challenged by a retrospective study published by Müller et al. [13] with 363 patients and a 12-year follow-up. In their study, only two patients died secondary to diverticular disease during follow-up, which supports the concept that patients should be operated on to achieve relief of symptoms rather than to prevent lethal complications.

Choice of Surgical Approach and Procedure

For recurrent diverticulitis, elective sigmoid colectomy with resection below the recto-sigmoid junction and anastomosis to the upper rectum remains the gold standard. The standard for perforated diverticulitis in staged Hinchey III and IV stages was extensively discussed in recent years. Salem [14] performed a meta-analysis including 98 studies that reported on the surgical approach for patients with these stages. While sigmoid colectomy with primary anastomosis (with or without ileostomy) has a lower morbidity (23.5 vs 39.4%) and a lower mortality (9.9 vs 19.6%) compared with the Hartmann operation (including operations for reanastomosis), a prospective randomized trial is still lacking. Thus, although no selection bias was identified in this review, the evidence for the recommendation to perform a sigmoid colectomy with primary anastomosis even in Hinchey III and IV stages remains limited.

Technical Aspects of Surgery

Laparoscopic sigmoid colectomy was shown to be a feasible and an acceptable alternative to open sigmoid colectomy for recurrent diverticulitis in the past. Conversion rates, morbidity and mortality following laparoscopic sigmoid colectomy were shown to be volume-dependent [15]. The laparoscopic technique has the potential result in reduced complications, reduced hospital stay and better cosmetic results compared with the open operation; however, it also carries the potential for increased operative time and increased treatment costs [16]. As the available comparative, nonrandomized studies have a selection bias, definitive conclusions are not possible at this time; thus, we need to wait for the results of ongoing randomized-controlled trials before the superior technique can be determined.

Peri- and Postoperative Care

Several publications addressing the potential of fast-track surgery following surgery for colorectal cancer were published in recent years [17, 18]. No reports are available addressing specifically the peri- and postoperative care following sigmoid colectomy for recurrent diverticulitis. As care after surgery for cancer of the sigmoid colon is similar, multimodal rehabilitation, i.e. fast-track surgery after sigmoid colectomy for recurrent diverticulitis, is likely to have a comparable advantageous effect on patient recovery. Interestingly, Basse et al. [19] demonstrated in a recent study that the laparoscopic approach does not provide additional advantages regarding patient recovery compared with open surgery, when fast-track principles are strictly followed.

References

1. Schreyer AG, Furst A, Agha A, Kikinis R, Scheibl K, Schölmerich J, Feuerbach S, Herfarth H, Seitz J (2004) Magnetic resonance imaging based colonography for diagnosis and assessment of diverticulosis and diverticulitis. Int J Colorect Dis 19:474–480
2. Sakhnini E, Lahat A, Melzer E, Apter S, Simon C, Natour M, Bardan E, Bar-Meir S (2004) Early colonoscopy in patients with acute diverticulitis: results of a prospective pilot study. Endoscopy 36:504–507
3. Broderick-Villa G, Burchette RJ, Collins JC, Abbas MA, Haigh PI (2005) Hospitalization for acute diverticulitis does not mandate routine elective colectomy. Arch Surg 140:576–583
4. Cunningham MA, Davis JW, Kaups KL (1997) Medical versus surgical management of diverticulitis in patients under age 40. Am J Surg 174:733–735
5. Ambrosetti P, Morel P (1998) Actue left-sided colonic diverticulitis: diagnosis and surgical indications after successful conservative therapy of first time acute diverticulitis. Zentralbl Chir 123:1382–1385
6. Makela J, Vuolio S, Kiviniemi H, Laitinen S (1998) Natural history of diverticular disease: when to operate? Dis Colon Rectum 41:1523–1528
7. Chautems RC, Ambrosetti P, Ludwig A, Mermillod B, Morel P, Soravia C (2002) Long-term follow-up after first acute episode of sigmoid diverticulitis: is surgery mandatory? A prospective study of 118 patients. Dis Colon Rectum 45:962–966
8. Vignati PV, Welch JP, Cohen JL (1995) Long-term management of diverticulitis in young patients. Dis Colon Rectum 38:627–629
9. Spivak H, Weinrauch S, Harvey JC, Surick B, Ferstenberg H, Friedman I (1997) Acute colonic diverticulitis in the young. Dis Colon Rectum 40:570–574
10. Reisman Y, Ziv Y, Kravrovitc D, Negri M, Wolloch Y, Halevy A (1999) Diverticulitis: the effect of age and location on the course of disease. Int J Colorectal Dis 14:250–254
11. Guzzo J, Hyman N (2004) Diverticulitis in young patients: is resection after a single attack always warranted? Dis Colon Rectum 47:1187–1190
12. Farmakis N, Tudor RG, Keighley MR (1994) The 5-year natural history of complicated diverticular disease. Br J Surg 81:733–735

13. Müller MH, Glatzle J, Kasparek MS, Becker HD, Jehle EC, Zittel TT, Kreis ME (2005) Long-term outcome of conservative treatment in patients with diverticulitis of the sigmoid colon. Eur J Gastroenterol Hepatol 17:649–654
14. Salem LFD (2004) Primary anastomosis or Hartmann's procedure for patients with diverticular peritonitis? A systematic review. Dis Colon Rectum 47:1953–1964
15. Scheidbach HSC, Rose J, Konradt J, Gross E, Bärlehner E, Pross M, Schmidt U, Köckerling F, Lippert H (2004) Laparoscopic approach to treatment of sigmoid diverticulitis: changes in the spectrum of indications and results of a prospective, multicenter study on 1545 patients. Dis Colon Rectum 47:1883–1888
16. Purkayastha S, Constantinides VA, Tekkis PP, Athanasiou T, Aziz O, Tilney H, Darzi AW, Heriot AG (2006) Laparoscopic vs open surgery for diverticular disease: a meta-analysis of nonrandomized studies. Dis Colon Rectum 49:446–663
17. Kehlet H, Wilmore DW (2005) Fast-track surgery. Br J Surg 92:3–4
18. Schwenk W, Neudecker J, Raue W, Haase O, Müller JM (2005) "Fast-track" rehabilitation after rectal cancer resection. Int J Colorectal Dis 9:1–7
19. Basse L, Jakobsen DH, Bardram L, Billesbolle P, Lund C, Mogensen T, Rosenberg J, Kehlet H (2005) Functional recovery after open versus laparoscopic colonic resection: a randomized, blinded study. Ann Surg 241:416–423

The EAES Clinical Practice Guidelines on Laparoscopic Resection of Colonic Cancer (2004)

Ruben Veldkamp, M. Gholghesaei, H. Jaap Bonjer, Dirk W. Meijer, M. Buunen, J. Jeekel, B. Anderberg, M. A. Cuesta, Alfred Cuschieri, Abe Fingerhut, J. W. Fleshman, P. J. Guillou, E. Haglind, J. Himpens, Christoph A. Jacobi, J. J. Jakimowicz, Ferdinand Koeckerling, Antonio M. Lacy, Emilio Lezoche, John R. T. Monson, Mario Morino, Edmund A. M. Neugebauer, S. D. Wexner, R. L. Whelan

Introduction

Laparoscopic surgery for colon cancer remains controversial. Because of early reports of port site metastases, many surgeons refrained from following the laparoscopic approach to colon cancer, despite evidence from experimental tumor biology studies that have indicated clear oncological benefit of laparoscopic surgery.

Multi-center clinical trials randomizing patients with colon cancer to either laparoscopic or open resection were initiated in the mid-1990s to assess the oncological safety of laparoscopic surgery. Because a minimum follow-up period of 3 years is required to establish cancer-free survival rates, none of these ongoing randomized trials has yet accumulated sufficient data that would enable reliable and definitive assessment of laparoscopic colectomy for cancer.

This consensus conference (CC) addresses only colon cancer. Rectal cancer has been excluded because the available experience with laparoscopic surgery for rectal cancer is limited and because the treatment of rectal cancer differs from that of colon cancer in many respects.

The objectives of the consensus conference were:

1. To establish the preferred diagnostic procedures, selection of patients, and surgical technique of laparoscopic resection of colon cancer
2. To assess the radicality, morbidity, hospital stay, costs, and recovery from laparoscopic resection of colon cancer
3. To define standards and optimal practice in laparoscopic colon cancer surgery and provide recommendations/statements that reflect what is known and what constitutes good practice.

Methods

The consensus recommendations and statements are based on a systematic review of the literature and a consensus development conference (CDC) held in Lisbon, Portugal, during the 2002 congress of the EAES. They are summarized in the "Appendix."

A panel of experts in both open and laparoscopic surgery were recruited for the CDC and to assist in the formulation of the consensus. Each expert had to complete independently a detailed questionnaire on laparoscopic resection of colon cancer, participate in the CDC, and review the consensus document. A reference list with accompanying abstracts was provided to the experts, who were asked to provide details of published articles not included in the bibliography that had been sent to them. The questionnaire covered key aspects of laparoscopic resections of colon cancer. The personal experience of the experts, their opinions, or references drawn from the literature search formed the basis for completion of the questionnaire. In parallel, the questions were also addressed by performing a systematic review of the relevant literature.

The systematic review was based on a comprehensive literature search of Medline, Embase, and the Cochrane Library. The following query was used to identify relevant articles: (colectom* OR hemicolectom* OR colon resection) AND (laparoscop* OR endoscop* OR minimal* invasive) AND (colorect* OR colon OR intestine, large) AND (malignanc* OR cancer OR adenocarcinoma* OR carcinoma* OR tumor* OR tumour* OR metastas* OR neoplas*) NOT (FAP OR familial adenomatous polyposis OR HNPCC OR hereditary nonpolyposis OR inflammatory bowel disease OR ulcerative colitis OR Crohn* OR diverticulitis). Only the terms colon cancer and laparoscopy were used in the Cochrane search because the previous query was too restricted and hence inappropriate for the Cochrane database. Relevant articles were first selected by title; their relevance to the objectives of the consensus conference was then confirmed by reading the corresponding abstracts. Missing articles were identified by hand searches of the reference lists of the leading articles and from articles brought to the attention of the organizing group by the experts. The primary objective of the search was to identify all clinically relevant randomized controlled trials (RCT). However, other reports (e.g., using concurrent cohort, external, or historical control), population-based outcomes studies, case series, and case reports were also included. All articles were categorized by two reviewers (R. Veldkamp and H. J. Bonjer) according to the quality of data and evidence they provided (Table 8.1).

The systematic review of the literature provided evidence on extent of the resection, morbidity, mortality, hospital stay, recovery, and costs of laparoscopic colon cancer surgery. Regrettably, the level of evidence of articles on

Table 8.1. A method for grading recommendations according to scientific evidence

Grade of recommen-dation	Level of evidence	Possible study designs for the evaluation of therapeutic interventions
A	1 a	Systematic review (with homogeneity) of RCT
	1 b	Individual RCT (with narrow confidence interval)
	1 c	All or none case series
B	2 a	Systematic review (with homogeneity) of cohort studies
	2 b	Individual cohort study (including low-quality RCT)
	2 c	"Outcomes" research
	3 a	Systematic review (with homogeneity) of case-control studies
	3 b	Individual case-control study
C	4	Case series (and poor-quality cohort and case-control studies)
D	5	Expert opinion without explicit critical appraisal, or based on physiology, bench research or "first principles," animal studies

From Sackett DL, Straus SE, Richardson WS, Rosenberg W, Haynes RB (2000) Evidence-based medicine: how to practice and teach EBM. 2nd ed. Churchill Livingstone, London
RCT randomized controlled trial(s)

surgical technique is low according to the Cochrane classification, indicating that surgical techniques are difficult to evaluate scientifically because many important aspects – e.g., multilimb coordination, dexterity, tactile and visual appreciation of anatomical structures, and surgical experience – cannot be measured objectively.

Analysis of the completed questionnaires and the information culled from the systematic review as outlined above formed the basis for the formulation of the draft consensus document, which was reviewed by the experts 3 weeks before the CDC in Lisbon, when all the panelists met for the first time on 2 June 2002. All statements, recommendations, and clinical implications with grades of recommendation were discussed during a 6-h session in terms of the prevailing internal (expert opinion) and external evidence. The following day, the consensus document with its clinical implications was presented to the conference audience by all panelists for public discussion. All suggestions from the audience were discussed, and the consensus document was modified where appropriate. In the following months, the consensus proceedings were published online on the Internet page of the EAES. All members of the EAES were invited to comment on the consensus proceedings on a forum Web page. Sixteen surgeons commented on the consensus proceedings through the Internet forum. The modified final consensus document was approved by all the panelists before publication.

Preoperative Evaluation and Selection of Patients

Preoperative Imaging

In current practice, the same preoperative workup is done prior to both laparoscopic and conventional colectomies. Metastatic spread of colonic cancer is commonly investigated by ultrasonography of the liver and plain radiography of the chest. Colonoscopic biopsy specimens from the tumor are taken in most patients to confirm the presence of cancer. However, colonoscopy does not accurately localize the lesion [1]. Abdominal CT imaging to assess the size of the tumor and possible invasion of adjacent tissues is performed selectively at some European centers and more extensively in the USA.

The size of the colonic tumor is one of the important criteria for establishing the suitability of laparoscopic resection. The atraumatic and protected removal of a tumor that has been mobilized laparoscopically requires an incision of the abdominal wall. The laparoscopic approach is not indicated when the size of this incision for extraction approximates the size of a conventional laparotomy. Hence, preoperative knowledge about the size of the tumor improves selection and reduces the need for conversion.

Barium enema studies provide reliable data on the localization of colon cancer but do not show invasion of the tumor in the colonic wall or surrounding structures [2]. Conventional CT of the colon can also provide information about the localization of the tumor. In the near future, more advanced radiologic techniques, such as virtual colonoscopy, may be able to assess the site of the tumor more precisely [3, 4].

Cancerous invasion of organs adjacent to the colon can be detected by CT. However, the accuracy of preoperative staging of colon cancer by CT varies from 40 to 77% [3] because of the limited soft tissue contrast of CT, which impairs assessment of mural invasion by the tumor. The importance of tumor size and infiltration of surrounding structures is documented by a review of the causes of conversion during laparoscopic colonic surgery which indicated that almost 40% of conversions were due to a bulky or adherent tumor (see "Conversion Rate").

Laparoscopy has the potential to assess tumor invasion of adjacent organs, but there are no published reports on the value of laparoscopic staging in the workup and selection of patients for open or laparoscopic resection of colon cancer as distinct from its established use in gastric, pancreatic, and esophageal tumors.

Recommendation 1: Preoperative imaging

Preoperative imaging studies of colon cancer to assess the size of the tumor, possible invasion of adjacent structures, and localization of the tumor are recommended in laparoscopic surgery for colon cancer (level of evidence: 5, recommendation: grade D).

Contraindications

Age

The experts agreed that age is not a contraindication. This view is supported by a subanalysis of a case series by Delgado et al. [5], who reported significantly lower morbidity after laparoscopic resection compared to open colectomy in patients over 70 years old. Schwandner et al. [6] performed a subanalysis of 298 patients undergoing laparoscopic or laparoscopic-assisted colorectal procedures. There were no statistically significant differences among the younger, middle aged, and older patients in terms of conversion rate (3.1 vs 9.4 vs 7.4%, respectively), major complications (4.6 vs 10.1 vs 9.5%, respectively), and minor complications (12.3 vs 15.% vs 12.6%, respectively). However, duration of surgery, stay in the intensive care unit, and postoperative hospitalization were significantly longer in patients older than 70 years ($p < 0.05$). Complications reported in case series involving elderly patients after laparoscopic cholecystectomy seem to compare favorably with open cholecystectomy studies [7, 8].

Statement 2: Contraindications: age

Age only is not a contraindication for laparoscopic resection of colon cancer (level of evidence: 2b).

Cardiopulmonary Condition

Cardiopulmonary consequences of the pneumoperitoneum were thoroughly reviewed in the EAES consensus statement of 2002 [9]. Relevant parts of this consensus have been enclosed in the current consensus. Decreased Cardiopulmonary function is not regarded a contraindication to laparoscopic resection of colon cancer.

Cardiovascular effects of pneumoperitoneum occur most often during its induction, and this should be considered when the initial pressure is raised for the introduction of access devices. In ASA I–II patients, the hemodynamic and circulatory effects of a 12–14 mmHg capnoperitoneum are generally not clinically relevant (grade A). Due to the hemodynamic changes in ASA III–IV patients, however, invasive measurement of blood pressure or circulating volume should be considered (grade A). These patients also should receive adequate preoperative volume loading (grade A), beta-blockers (grade A), and intermittent sequential pneumatic compression of the lower limbs, especially in prolonged laparoscopic procedures (grade C). If technically feasible, gasless or low-pressure laparoscopy might be an alternative for patients with limited cardiac function (grade B). The use of other gases (e.g., helium) showed no clinically relevant hemodynamic advantages (grade A).

Carbon dioxide (CO_2) pneumoperitoneum causes hypercapnia and respiratory acidosis. During laparoscopy, monitoring of end-tidal CO_2 concentration is mandatory (grade A), and minute volume of ventilation should be increased in order to maintain normocapnia. Increased intraabdominal pressure and head-down position reduce pulmonary compliance and lead to ventilation–perfusion mismatch (grade A). In patients with normal lung function, these intraoperative respiratory changes are usually not clinically relevant (grade A). In patients with limited pulmonary reserves, capnoperitoneum carries an increased risk of CO_2 retention, especially in the postoperative period (grade A). In patients with cardiopulmonary diseases, intra- and postoperative arterial blood gas monitoring is recommended (grade A). Lowering intraabdominal pressure and controlling hyperventilation reduce respiratory acidosis during pneumoperitoneum (grade A). Gasless laparoscopy, low-pressure capnoperitoneum, or the use of helium might be an alternative for patients with limited pulmonary function (grade B). Laparoscopic surgery preserves postoperative pulmonary function better than open surgery (grade A).

Recommendation 3:
Contraindications: cardiopulmonary status

Invasive monitoring of blood pressure and blood gases is mandatory in ASA III–IV patients (recommendation: grade A, no consensus: 91% agreement among experts). Low-pressure (less than 12 mm Hg) pneumoperitoneum is advocated in ASA III–IV patients (recommendation: grade B).

Obesity

Intraoperative ventilation of obese patients is more often problematic than in normal-weight patients, largely because the static pulmonary compliance of obese patients is 30% lower and their inspiratory resistance is 68% higher than normal [10]. The respiratory reserve of obese patients is thus reduced, with a tendency to hypercarbia and respiratory acidosis.

Obesity also reduces the technical feasibility of the laparoscopic approach. In obese patients, anatomical planes are less clear. This increases the level of difficulty of the dissection and prolongs operation time. Retraction of the small intestine and fatty omentum are more difficult and prevent easy exposure of the vascular pedicle at the base of the colonic mesentery in all parts of the colon. The routine use of hand-assisted laparoscopy may facilitate this.

Pandya et al. [11] have shown that the conversion rate is higher in patients with a body mass index (BMI) above 29 due to increased technical difficulties. A similar conclusion was reached by Pikarsky et al. who reported a higher conversion rate in patients with a BMI above 30 [12].

There is insufficient evidence in the literature to indicate which method should be preferred. Also, in conventionally operated patients, complication rates rise with increasing BMI. In particular, ventilatory complications and wound infections are encountered in these patients. We found no study comparing laparoscopic to open colon-cancer surgery in the obese. For laparoscopic cholecystectomy, many studies have demonstrated similar complication rates after open and laparoscopic surgery [13–15, 17, 18].

Statement 4: Contraindications: obesity

Obesity is not an absolute contraindication, but the rates of complication and conversion are higher at a BMI above 30 (level of evidence: 2c, no consensus: 93% agreement among experts).

Characteristics of the Tumor

Radical resection of colonic cancer is essential for cure. Atraumatic manipulation of the tumor and wide resection margins (longitudinal and circumferential) are the basic elements of curative surgery [19]. Laparoscopic radical resection of locally advanced colorectal tumors is problematic because adequate laparoscopic atraumatic dissection of bulky tumors is difficult. Furthermore, laparoscopic resection of adjacent involved organs or the abdominal wall compounds the technical problem. Hence, the role of laparoscopic surgery in patients with T4 cancers remains controversial. The majority of the experts consider T4 colonic cancer an absolute contraindication to laparoscopic resection; en bloc laparoscopic resection is possible only in a limited number of patients. The routine use of hand-assisted laparoscopy may change this in the future.

The laparoscopic approach is useful for palliative resections of colonic cancer. Most experts do not consider peritoneal carcinomatosis to be a contraindication for laparoscopic surgery.

Recommendation 5:
Contraindications: tumor characteristics

Potentially curative resections of colon cancer suspected of invading the abdominal wall or adjacent structures should be undertaken by open surgery (level of evidence: 5, recommendation: grade D, no consensus: 83% agreement among experts).

Adhesions

Adhesions account for 17% of all conversions. However, prior abdominal operation appears to play a less important role in the completion rate of laparoscopic colon resection, as reported by Pandya et al. [11]. In this study, conversion rates did not differ between patients who had previous abdominal operation and those who did not. In this series of 200 patients, 52% of whom had had a previous laparotomy, only five required conversion to laparotomy because of extensive intraabdominal adhesions. Hamel et al. [20] compared the morbidity rate following right hemicolectomy between patients with and without prior abdominal operation. The complication rates for the two groups were similar despite the presence of more adhesions in the previously operated group.

To our knowledge, no studies have been published comparing laparoscopic to open surgery for patients with previous abdominal operation.

Statement 6: Contraindications: adhesions

Adhesions do not appear to be a contraindication to laparoscopic colectomy (level of evidence: 4).

Localization

Half the experts do not recommend laparoscopic resections of the transverse colon and the splenic flexure. The omentum, which is adherent to the transverse colon, renders dissection of the transverse colon difficult. Mobilization of a tumor at the splenic flexure can be very demanding.

Operative Technique

Anesthesia

Nitrous oxide, when employed as inhalational anesthetic, does not cause intestinal distention assessed by girth of transverse colon and terminal ileum at the beginning and end of the procedure [21]. The first study investigating the usefulness of nitrous oxide during laparoscopic surgery was completed by Taylor et al. [22]. In one group, isoflurane with 70% N_2O in oxygen (O_2) was used, in the other; isoflurane in an air/O_2 mixture was used during laparoscopic cholecystectomy. No significant intraoperative differences were found between the two groups with respect to operating conditions or bowel distension. However, the consequences of the use of nitrous oxide during longer laparoscopic procedures have not been investigated.

Most experts employ general anesthesia without epidural analgesia.

Pneumoperitoneum

Recommendations regarding the creation of a pneumoperitoneum are given in the EAES consensus statement of 2002 [9].

Trocar Positions

Positioning of the trocars is based on the experience and preference of the individual surgeon. For right hemicolectomies, 50% of experts use four trocars, 30% use three trocars, and 20% use five trocars. Most of them extract the specimen through an incision made at the site of the umbilical trocar. At the umbilicus, a 10–12-mm trocar is placed. A 10-mm trocar is placed suprapubically and another trocar in the epigastric region by 70% of authors. Some experts place a 5-mm trocar at the left iliac fossa or at the right subcostal space.

For left hemicolectomy and for sigmoid resection, trocars are positioned at almost the same sites. Thirty percent of experts perform these procedures using a hand-assisted technique. Five trocars are used by more than 70% of experts. A 10–12-mm trocar is placed at the umbilicus; two 10-mm trocars are placed by 80% of experts in the right iliac fossa and in the right suprapubic region. The incision for specimen extraction is made at the left iliac fossa, or, if the hand-assisted technique is used, the specimen is extracted through the hand port incision, usually in the upper lateral abdomen. For left hemicolectomy, the specimen is extracted through a suprapubic incision or through an incision at the left iliac fossa.

Statement 7: Placement of trocars

Placement of trocars is based on the experience and the preference of the individual surgeon (level of evidence: 5).

Camera

There is unanimous agreement about the use of a threechip camera, because of its better resolution. The laparoscope can be 30° or 0°, depending on the surgeon's preference. Two experts use a flexible videolaparoscope. The camera is hand-held by most experts. Mechanical and robotic devices are available, but they are used by less than 10% of experts.

Recommendation 8: Videoscopic Image

High-quality videoscopic imaging is strongly recommended (level of evidence: 5, recommendation: grade D).

Prevention of Port Site Metastasis

Port site metastases after laparoscopic resection of colon cancer have caused great concern in the surgical community. Therefore, the causative mechanisms in the occurrence of port site metastases has become an important subject for experimental research. Many mechanisms have been proposed and have been subject of extensive research [23]. However, so far no conclusive pathogenesis of port site metastases has been established. We will discuss the most common preventive measures for port site metastases and their pathogenesis. No levels of evidence and grades of recommendation are given for each individual measure because most evidence is derived from experimental research and there is no consensus among the experts on which measures to use.

Surgical Experience

The incidence of port site metastases has decreased dramatically with growing experience. The initial incidence of port site metastases of 21% has dropped to less than 1% (see "Port Site Metastases After Laparoscopic Colectomy"). Surgical experience thus appears the main determinant for the occurrence of port site metastases.

Wound Protectors

Experimental studies have shown that tumor growth is increased at the site of extraction of a malignant tumor [24]. All experts protect the abdominal wall or place the specimen in a plastic bag prior to extraction to prevent tumor cell implantation and growth. However, port site recurrences have been reported after extraction of a right colonic cancer that was placed in a plastic bag [25]. Therefore, wound protection is considered safer.

Gasless Laparoscopy

In view of the possibility that a positive pressure pneumoperitoneum may be responsible for wound tumor deposits, some surgeons have suggested the use of gasless laparoscopy. In this respect, experimental findings on gasless laparoscopy are controversial. Bouvy et al. [24] and Watson et al. [26] reported a significant decrease in the occurrence of port site metastasis when gasless laparoscopy was used in an animal model. Gutt et al. [27] and Iwanaka et al. [28] could not confirm these observations. Wittich et al. [29] reported in an experimental study that tumor growth was proportional to the insufflation pressure. Hence, low insufflation pressures may reduce the risk of dissemination.

Different Types of Gas

Carbon dioxide attenuates the local peritoneal immune response, which might enhance the risk of tumour cell implantation and tumor growth in the traumatized tissues [28, 30–34]. Neuhaus et al. [35], Jacobi et al. [36], and Bouvy et al. [37] assessed tumor growth in animals after abdominal insufflation with different gases. Only helium significantly reduced the rate of wound metastasis. However, the clinical implications of the use of helium in humans have not been explored fully.

Wound Excision

Because cancer cells can implant in wounds during surgery, it might be expected that excision of the wound edges would reduce the rate of neoplastic wound recurrences. This has not been confirmed in animal studies. Wu et al. [38] reported a reduction in port site metastases rates from 89 to 78% after wound excision, whereas Watson et al. reported that wound excision was followed by a significant increase of wound recurrence [39].

Irrigation of Peritoneal Space and Port Site

Irrigation of the peritoneal cavity with various solutions to reduce the incidence of peritoneal and port site metastases has been studied mostly in animal models. These studies have shown that peritoneal irrigation with povidone-iodine [40, 41], heparin [42], methotrexate [40], and cyclophosphamide [28] all reduced the rate of port site metastasis. Intraperitoneal tumor growth and trocar metastases were suppressed by the use of taurolidine in a rat model [36, 43, 44]. Eshraghi et al. [45] irrigated the port sites with distilled water, saline, heparin, and 5-FU. They found that 5-FU reduced the recurrence rate. Half of the experts irrigate the port sites with either betadine, distilled water, or tauroline.

Trocar Fixation

Tseng et al. [46] showed in an experimental study that gas leakage along a trocar ("chimney effect") and tissue trauma at the trocar site predisposed to tumor growth. However, the chimney effect has never been validated clinically.

Aerosolization

In experimental studies [47, 48], aerosolization occurs only when very large numbers of tumor cells are present in the abdominal cavity. The clinical significance of the aerosolization of tumor cells has not been proven. Some experts advocate desufflation of the pneumoperitoneum at the end of the operation before removal of the ports.

No-Touch Technique

The no-touch technique is based on the risk of dislodging tumor emboli during manipulation of the colorectal carcinoma. The value of the no-touch technique in colon surgery remains controversial. An improvement in the 5-year survival was reported by Turnbull et al. [49] in a retrospective analysis. In the only prospective randomized trial, which evaluated 236 patients, Wiggers et al. [50] showed that the no-touch technique did not impart a significant 5-year survival advantage. The absolute 5-year survival rates were 56.3 and 59.8% in the conventional arm and no-touch surgical groups, respectively. In the conventional group, more patients had liver metastases and the time to metastasis was shorter, but differences in survival were not statistically significant.

Bowel Washout

Studies have shown that viable tumor cells exist in the lumen of the colon and rectum. Rectal washout may thus reduce risk of recurrence, but the potential benefit remains unproven [19]. Exfoliated tumor cells have been detected in resection margins, rectal stumps, and circular stapling devices [51–53]. Furthermore, the viability and proliferative and metastatic potential of exfoliated malignant colorectal cells have been confirmed [52, 53]. Several washout solutions, including normal saline, have been shown to eliminate exfoliated malignant cells in the doughnut of rectal tissue from circular staplers [54]. Despite these observations, there is no conclusive evidence that bowel washouts reduce local recurrence and hence no data to support their use in surgery for colon cancer.

Statement 9: Preventive measures for port site metastasis

Proper surgical technique and practice reduce the likelihood of port site metastasis (level of evidence: 5).

Tumor Localization

Preoperative tumor localization is important in the laparoscopic resection of colonic cancer because intraoperative localization by palpation of the colon for tumors that are not visible on the serosal side is not possible unless the hand-assisted laparoscopic surgery (HALS) technique is used. The risk of incorrect tumor localization includes resection of the wrong bowel segment or less than radical resection because of insufficient proximal or distal margins [55–57].

Many colonoscopic techniques are used for marking the site of a tumor. Two of these, metal clip placement [58, 59] and tattooing [60, 61], are most commonly used. Tumor localization is advisable except for tumors located near the ileo-cecal valve, which forms a clear landmark during colonoscopy [62]. Special equipment is needed for clip placement. Before surgery, plain abdominal radiography is performed to exclude the migration of clips. During surgery, the clips are identified by intraoperative ultrasound or fluoroscopy. Hence, this is an expensive and time-consuming technique [63], although it is very reliable [59, 64].

Intra-operative colonoscopy is an alternative modality to localize the colonic lesion. However, this technique can induce distention of the colon and small bowel, particularly in right-sided lesions [65]. The colonoscopic tattooing technique with india ink or methylene blue is efficient. Tattoo injection with ink can be carried out at the time of the first colonoscopy because ink remains in place for several weeks. It is important to inject the dye in all quadrants, at an angle of 45°, and to mark the oral and aboral margins of the lesion. A thick omentum or tattooing along the mesocolic margin can mask a tattoo such that localization fails. Reported success rates for detection of the tumor after tattooing vary between 78.6 and 98% [61, 66]. The reported morbidity rate for tattooing is 0.22% [67]. In this review, only one patient was found in whom overt clinical complications developed. Injection into the peritoneal space has been reported in 0.5–8% [63, 68].

Recommendation 10: Intraoperative localization of tumor

Preoperative tattooing of small colonic tumors is advised. The alternatives are intraoperative colonoscopy, or pre-operative colonoscopic clipping followed by peroperative fluoroscopy, or ultrasonography (level of evidence: 5, recommendation: grade D).

Hand-Assisted or Laparoscopic-Assisted Approach

Basically, three different techniques are described for laparoscopic colon resection: totally laparoscopic, laparoscopic-assisted, and hand-assisted colectomy.

During totally laparoscopic procedures, the resected specimen is removed through the anus. It can be performed during low anterior resection or sigmoidectomy. The anastomosis is done laparoscopically using a circular stapler introduced through the anus. Totally laparoscopic procedures have been abandoned, largely because early experience indicated a high recurrence rate at the extraction site and no apparent advantage [69].

In laparoscopic-assisted colon resection, part of the procedure is performed in an open fashion through an incision of the abdominal wall made for the extraction of the resected specimen. This is the most common procedure for all colectomies.

Hand-assisted laparoscopic surgery (HALS) is an alternative to laparoscopically assisted colectomy. This procedure enables the surgeon to use his or her hand, with the dual benefit of magnified view and restoration of the tactile sense by the internal hand, which also provides atraumatic retraction and effective control of sudden bleeding. In addition, the internal hand is able to locate small tumors that are not visible from the serosal aspect.

With the early hand access devices, maintenance of the pneumoperitoneum was difficult, but this problem has been resolved with the second generation of hand access devices [70]. HALS appears to be at least as effective as the laparoscopically assisted technique in terms of operative time, conversion rate, and postoperative outcome [71]. Only two experts use HALS for laparoscopic colectomy.

Dissection of Mesocolon

Most experts dissect the mesocolon before taking down the lateral attachments of the colon. Fifty-four percent of experts use a vascular stapling device, 27% employ an external knotting technique, and 18% use clips to ligate the large-caliber mesocolic vessels. Most experts dissect the mesocolon from medially to laterally over Toldt's fascia. All agree that the surgeon must know both approaches to be able to deal with a difficult problem during the procedure.

For right hemicolectomy, the mobilization of the bowel is always performed laparoscopically. Dissection of the mesocolon and bowel transection can both be performed laparoscopically or after the colon has been exteriorized. Transection of the ileum is performed laparoscopically by 71% of experts. Aboral transection of the colon, as well as the anastomosis, is performed after exteriorization. In left hemicolectomy, dissection of the mesocolon, mobilization of the colon, and transection of the aboral colon are done laparoscopically. The anastomosis is performed using a circular stapler introduced through the anus by 66% of experts. Others perform a stapled or hand-sewn anastomosis after exteriorization of the colon. No preference exists for either end-to-end, end-to-side, or side-to-side anastomosis.

Sigmoidectomy involves the same steps as left hemicolectomy, but all experts use a circular stapler for the anastomosis.

Recommendation 11: Dissection of mesocolon

Dissection of the mesocolon from medial to lateral is the preferred approach in laparoscopic colon surgery (level of evidence: 5, recommendation: grade D).

Learning Curve

"Learning curve" can be defined in various ways. Simons et al. considered the learning curve completed when the operative time stabilizes and does not vary by more than 20 min [72]. Schlachta et al. [73] demonstrated that operating time, intraoperative complications, and conversion rates decline after the performance of 30 colorectal resections. Bennett et al. [74] reported that experience plays an important role in reducing complication rates and has less impact on reducing the operating time. Lezoche et al. reported that the conversion rate dropped from 17 to 2% after 30 laparoscopic colectomies [75]. Many surgeons consider the learning curve for laparoscopic colonic resection to be longer than that for laparoscopic cholecystectomy.

Intraoperative Results of Laparoscopic Resection of Colon Cancer

Conversion Rate

Reported conversion rates in laparoscopic surgery depend on the definition of conversion, the selection of patients, and the experience of the surgeon. Conversion rates between 4 and 28% have been reported in comparative studies (Table 8.2).

There is currently no standardized definition of conversion. In most studies, an operation is considered to be converted when a laparoscopic procedure was commenced but could not be completed by this approach. In two studies, a diagnostic laparoscopy was performed before every operation to establish the feasibility of a laparoscopic resection [76, 77]. If laparoscopy indicated that resection would not be possible, open surgical resection was performed. These operations were not considered as converted. In two case series, high conversion rates of 41 and 48% were reported [78, 79]. Both studies reflected a very early experience with laparoscopic surgery, and no attempt was made to select patients according to weight, tumor stage, or number of previous abdominal operations. None of the other case series that have been reviewed reported higher conversion rates [56, 76, 80–83].

In a study by Lezoche et al. [84], conversion rates were calculated for the first 30 patients operated laparoscopically and for the consecutive 26 patients. The conversion rate in the early experience group was 16.8%, whereas in the subsequent group it was 1.8%; this finding underscores the importance of experience in reducing the conversion rate. This finding was confirmed by several other reports analyzing early and later experiences with laparoscopic colon surgery [11, 56, 81, 85]. All found a clear decrease in the number of conversions as more operations were performed.

Laparoscopic colectomies are converted for a variety of reasons. Locally advanced bulky or invasive tumors, adhesions, and technical problems account for most conversions (Table 8.2). Because many conversions are for invasive or bulky tumors, improved preoperative selection of patients based on more accurate clinical staging may decrease conversion rates. Preoperative CT or MRI scanning can provide more information on the localization of the tumor and the invasion of surrounding structures.

Statement 12: Conversions

Laparoscopic colectomy is converted to open surgery in 14% (0–42%) of cases. The most common causes of conversion are tumor invasion of adjacent structures or bulky tumor, adhesions, and technical failure (level of evidence: 3a).

Duration of Surgery

In general, laparoscopic resection of colonic cancer takes longer to perform than open resection. Although operating time decreases with increasing experience [75, 78, 81, 84, 86], it is difficult to compare operating times between open and laparoscopic resections for colon cancer because most studies include a wide variety of procedures and do not specify per type of resection performed. Studies that included rectal procedures reported longer operating times [77, 87, 88].

Reported operating times vary between 140 and 251 min for laparoscopic colorectal resections and 120 and 175 min for open surgery (Table 8.3). In some studies, benign lesions were also included [77], and rectal procedures

Table 8.2. Reported conversion rates in studies on laparoscopic resection of colorectal cancer

Study	n	Conversion rate	Cause
1			
Weeks et al. [115]	58/228	25	1 advanced disease, 3 positive margins, 10 inability to visualize structures, 4 inability to mobilize colon, 12 adhesions, 4 intraoperative complications, 2 associated complicating disease, 12 other
Schwenk et al. [111]	0/30	0	After diagnostic laparoscopy
Milsom et al. [77]	4/59	7	2 bowel distension, 2 tumor too low, 1 adhesions
Delgado et al. [5]	18/129	14	15 invasion of adjacent organs, 1 adherence, 2 NS
Curet et al. [87]	7/25	28	3 tumor fixation to adjacent organs, 3 extensive adhesions, 1 abscess around ureter
Stage et al. [94]	3/18	17	3 extensive tumor growth
Lacy et al. [93]	4/25	16	4 invasion of small bowel
3			
Lezoche et al. [84]	6/140	4	2 hemorrhage, 2 anastomotic defects, 1 obesity, 1 inadequate splenic flexure mobilization
Feliciotti et al. [126]	5/104	4.8	2 anastomotic defects, 1 obesity, 1 inadequate splenic flexure mobilization, hemorrhage
Bouvet et al. [88]	38/91	42	12 adhesions, 8 poor exposure, 5 extensive tumor growth, 3 excessive procedure time, 2 bleeding, 2 inability to identify the ureter, 1 inadequate distal margin, 1 equipment failure, 4 combination of factors
Hong et al. [112]	12/98	12	5 adherence, 5 size of tumor, 2 adhesions
Psaila et al. [117]	3/25	12	NS
Khalili et al. [90]	6/80	8	3 extensive tumor, 2 adhesions, 1 intraoperative bleed
Pandya et al. [11]	47/200	23.5	6 hypercarbia, 2 unclear anatomy, 2 stapler misfiring, 5 too ambitious, 6 bleeding, 7 cystotomy, 2 enterotomy, 5 adhesions, 3 obesity, 10 size/invasion tumor, 5 phlegmon
Bokey et al. [95]	6/34	18	1 injury cecum, 1 adhherence, 1 adhesions, 1 hypercapnia, 2 lack of progress
Franklin et al. [116]	8/192	4.2	7 large invasive tumor, 1 bleed
Santoro et al. [114]	0/50	0	–
Leung et al. [92]	8/50	4	2 adhesions, 2 bleeding, 3 large/invasive tumors, 1 low tumor
Van Ye et al. [99]	1/15	6.7	1 adhesions
Leung et al. [104]			

Table 8.2 (continued)

Study	n	Conver-sion rate	Cause
4			
Schiedeck et al. [152]	25/399	6.3	NS
Bokey et al. [103]	9/66	14	2 lack of progress, 2 adherence, 1 adhesions, 1 cecal injury, 1 hypercapnia, 1 ureter not identified, 1 bleed
Fleshman et al. [163]	58/372	15.6	NS
Franklin et al. [154]	3/50	6	3 bulky/invasive tumor
Poulin et al. [155]	12/131	9	6 fixed tumor, 3 adhesions, 1 oncologic resection impossible, 1 hemorrhage, 1 perforation of small bowel
Leung et al. [108]	54/201	26.9	22 conversions after diagnostic laparoscopy (not further specified) Invaisve or bulky tumor: 36% Adhesions: 18% Technical problem: 22% (12 lack of progress, 18 poor exposure, 8 hypercarbia, 6 anastomotic problem, 2 bowel distension, 6 inadequate mobilization, one equipment failure)
Total	395/2812	14%	Bleed: 7% Safe oncologic resection impossible: 2% Visceral injury: 3% Obesity: 2% Others: 10%

NS not specified

were excluded in only one RCT [89]. In two RCT [77, 87] and in five nonrandomized comparative studies, the intention-to-treat principle was violated [75, 88, 90–92], resulting in selection bias, possibly favoring the laparoscopic group.

Statement 13: Duration of surgery

Laparoscopic colectomy requires more operating time than open colectomy (level of evidence: 2 a).

Statement 14: Extent of resection

For a laparoscopic oncological resection to be as safe as an open resection, the extent of resection of colonic and lymphatic tissue should not differ from that of open colectomy. All RCT report similar numbers of lymph nodes harvested in laparoscopic and open surgical specimens. Also, the length of

Table 8.3. Duration of surgery

Study	Laparoscopic	Open	p value
2			
Lacy et al. [89]	142±52	118±45	0.001
Hewitt et al. [102]	165 (130–300)	107.5 (90–150)	0.02
Milsom et al. [77]	200±40	125±51	<0.0001
Delgado et al. [5]	<70 years: 144±40	122±45	0.005
	>70 years: 150±60	119±51	0.001
Curet et al. [87]	210 (128–275)	138 (95–240)	<0.05
Stage et al. [94]	150 (60–275)	95 (40–195)	0.05
Lacy et al. [93]	148.8±45.5	110.6±49.3	0.006
Schwenk et al. [156]	219±64	146±41	<0.01
3			
Lezoche et al. [84]	RHC 190 (90–330)	140 (90–280)	0.03
	First 30: 226 (140–330)		
	Last 20: 153 (90–240)	190 (130–340)	0.04
	LHC 240 (150–480)		
	First 30: 260 (150–480)		
	Last 20: 210 (150–320)		
Bouvet et al. [88]	240 (150–516)	150 (60–376)	<0.01
Fukushima et al. [150]	231±23	169±20	NS
Hong et al. [112]	140±49.5	129±53.5	NS
Psaila et al. [117]	179±41	123±41	<0.05
Khalili et al. [90]	161±7	163±8	NS
Lezoche et al. [75]	Overall 251 (90–480)	175 (90–340)	<0.001
	RHC 203 (90–330)	140 (90–280)	<0.001
	LHC 282 (150–480)	190 (130–340)	<0.001
Marubashi et al. [91]	RHC 211.9 (134–330)	148.7 (104–173)	<0.05
Leung et al. [92]	196±44.4	150±61.1	<0.001

Results given as mean±standard deviation (*SD*) or median (range).
NS not significant, *RHC* right hemicolectomy, *LHC* left hemicolectomy

the retrieved bowel segments and tumor-free margins were comparable [5, 77, 87, 93, 94] (Table 8.4).

In nonrandomized comparative studies, no differences between open and laparoscopic groups were found for number of lymph nodes, length of the retrieved specimen, tumor-free proximal and distal margins, and total length of specimen. In two studies, a smaller distal resection margin was recorded [88, 95]. However, in these studies, the mean distal tumor-free resection margins were still 6 and 10 cm, respectively, which is oncologically acceptable.

There are reports of laparoscopic colon resections not containing the primary tumor or missing a synchronous second colonic carcinoma [55–57]. This type of result underscores the importance of tumor localization by either tattooing the tumor with ink or intraoperative colonoscopy.

The extent of laparoscopic lymphadenectomy and bowel resection is similar to those obtained by open colectomy (level of evidence: 2 b).

Table 8.4. Number of lymph nodes and extent of resection

Study	No. of lymph nodes Laparoscopic	Resection margins (cm) Open	p value	Laparoscopic	Open	p value
2						
Milsom et al. [77]	19 [a]	25	–	Clear in all	Clear in all	
Delgado et al. [5]	<70 years 9.6	10.5	NS			
	>70 years 12.2	10.5	NS			
Curet et al. [87]	11	10	NS	Length 26	25	–
Stage et al. [94]	7	8	–	Margins 4	4	
Lacy et al. [93]	13	12.5	NS			
3						
Lezoche et al. [84]	RHC 14.2	13.8	NS	Length 28.3	29.1	NS
	LHC 9.1	8.6	NS	Length 22.9	24.1	NS
				LHC TFM 5.2	5.3	NS
Bouvet et al. [88]	8	10	NS	Prox 10	10	NS
				Dist 6	9	0.03
Hong et al. [112]	7	7	NS	Dist 7.9	7.2	NS
Koehler et al. [113]	14	11	–	Length 24.1	22.6	–
				Prox 13.2	10.1	–
				Dist 7.9	8.6	–
Psaila et al. [117]	7.0	7.7	NS			
Khalili et al. [90]	12	16	–			
Lezoche et al. [75]	10.7	11	NS	Length 26.8	29.4	NS
				LHC TFM 5.2	5.3	NS
Marubashi et al. [91]			.	LoD 1.7	2.25	<0.01
Bokey et al. [95]	17	16	NS	Prox 10.1	11.0	NS
				Dist 10.0	13.4	0.03
Franklin et al. [116]	NA	NA	NS	NA	NA	NS
Santoro et al. [114]						
Leung et al. [92]	9 [a]	8 [a]		Dist 3 [a]	3.5 [a]	

Results are given as the mean
NS not significant, NA not available, Length length of resected specimen, Prox proximal re-section margin, Dist distal resection margin, TFM tumor-free margin, LoD level of dissection
[a] Median

Clinical Outcome

Short-Term Outcome

Morbidity

The reported morbidity and mortality rates for open conventional colorectal surgery range from 8 to 15% and from 1 to 2%, respectively [96]. Serious complications include anastomotic leakage, bowel obstruction, and abdominal and pulmonary infection.

Table 8.5 summarizes the studies describing morbidity following laparoscopic colectomy. Data from the RCT indicated a significantly lower overall complication rate after laparoscopic surgery [5, 89, 93]. In a subset analysis comparing laparoscopic to open resection, reduction of postoperative morbidity after laparoscopic resection was more pronounced than in patients under 70 years of age [5].

Table 8.5. Morbidity

Study	Laparoscopic (%)	Open (%)	p value
2			
Lacy et al. [89]	11	29	0.001
Milsom et al. [77]	15	15	NS
Delgado et al. [5]	10.9	25.6	0.001
	<70 years 11.4	20.3	NS
	>70 years 10.2	31.3	0.0038
Curet et al. [87]	1.5	5.28	NS
Stage et al. [94]	11	0	–
Lacy et al. [93]	8	30.8	0.04
Schwenk et al. [111]	7	27	0.08
3			
Lezoche et al. [84]	RHC 1.9	2.3	NS
	LHC 7.5	6.3	NS
Bouvet et al. [88]	24	25	NS
Hong et al. [112]	Major 15.3	14.6	NS
	Minor 11.2	21.5	0.029
Khalili et al. [90]	19	22	NS
Lezoche et al. [75]	13	14.3	NS
	Minor 3.6	7.5	NS
	Major 9.4	6.8	NS
Marubashi et al. [91]	27.5	25	–
Bokey et al. [95]	NA	NA	NS
Franklin et al. [116]	Early 17	23.8	NA
	Late 5.2	8.9	
Santoro et al. [114]	Early 28	28	–
	Late 12	0	
Leung et al. [92]	26	30	NS

NS not significant

Table 8.6. Complication rates in an analysis of 11 studies

Complication	n	Percentage
Wound infections	30	5.7
Respiratory	16	3.1
Cardiac	15	2.9
Hemorrhage	10	1.9
Anastomotic leaks	8	1.5
Urinary tract infections	3	0.6
Small bowel perforations	3	0.6
Port site herniation	2	0.4
Hematoma	2	0.4
Septicemia	1	0.2
Peritonitis	1	0.2
Anastomotic stricture	1	0.2
Anastomotic edema	1	0.2
Hypoxia	1	0.2
Acute renal failure	1	0.2
Uncompensated renal insufficiency	1	0.2
Urinary retention	1	0.2
Deep vein thrombosis	1	0.2
Small bowel obstructions	1	0.2
Phlebitis	1	0.2
Intraabdominal abscesses	1	0.2

Morbidity of laparoscopic resection of colonic cancer has not been reported in sufficient detail by most authors [97]. Specific complications of laparoscopic surgery involve vascular and visceral injuries, trocar site hernias [98, 99], and transection of the ureter [79]. Vascular injuries may be caused by blind introduction of the Veress needle or first trocar [78, 79, 97, 100]. Winslow et al. reported incisional hernias at the extraction site in 19% after laparoscopic colectomy, whereas incisional hernias occurred in almost 18% after open colectomy [101].

Experience is an important factor in preventing complications, as shown in three studies that reported lower morbidity with increasing experience [56, 74, 85]. Arecent systematic review [96] analyzed morbidity as reported in 11 studies [92–94, 102–109] (Table 8.6). The infectious complications of laparoscopic colectomy have not been assessed by large-scale prospective randomized studies. Wound infection at the extraction site was encountered in 14% of patients after laparoscopic colectomy vs 11% of patients after open colectomy [101].

Statement 15: Morbidity

Morbidity after laparoscopic colectomy does not differ from that after open colectomy (level of evidence: 2b).

Mortality

Mortality rates, defined as death within 30 days after surgery, are similar for both open and laparoscopic colectomy. However, no randomized controlled trials on laparoscopic vs open colectomy have yet been conducted with sufficient numbers to distinguish small differences. In two RCT, a 0% mortality rate was reported for both open and laparoscopic procedures [102, 110]. In the RCT by Schwenk et al. [111], one death occurred in the conventional group and none in the laparoscopic group. In another RCT, three deaths occurred, but this study failed to report to which group these patients were assigned to and the causes of death [94].

In nonrandomized reports, mortality was reported in only five studies [95, 104, 112–114]. None of these studies showed any significant differences between the open and laparoscopic groups, although the cohorts were too small to detect small differences.

Statement 16: Mortality

Mortality of laparoscopic colectomy appears similar to that of open colectomy (level of evidence: 2b).

Recovery

Length of Hospital Stay

Many factors determine length of hospital stay after surgery, and length of stay differs by country and hospital. Clinical condition of the patient is only one such factor. Type of insurance, social and economic status, and perception of postoperative recovery by both surgeon and patient are also important factors. Table 8.7 summarizes all studies comparing length of hospital stay after laparoscopic and open colectomy for cancer. The COST trial reported by Weeks et al. [115] is currently the multicenter RCT with the highest power and most published data. In this trial, a highly significant shorter hospital stay was found after laparoscopic colectomy (5.6 ± 0.26 vs 6.4 ± 0.23 days, $p < 0.001$), even though the analysis was performed on an intention-to-treat basis and patients converted to open operation were included in the laparoscopic group.

Six other RCT reported on length of hospital stay [5, 77, 87, 93, 94, 102]. In four RCT, a significant earlier hospital discharge was reported for the laparoscopic group [5, 87, 93, 94]. In one RCT with a sample size of 16, no statistical analysis was performed [102]. Median and range of length of hospital stay did not differ in this study (6 days [5–7] vs 7 days [4–9]). In one RCT, the difference was not significant [77].

Table 8.7. Length of hosipital stay (in days)

Study	Laparoscopic	Open	p value
1			
Weeks et al. [115]	5.6±0.26	6.4±0.23	<0.001
2			
Hewitt et al. [102]	6 (57)	7 (4–9)	–
Milsom et al. [77]	6.0 (3–37)	7.0 (524)	NS
Delgado et al. [5]	<70 years 5	7	0.0001
	>70 years 6	7	0.0009
Curet et al. [87]	5.2	7.3	<0.05
Stage et al. [94]	5 (3–12)	8 (5–30)	0.01
Lacy et al. [93]	5.2±1.2	8.1±3.8	0.0012
3			
Lezoche et al. [84]	RHC 9.2	13.2	0.001
	LHC 10.0	13.2	0.001
Bouvet et al. [88]	6 (2–35)	7 (4–52)	<0.01
Hong et al. [112]	6.9±5.4	10.9±9.3	0.003
Koehler et al. [113]	8.1 (6–14)	15.3 (9–23)	–
Psaila et al. [117]	10.7±4.7	17.8±9.5	0.001
Khalili et al. [90]	7.7±0.5	8.2±0.2	NS
Lezoche et al. [75]	10.5	13.3	0.027
Marubashi et al. [91]	18.7	35.8	<0.0001
Franklin et al. [116]	<50 years 5.2	9.35 (517)	–
	(2.0–9.2)	12.85 (941)	
	>50 years 7.84		
	(448)		
Leung et al. [92]	6 (3–22)	8 (3–28)	<0.001

Results given as mean±SD or median (range)
NS not significant

In the nonrandomized comparative studies, hospital stay after laparoscopic surgery varies from 5.7 to 18.7 days and between 8 and 35.8 days after
open surgery [75, 84, 88, 90–92, 112, 113, 116, 117]. In all these studies, hospital stay was shorter in the laparoscopic group, although in three studies the
differences were not significant [90, 113, 118]. Differences in hospital stay between laparoscopic and open colectomy groups vary from 1 to 7 days.

A recent article by Wilmore et al. [119] reviewed fast-track surgery for
open procedure. Fast-track surgery is a multimodal approach that combines
various techniques used in the perioperative care of patients to achieve a faster recovery and discharge after surgery. Methods include epidural or regional anesthesia, optimal pain control, early enteral feeding, and early mobilization. This Danish research group managed to shorten the postoperative hospital stay to 2 days after conventional open colectomy. So far, this approach
has not been studied for patients undergoing the laparoscopic resection of
colon cancer.

Statement 17: Length of hospital stay

Hospital stay after laparoscopic resection of colon cancer is shorter than after open colectomy (level of evidence: 1 a).

Postoperative Pain

Postoperative pain is an endpoint that impacts on the perceived health status, quality of life, hospital stay, and resumption of normal activities. In general, less postoperative pain is perceived after endoscopic surgery than after open surgery. In one RCT, statistically significantly less pain at rest after laparoscopic resection of colonic cancer was observed for 30 days or fewer postoperatively, when compared to open colectomy [94]. Also pain during mobilization was reported to be less severe. The number of patients included in this trial, however, was limited and the methodology used was flawed because the intention-to-treat principle was violated. Similar results were obtained by another RCT [113]. This study showed differences in pain at rest and during mobilization for 12 days or fewer, but these differences were not significant. In a recent RCT, postoperative pain was analyzed using the Symptoms Distress Scale, which includes self-reported symptoms such as pain, along with the duration of use of analgesics [115]. In this study, only a shorter duration of use of analgesics was observed in the laparoscopic arm.

Statement 18: Pain

Pain is less severe after laparoscopic colectomy (level of evidence: 2 a).

Postoperative Analgesia

The need for analgesics after surgery can be measured in several ways. Table 8.8 summarizes all studies comparing postoperative analgesia after laparoscopic or open resection of colon cancer. Some authors assessed the number of pills or injections per day [75, 77, 92], whereas others recorded the number of days the patient needed analgesics [91, 95, 112]. In the COST trial, patients in the laparoscopic arm required parenteral and oral analgesics for a shorter period of time [115]. In another RCT, significantly less morphine was used in the laparoscopic groups only on the 1st postoperative day [77]. In all other studies, the laparoscopic group used fewer analgesics, although the difference was not always significant [75, 91, 92, 95, 102, 112, 120].

Table 8.8. Postoperative analgesia

Study			Laparoscopic	Open	p value
1					
Weeks et al. [115]	Oral (days)		2.2±0.15	1.9±0.15	0.03
	Parenteral (days)		4.0±0.16	3.2±0.17	<0.001
2					
Milsom et al. [77]	Morphine	Day 1	0.78±0.32	0.92±0.34	0.02
		Day 2	0.4 ±0.29	0.50±0.31	NS
		Day 3	0.39±0.32	0.36±0.24	NS
Schwenk et al. [120]	PCA (morphine)	Cumulative dose until day 4	0.78 (0.24–2.38)	1.37 (0.71–2.46)	<0.01
Hewitt et al. [102]	Morphine	Cumulative dose until day 2	27 (0–60)	62 (28–88)	0.04
3					
Hong et al. [112]	Days till stop iv or im analgesia		2.7±1.5	3.2±2.0	0.021
Lezoche et al. [75]	Analgesics in percentage of patients	Day 1	75%	98%	<0.001
		Day 2	49%	91%	0.001
		Day 3	10%	71%	<0.001
		Day 4	0.7%	49%	<0.001
		Day 5		21%	
Marubash et al. [91]	Days till stop epidural No. of pills		2.98 1.49	4.04 2.68	<0.05 NS
Bokey et al. [95]	Days till stop (parental analgesia)		4.4	4.9	NS
Leung et al. [92]	No. of injections		3 (0–16)	6 (0–32)	<0.001

NS not significant
Results given as mean±SD or median (range)

Statement 19: Postoperative use of analgesics

Less analgesia is needed after laparoscopic colectomy than after open co-lectomy (level of evidence: 1b).

Gastrointestinal Function

Resumption of intestinal function can be measured by several parameters: time to first bowel movement, first passage of flatus or defecation (Table 8.9), and time to resume intake of liquid or solid foods (Table 8.10). In the RCT, data on passage of first flatus and defecation are consistent with a faster re-

Table 8.9. Gastrointestinal function

Study	Flatus/defecation (days)			Bowel movement		
	Laparo-scopic	Open	p value	Laparo-scopic	Open	p value
2						
Lacy et al. [89]				36±31	55±40 h	0.001
Milsom et al. [77]	3 (0.8–8)	4 (0.8–14)	0.006	4.8 (1.5–8)	4.8 (1.5–14.5)	NS
Delgado et al. [5]				<70 years 35±36 >70 years 37±19	53±26 57±33	0.0007 0.0005
Lacy et al. [93]	35.5± 15.7 h	71.1± 33.6 h	0.0001			
Schwenk et al. [156]	50±19	79±21	<0.01	70±32	91±22	<0.01
3						
Lezoche et al. [84]	Flatus RHC 2.9 LHC 2.7 Defecation 3.5 3.8	3.0 3.5 4.0 5.2	NS <0.0001 <0.0001 <0.0001			
Hong et al. [112]	3±1.7	4.1±1.8	<0.0001	3.5±2	4.9±2.1	<0.0001
Koehler et al. [113]	3.4 (2–5)	5.8 (3–7)	–			
Lezoche et al. [75]	3.0	3.7	NS	3.4	4.5	0.036
Marubashi et al. [91]	2.1	3.75	<0.0001			
Bokey et al. [95]	4.5	4.4	NS	4.9	5.5	NS

Results given as mean±SD or median (range)
NS not significant

covery in the laparoscopic group. In two studies, the differences were not significant [75, 103]. In all RCT, first bowel movement and resumption of diet were earlier after laparoscopic colorectal surgery.

Statement 20: Gastrointestinal function and start of postoperative oral intake

Gastrointestinal function recovers earlier after laparoscopic colectomy (level of evidence: 2b).

Pulmonary Function

Laparoscopic surgery causes less impairment of pulmonary function, enabling faster recovery. Postoperative pulmonary function after laparoscopic cholecystectomy, as compared to the open counterpart, is improved [121].

Table 8.10. Start of postoperative oral intake

Study	Parameter	Laparoscopic	Open	p value
2				
Lacy et al. [89]	Oral intake	54±42	85±67	0.001
Delgado et al. [5]	Oral intake	<70 years	59±33	0.0001
		50±45	81±48	0.002
		>70 years		
		59±33		
Curet et al. [87]	Clear liquids	2.7	4.4	<0.05
	Regular diet	4.1	5.8	<0.05
Lacy et al. [93]	Oral intake	50.9±20	98.8±48.6	0.0001
Schwenk et al. [156]	Regular diet	3.3±0.7	5.0±1.5	<0.01
3				
Hong et al. [112]	Fluids	2.1±1.8	4.0±2.0	<0.0001
	Solid food	5.2±3.1	7.1±2.8	<0.0001
Koehler et al. [113]	Regular diet	3.2 (2–6)	6.2 (4–10)	–
Khalili et al. [90]	Oral intake	3.9±0.1	4.9±0.1	0.001
Lezoche et al. [75]				
Marubashi et al. [91]	Oral intake	5.13	10.04	<0.0001
Bokey et al. [95]	Fluids	4.3	4.2	NS
	Full diet	6.9	7.6	NS
Leung et al. [92]	Normal diet	4 (2–20)	4 (3–17)	NS
Van Ye et al. [99]	Normal diet	4.8	7.2	0.001

Results given as mean±SD at median (range)
NS not significant

Postoperative pulmonary function after colorectal resection has been investigated in an RCT by Schwenk et al. [111]. Parameters shown in Table 8.11 were measured preoperatively and at different time points postoperatively. Forced vital capacity and forced expiratory volume were more profoundly impaired in patients who underwent conventional resections than in the laparoscopic group. Similar results were found for the peak expiratory flow and the midexpiratory phase of the forced expiratory flow. Also, the postoperative oxygen saturation was lower in the conventional group than in the laparoscopic group. Two pneumonias occurred in the conventional group vs none in the laparoscopic group. The difference was not significant, but the sample size of the study was only 30 patients.

Postoperative pulmonary function was investigated in two other RCT. Milsom et al. [122] found a significantly earlier postoperative recovery of pulmonary function after laparoscopic surgery. The RCT conducted by Stage et al. [94] showed no significant differences between the two groups in pulmonary function.

Table 8.11. Postoperative pulmonary function

Study	Parameter	Laparoscopic	Open	p value
1				
Schwenk et al. [111]	FVC (p.o. day 1)	2.59 ± 1.11	1.73 ± 0.60	<0.01
	FEV1 (p.o. day 1)	1.80 ± 0.80	1.19 ± 0.51	<0.01
	PEF (p.o. day 1)	3.60 ± 2.22	2.51 ± 1.37	<0.05
	FEF 25–75% (p.o. day 1)	2.67 ± 1.76	1.87 ± 1.12	<0.05
	SaO2 (%) (p.o. day 1)	93.8 ± 1.9	92.1 ± 3.3	
2				
Milsom et al. [77]	FEV1 and FVC (days till 80% recovery of pre-operative values)	3.0	6.0	0.01
Stage et al. [94]	FEV1	NA	NA	NS
	FVC	NA	NA	
	PEF	NA	NA	

Results given as mean ± SD or median (range)
p.o. postoperative, *NS* not significant, *FVC* forced vital capacity, *FEV1* forced expiratory volume in 1, *PEF* peak expiratory flow, *FEF 25–75%* forced expiratory flow at 25–75% of forced vital capacity, *SaO₂* arterial oxygen saturation

Statement 21: Postoperative pulmonary function

Postoperative pulmonary function is less impaired after laparoscopic resection of colon cancer (level of evidence: 1b).

Return to Work and Daily Activities

The parameters of early recovery are strongly influenced by societal and economic organization of health care within a community. This may explain the wide variability between studies. Only in randomized trials can one assume that these factors are evenly distributed in both groups. None of the available randomized trials addressed this topic.

Long-Term Outcome of Laparoscopic Colectomy

Recently, Lacy et al. [89] published the results of their single-center randomized controlled trial on laparoscopic curative resection of colon cancer. In this study of 219 patients, 111 underwent laparoscopic colectomy. A significantly better 3-year cancer-related survival was found in the laparoscopically operated patients than in the open group (91 vs 79%, respectively). This difference in survival could be attributed mainly to the markedly better survival

Table 8.12. Overall survival rates

Study	Follow-up	Laparoscopic (%)	Open (%)	p value
2				
Lacy et al. [89]	43 months	82	74	NS
3				
Leung et al. [104]	21.4 months (median)	90.9 (n=28)	55.6 (n=56)	NS
Leung et al. [92]	32.8 months (median)	67.2 (n=50)	64.1 (n=50)	NS
Khalili et al. [90]	19.6 months	87.5 (n=80)	85 (n=90)	NS
Santoro et al. [114]	5 years	72.3 (n=50)	68.8 (n=50)	NS
Hong et al. [112]	Lap 30.6 months Open 21.6 months	NA (n=98)	NA (n=219)	NS
4				
Delgado et al. [157]	42 months	AR 83, SR 87 (n=31)		
Cook and Dehn [158]	Until patient's death	20 (n=5)		
Hoffman et al. [159]	2 years	Node–: 92 (n=89) Node +: 80%		
Molenaar et al. [160]	3 years	All: 59, by Dukes' stage (n=35): A=86, B=66, C=68, D=0		
Quattlebaum et al. [161]	8 months	90 (n=10)		
Poulin et al. [155]	Stages I–III: 24 months Stage IV: 9 months	81		

NS not significant, *AR* anterior resection, *SR* sigmoid resection

in stage III colon cancer patients. Follow-up data of large multicenter randomized controlled trials the (CLASICC [123], COST [124], and COLOR [125] trials) will provide a more definitive assessment of survival after laparoscopic vs open colon resections.

In smaller nonrandomized comparative studies, no significant differences in disease-free and overall survival have been observed between open and laparoscopic patient groups (Tables 8.12, 8.13). No significant differences were found between open and laparoscopically operated patients in a nonrandomized matched control study with 5-year follow-up [104]. Another study using historical controls also showed no difference in long-term survival, with survival rates of 64.1 and 67.2% in the open and laparoscopic arms, respectively [92]. In a further six comparative studies, no differences of overall survival were found between laparoscopic and open resections of colon cancer [84, 88, 112, 114, 116, 126].

Table 8.13. Disease-free survival rates

Study	Follow-up	Laparoscopic (%)	Open (%)	p value
2				
Lacy et al. [89]	43 months	91	79	0.03
3				
Leung et al. [104]	5 years	95.2	74.7	NS
Leung et al. [92]	4 years	80.5	72.9	NS
Feliciotti et al. [126]	48.9 months	86.5	86.7	NS
Lezoche et al. [84]	42.2 months	RHC 78.3	75.8	NS
	42.3 months	LHC 94.1	86.8	
Bouvet et al. [88]	26 months	93	88	NS
Santoro et al. [114]	NA	73.2	70.1	NS
Hong et al. [112]	Lap 30.6 months	NA	NA	NS
	Open 21.6 months			
Franklin et al. [116]	5 years	87	80.9	NS
4				
Delgado et al. [157]	42 months	AR: 78		
		SR: 70		
Hoffman et al. [159]	2 years	Node–: 96		
		Node +: 79		

NS not significant

Statement 22: Overall and cancer-related disease-free survival

Cancer-related survival after laparoscopic resection appears to be at least equal to open resection (level of evidence: 2 a).

Port Site Metastases After Laparoscopic Colectomy

Early reports of port site metastases after laparoscopic resection of colonic cancer generated considerable concern in the surgical community in the early 1990s. Initial enthusiasm for the laparoscopic approach to colon cancer was replaced by skepticism. Abdominal wall recurrence after open colectomy was considered to be rare – approximately 0.7% according to a retrospective study by Hughes et al. [127]. However, Cass et al. reported abdominal wall recurrence in 2.5% of patients after open resection of colon cancer [128], and Gunderson et al. showed that two-thirds of abdominal wall recurrences are missed by physical examination of the abdominal wall [129]. At second-look laparotomy 3 months after the open curative resection of colon cancer, 3.3% of patients suffered a recurrence in the abdominal wall.

In the literature on laparoscopic resection of colon cancer published before 1995, high incidences of port site metastasis were reported, ranging from 0.6 to 21% [130–133]. In a review of data from reports on laparoscopic resection of colon cancer published later, a much lower rate of 0.85% was recorded in an analysis of 1,769 operation [23]. Wittich et al. [134] analyzed data from 16 studies, including a total of 3,547 patients, 30 of whom (0.85%) developed port site metastases. In a recent systematic review, 11 port site metastases were found in 1,114 operations, translating to an incidence of 1% [96]. The high incidences of port site metastasis in early reports on laparoscopic surgery appear to reflect inexperience with the technique, such that an oncologically appropriate operation was not performed. The details of the published port site metastases are shown in Tables 8.14 and 8.15.

Table 8.14. Port site metastasis after resection of colorectal carcinoma

Study	Design	n	Follow-up	PSM
Lacy et al. [89]	RCT	111	Median 43	1
Milsom et al. [77]	RCT	42	Median 18	0
Lacy et al. [110]	RCT	31	21	40
Ballantyne [162]	Registry	498	NA	3
Fleshman et al. [163]	Registry	372	NA	4 (1.3%)
Rosato et al. [164]	Registry	1071	NA	10 (0.93%)
Vukasin et al. [165]	Registry	480	>12	5 (1.1%)
Schledeck et al. [152]	Registry	399	Mean 30	1 (0.25%)
Leung et al. [108]	Prospective	217	Mean 19.8	1 (0.65%)
Poulin et al. [155]	Prospective	172	Mean 24	0
Franklin et al. [116]	Prospective	191	>30	0
Bouvet et al. [88]	Prospective	91	26	0
Feliciotti et al. [126]	Prospective	158	Mean 48.9	2
Bokey et al. [103]	Retrospective	66	Median 26	1 (0.6%)
Fielding et al. [86]	Retrospective	149	NA	2 (1.5%)
Gellman et al. [166]	Retrospective	58	NA	1 (1.7%)
Hoffman et al. [159]	Retrospective	39	24	0
Huscher et al. [80]	Retrospective	146	Mean 15	0
Leung et al. [92]	Retrospective	50	>32	1
Khalili et al. [90]	Retrospective	80	Mean 21	0
Kwok [167]	Retrospective	83	NA	2 (2.5%)
Leung et al. [108]	Retrospective	179	Mean 19.8	1 (0.65%)
Lord et al. [98]	Retrospective	71	Mean 16.7	0
Lumley et al. [82]	Retrospective	103	NA	1 (1.0%)
Khalili et al. [90]	Retrospective	80	Mean 19.6	0
Guillou et al. [168]	Retrospective	59	NA	1 (1.7%)
Larach et al. [56]	Retrospective	108	Mean 12.6	0
Croce et al. [169]	Retrospective	134	NA	1 (0.9%)
Kawamura et al. [170]	Retrospective	67 (gasless)	NA	0
		5305		38 (0.72%)

PSM port site metastases

Table 8.15. Case reports on port site metastasis

Study	Year	Duke's stage	Months to recurrence
Alexander et al. [171]	1993	C	3
O'Rourke et al. [172]	1993	B	10
Walsh et al. [173]	1993	C	6
Fusco et al. [174]	1993	C	10
Cirocco et al. [175]	1994	C	9
Nduka et al. [176]	1994	C	3
Prasad [176]	1994	B	6
		A	26
Berends et al. [130]	1994	B	NA
		C	NA
		D	NA
Lauroy [177]	1994	A	9
Ramos et al. [178]	1994	C	NA
		C	NA
		C	NA
Cohen et al. [179]	1994	B	3
		B	6
		C	6
		C	9
		C	12
Jacquet et al. [180]	1995	B	10
		B	9
Montorsi et al. [25]	1995	B	2

Statement 23: Port site metastasis

The incidence of port site metastases after laparoscopic colectomy is below 1% (level of evidence: 2c).

Quality of Life

Health-related quality of life associated with laparoscopic colon resection for malignancy has been addressed only by Weeks et al. [115]. The investigators used the Symptoms Distress Scale, Quality of Life Index (QLI), and a global rating scale. The only statistically significant difference reported was the global rating scale score 2 weeks postoperatively ($p=0.009$). In this study, both the global rating scale and the QLI were not employed during the first two postoperative weeks, despite the probability that differences in quality of life are likely to be most evident and most pronounced in the early days after surgery.

Costs

The issue of costs associated with the implementation of health care technologies is of increasing importance. Not only are financial demands on health care increasing, but at the same time health budgets are limited. Currently, there are no prospective cost-effectiveness evaluations available for laparoscopic colon resection. Some evaluations are currently being conducted alongside large multicenter RCT. In the CLASICC [123], COST [124], and COLOR [125] trials, cost-effectiveness of the two approaches is being evaluated. Such analyses include both direct costs (costs primarily associated with treatment) and indirect costs (costs secondarily related to disease or treatment).

Direct Costs

In-hospital costs need to be carefully evaluated. In a retrospective review, the in-hospital costs of laparoscopically assisted right hemicolectomy were compared to the costs of open colectomy [135]. Costs were collected only from the time of operation until the time of discharge and thus reflected only hospital costs. This study reported higher direct costs for laparoscopic hemicolectomy than for open hemicolectomy due to increased operating time and the use of disposables (AUD 9,064 vs AUD 7,881, respectively). A review of the hospital costs of laparoscopic colectomy concluded that the shorter hospital stay in the laparoscopy arm more than compensated for the increased operating room costs, resulting in lower total hospital costs for laparoscopic colectomy (USD 9,811 vs USD 11,207) [136]. This evaluation included operations for both benign and malignant disease of the colon. In a prospective study, direct in-hospital costs for laparoscopic colectomy were also lower than those for open surgery (DEM 5,400 vs DEM 7,500) [113]. However, this large study included operations for both benign and malignant colorectal disease and violated the intention-to-treat principle.

Out-of-Hospital Costs

Out-of-hospital costs, such as visits to outpatient clinics, home care, and visits to family doctors, have not yet been estimated for laparoscopic colectomy.

Indirect Costs

The preferred method of cost analysis is to evaluate cost-effectiveness from a societal perspective. This implies the measurement of indirect costs. The most important indirect costs are incurred from patients who are employed but are unable to work, causing loss of productivity. One might argue that a faster recovery would lead to patients returning to work earlier. Koehler et al. reported that such costs were lower for laparoscopic colectomy (DEM 1,600) than for open colectomy (DEM 2,200).

Cost-Effectiveness

For policy making and the implementation of new techniques, one must assess both the costs associated with this technique as well as the effects of this technique and its widespread safe applicability. Survival is the most important endpoint after the resection of colon cancer. The differences in costs between laparoscopic and open colorectal surgery have to be assessed in the context of survival rates obtained by the two approaches. The next endpoint in order of importance is quality of life. The calculation of quality-adjusted life years combines both. No cost-effectiveness studies have been reported.

Statement 24: Costs

The operative costs for the laparoscopic resection of colon cancer are higher because of a longer operating time and the use of more expensive (disposable) devices (level of evidence: 3 b).

Postoperative Stress Response

Stress Response After Laparoscopy

Laparoscopic surgery induces less trauma than conventional surgery and is thus likely to depress the immune response to a lesser extent. The preservation of the peritoneal and systemic immune system is important to prevent infections, sepsis, and the implantation of tumor cells to the traumatized tissues. In general, open surgery appears to inflict a greater nonspecific depression of the immune response than the laparoscopic approach.

Carbon dioxide pneumoperitoneum may impair the local immunity of the peritoneal lining. Peritoneal macrophages produce less cytokines [31, 32], and their intrinsic function (phagocytosis) [137, 138] diminishes on exposure to carbon dioxide insufflation.

Systemic immunity is depressed to a lesser extent by laparoscopic surgery than conventional open surgery. Both experimental and clinical studies on delayed-type hypersensitivity (DTH) response [139, 140], production of cytokines [141], and expression of HLA-DR receptors [139, 142] have confirmed this.

Stress Response During Colectomy

It has been suggested that survival may be improved if immunosupression induced by surgery could be reduced or eliminated [143]. The acute-phase response is a good index of the immune status of patients. Production of acute-phase proteins by hepatocytes often increases 1,000-fold, as does C-reactive protein (CRP) after tissue injury. This reaction of liver cells is induced by corticoids and cytokines, of which interleukin-6 (IL-6) is the main activator. During recovery, the levels of acute-phase proteins normalize. This acute-phase reaction has been measured in most studies by monitoring the levels of IL-6 and CRP (Tables 8.16, 8.17).

Most studies demonstrated lower IL-6 levels after laparoscopic colorectal resection compared with open conventional surgery [102, 142, 144–149]. Only one study reported a significant raise in IL-6 serum level after laparoscopic sigmoidectomy [150]. Although IL-6 was lower after laparoscopic colectomy, studies have shown conflicting CRP data (Table 8.17).

In addition to cytokines, other cell-related parameters, such as DTH and CD4/CD8 markers, have been assessed after laparoscopic colectomy, with no significant changes reported between laparoscopic and open colorectal surgery [102, 151].

Table 8.16. Measurements of plasma interleukin-6 (IL-6) levels (pg/ml)

Study	Preoperative	Laparoscopic	Open	p value
1–2				
Ordemann et al. [142]	NA	Significantly lower after laparoscopy		<0.01
Schwenk et al. [144]	4.25 (3.4–7.7)	34.0 (25.6–48.7)	50.5 (39.8–75.7)	0.03
Hewitt et al. [102]	NA	173±156	313±294	0.25
Wu et al. [145]	NA	83±7	105±33	<0.05
3				
Sietses et al. [146]	1.75±1.64	85.6±82.3	132.1±143.8	NS
Fukushima et al. [150]	NA	Significantly higher after laparoscopy		<0.05
Delgado et al. [149]	NA	239.5 (49.1–645.7)	372.7 (31.4–3.226)	<0.05
Nishiguchi et al. [147]	NA	Significantly lower after laparoscopy		<0.05

Results given as mean±SD or median (range)
NS not significant

Table 8.17. Measurements of plasma C-reactive protein (mg/dl)

Study	Preoperative	Laparoscopic	Open	p value
1–2				
Schwenk et al. [144]	NA	40 (33.0–49.4)	61.2 (52.0–77.9)	0.002
Wu et al. [145]	6.4	NA	NA	NS
3				
Fukushima et al. [150]	NA	NA	NA	NS
Delgado et al. [149]	NA	6.9±4.5	9.1±4.8	0.01
Nishiguchi et al. [147]	NA	Significantly lower after laparoscopy		0.05

Results given as mean±SD or mean (range)
NS not significant

Statement 25: Stress response

Stress response after laparoscopic colectomy is lower (level of evidence: 1 b).

Table 8.18. Summary of all statements and recommendations

	No.	Statements and recommendations	Level of evidence	Grade of recommendation
Preoperative evaluation and selection of patients				
Recommendation	1	Preoperative imaging studies of colon cancer to assess the size of the tumor, possible invasion of adjacent structures, and localization of the tumor are recommended in laparoscopic surgery for colon cancer	5	D
Statement	2	Age only is not a contraindication for laparoscopic resection of colon cancer	2 b	–
Recommendation	3	Invasive monitoring of blood pressure and blood gases is mandatory in ASA II–IV patients (no consensus: 91% agreement among experts). Low-pressure (< 12 mmHg) pneumoperitoneum is advocated in ASA II–IV patients		A B

Table 8.18 (continued)

	No.	Statements and recommendations	Level of evidence	Grade of recommen-dation
Statement	4	Obesity is not an absolute contraindication, but the rates of complications and conversions are higher at BMI > 30 (no consensus: 93% agreement among experts)	2c	–
Recommendation	5	Potentially curative resections of colonic cancer suspected of invading the abdominal wall or adjacent structures should be undertaken by open surgery (no consensus: 83% agreement among experts)	5	D
Statement	6	Adhesions do not appear to be a contraindication to laparoscopic colectomy	4	–
Operative technique				
Statement	7	Placement of trocars is based on the experience and the preference of the individual surgeon	5	–
Recommendation	8	High-quality videoscopic imaging is strongly recommended	5	D
Statement	9	Proper surgical technique and practice reduces the likelihood of port site metastasis	5	–
Recommendation	10	Preoperative tattooing of small colon tumors is advised. The alternatives are intra-operative colonoscopy or preoperative colonoscopic clipping followed by pre-operative fluoroscopy or ultrasonography	5	D
Recommendation	11	Dissection of the mesocolon from medial to lateral is the preferred approach in laparo-scopic colonic surgery. Intra-operative results of laparo scopic resection of colon cancer	5	D

67. Nizam R, et al. (1996) Colonic tattooing with India ink: benefits, risks, and alternatives. Am J Gastroenterol 91:1804–1808
68. Park SI, et al. (1991) Colonic abscess and focal peritonitis secondary to india ink tattooing of the colon. Gastrointest Endosc 37:68–71
69. Bernstein MA, et al. (1996) Is complete laparoscopic colectomy superior to laparoscopic assisted colectomy? Am Surg 62:507–511
70. Kurian MS, et al. (2001) Hand-assisted laparoscopic surgery: an emerging technique. Surg Endosc 15:1277–1281
71. Bemelman WA, et al. (1996) Laparoscopic-assisted colectomy with the dexterity pneumo sleeve. Dis Colon Rectum 39(10 Suppl):S59–S61
72. Simons AJ, et al. (1995) Laparoscopic-assisted colectomy learning curve. Dis Colon Rectum 38:600–603
73. Schlachta CM, et al. (2001) Defining a learning curve for laparoscopic colorectal resections. Dis Colon Rectum 44:217–222
74. Bennett CL, et al. (1997) The learning curve for laparoscopic colorectal surgery: preliminary results from a prospective analysis of 1194 laparoscopic-assisted colectomies. Arch Surg 132:41–44; discussion 45
75. Lezoche E, et al. (2000) Laparoscopic colonic resections versus open surgery: a prospective non-randomized study on 310 unselected cases. Hepatogastroenterology 47:697–708
76. Kwok SP, et al. (1996) Prospective evaluation of laparoscopicassisted large bowel excision for cancer. Ann Surg 223:170–176
77. Milsom JW, et al. (1998) Aprospect ive, randomized trial comparing laparoscopic versus conventional techniques in colorectal cancer surgery: a preliminary report. J Am Coll Surg 187:46–54; discussion 54–55
78. Falk PM, et al. (1993) Laparoscopic colectomy: a critical appraisal. Dis Colon Rectum 36:28–34
79. Dean PA, et al. (1994) Laparoscopic-assisted segmental colectomy: early Mayo Clinic experience. Mayo Clinic Proc 69:834–840
80. Huscher C, et al. (1996) Laparoscopic colorectal resection: a multicenter Italian study. Surg Endosc 10:875–879
81. Lauter DM, Froines EJ (2001) Initial experience with 150 cases of laparoscopic assisted colectomy. Am J Surg 181:398–403
82. Lumley JW, et al. (1996) Laparoscopic-assisted colorectal surgery: lessons learned from 240 consecutive patients. Dis Colon Rectum 39:155–159
83. Phillips EH, et al. (1992) Laparoscopic colectomy. Ann Surg 216:703–707
84. Lezoche E, et al. (2002) Laparoscopic vs open hemicolectomy for colon cancer. Surg Endosc 16:596–602
85. Marusch F, et al. (2001) Experience as a factor influencing the indications for laparoscopic colorectal surgery and the results. Surg Endosc 15:116–120
86. Fielding GA, et al. (1994) Laparoscopic colectomy. Surg Endosc 11:745–749
87. Curet MJ, et al. (2000) Laparoscopically assisted colon resection for colon carcinoma: perioperative results and long-term outcome. Surg Endosc 14:1062–1066
88. Bouvet M, et al. (1998) Clinical, pathologic, and economic parameters of laparoscopic colon resection for cancer. Am J Surg 176:554–558
89. Lacy AM, et al. (2002) Laparoscopy-assisted colectomy versus open colectomy for treatment of non-metastatic colon cancer: a randomised trial. Lancet 359:2224–2229
90. Khalili TM, et al. (1998) Colorectal cancer: comparison of laparoscopic with open approaches. Dis Colon Rectum 41:832–838
91. Marubashi S, et al. (2000) The usefulness, indications, and complications of laparoscopy-assisted colectomy in comparison with those of open colectomy for colorectal carcinoma. Surg Today 30:491–496
92. Leung KL, et al. (1997) Laparoscopic-assisted resection of rectosigmoid carcinoma: immediate and medium-term results. Arch Surg 132:761–764; discussion 765
93. Lacy AM, et al. (1995) Short-term outcome analysis of a randomized study comparing laparoscopic vs open coloctomy for colon cancer. Surg Endosc 9:1101–1105

94. Stage JG, et al. (1997) Prospective randomized study of laparoscopic versus open colonic resection for adenocarcinoma. Br J Surg. 84:391–396

95. Bokey EL, et al. (1996) Morbidity and mortality following laparoscopic-assisted right hemicolectomy for cancer. Dis Colon Rectum: 39(10 Suppl):S24–S28

96. Chapman AE, et al. (2001) Laparoscopic assisted resection of colorectal malignancies a systematic review. Ann Surg 234:590–606

97. Wexner SD, et al. (1993) Laparoscopic colorectal surgery: a prospective assessment and current perspective. Br J Surg 80:1602–1605

98. Lord SA, et al. (1996) Laparoscopic resections for colorectal carcinoma: a three-year experience. Dis Colon Rectum 39:148–154

99. Van Ye TM, Cattey RP, Henry LG (1994) Laparoscopically assisted colon resections compare favorably with open technique. Surg Laparosc Endosc 4:25–31

100. Bonjer HJ, et al. (1997) Open versus closed establishment of pneumoperitoneum in laparoscopic surgery. Br J Surg 84:599–602

101. Winslow ER, et al. (2002) Wound complication of laparoscopic vs open colectomy. 8th World Congress of Endoscopic Surgery, New York, NY, USA, Final program (S183), p 120

102. Hewitt PM, et al. (1998) Laparoscopic-assisted vs open surgery for colerectal cancer: comparative study of immune effects. Dis Colon Rectum 41:901–909

103. Bokey EL, et al. (1997) Laparoscopic resection of the colon and rectum for cancer. Br J Surg. 84:822–825

104. Leung KL, et al. (1999) Laparoscopic-assisted resection of rightsided colonic carcinoma: a case-control study. J Surg Oncol 71:97–100

105. Goh YC, Eu KW, Seow-Choen F (1997) Early postoperative results of a prospective series of laparoscopic vs open anterior resections for rectosigmoid cancers. Dis Colon Rectum 40:776–780

106. Tate JJ, et al. (1993) Propective comparison of laparoscopic and conventional anterior resection. Br J Surg. 80:1396–1398

107. Delgado Gomis F, et al. (1998) Early results of laparoscopic resection of colorectal cancer. Rev Esp Enferm Dig 90:323–334

108. Leung KL, et al. (1999) Laparoscopic-assisted resection of colorectal carcinoma: five-year audit. Dis Colon Rectum 42:327–332; discussion 332–333

109. Vara-Thorbeck C, et al. (1994) Indications and advantages of laparoscopy-assisted colon resection for carcinoma in elderly patients. Surg Laparosc Endosc 4:110–118

110. Lacy AM, et al. (1998) Port site metastases, and recurrence after laparoscopic colectomy: a randomized trial. Surg Endosc 12:1039–1042

111. Schwenk W, et al. (1999) Pulmonary function following laparoscopic or conventional colorectal resection: a randomized controlled evaluation. Arch Surg 134:6–12; discussion 13

112. Hong D, Tabet J, Anvari M (2001) Laparoscopic vs open resection for colorectal adenocarcinoma. Dis Colon Rectum 44:10–18; discussion 18–19

113. Kohler L, Holthausen U, Troidl H (1997) [Laparoscopic colorectal surgery – attempt at evaluating a new technology]. Chirurg 68:794–800; discussion 800

114. Santoro E, et al. (1999) Colorectal carcinoma: laparoscopic versus traditional open surgery. A clinical trial. Hepatogastroenterology 46:900–904

115. Weeks JC, et al. (2002) Short-term quality-of-life outcomes following laparoscopic-assisted colectomy vs open colectomy for colon cancer: a randomized trial. JAMA 287:321–328

116. Franklin ME Jr, et al. (1996) Prospective comparison of open vs laparoscopic colon surgery for carcinoma: five-year results. Dis Colon Rectum 39(10 Suppl):S35–S46

117. Psaila J, et al. (1998) Outcome following laparoscopic resection for colorectal cancer. Br J Surg 85:662–664

118. Franklin ME Jr, Rosenthal D, Norem RF (1995) Prospective evaluation of laparoscopic colon resection versus open colon resection for adenocarcinoma: a multicenter study. Surg Endosc 9:811–816

119. Wilmore DW, Kehlet H (2001) Management of patients in fast track surgery. BMJ 322:473–476
120. Schwenk W, Bohm B, Muller JM (1998) Postoperative pain and fatigue after laparoscopic or conventional colorectal resections: a prospective randomized trial. Surg Endosc 12:1131–1136
121. Hardacre JM, Talamini MA(2000) Pulmonary and hemodynamic changes during laparoscopy – are they important? Surgery 127:241–244
122. Milsom JW, et al. (1994) Use of laparoscopic techniques in colorectal surgery: preliminary study. Dis Colon Rectum 37:215–218
123. Stead ML, et al. (2000) Assessing the relative costs of standard open surgery and laparoscopic surgery in colorectal cancer in a randomised controlled trial in the United Kingdom. Crit Rev Oncol Hematol 33:99–103
124. Nelson H, Weeks JC, Wieand HS (1995) Proposed phase III trial comparing laparoscopic-assisted colectomy versus open colectomy for colon cancer. J Natl Cancer Inst Monogr 19:51–56
125. Anonymous (2000) COLOR: Dig Surg 17:617–622 126
126. Feliciotti F, et al. (2002) Results of laparoscopic vs open resections for colon cancer in patients with a minimum follow-up of 3 years. Surg Endosc 16:1158–1161
127. Hughes ES, et al. (1983) Tumor recurrence in the abdominal wall scar tissue after large-bowel cancer surgery. Dis Colon Rectum 26:571–572
128. Cass AW, Million RR, Pfaff WW (1976) Patterns of recurrence following surgery alone for adenocarcinoma of the colon and rectum. Cancer 37:2861–2865
129. Gunderson LL, Sosin H (1974) Areas of failure found at reoperation (second or symptomatic look) following "curative surgery" for adenocarcinoma of the rectum: clinicopathologic correlation and implications for adjuvant therapy. Cancer 34:1278–1292
130. Berends FJ, et al. (1994) Subcutaneous metastases after laparoscopic colectomy. Lancet 344:58
131. Ortega AE, et al. (1995) Laparoscopic Bowel Surgery Registry: preliminary results. Dis Colon Rectum. 38:681–685; discussion 685–686
132. Wexner SD, et al. (1995) Laparoscopic colorectal surgery–are we being honest with our patients? Dis Colon Rectum 38:723–727
133. Wexner SD, Cohen SM (1995) Port site metastases after laparoscopic colorectal surgery for cure of malignancy. Br J Surg 82:295–298
134. Wittich P, Bonjer HJ (2000) Port-site recurrences in laparoscopic surgery. In: Kockerling F (Port-site and wound recurrences in cancer surgery. Springer, Berlin Heidelberg New York, pp 12–20
135. Philipson BM, et al. (1997) Cost of open versus laparoscopically assisted right hemicolectomy for cancer. World J Surg 21:214–217
136. Musser DJ, et al. (1994) Laparoscopic colectomy: at what cost? Surg Laparosc Endosc 4:1–5
137. Gutt CN, et al. (1997) The phagocytosis activity during conventional and laparoscopic operations in the rat: a preliminary study. Surg Endosc 11:899–901
138. Chekan EG, et al. (1999) Intraperitoneal immunity and pneumoperitoneum. Surg Endosc 13:1135–1138
139. Kloosterman T, et al. (1994) Unimpaired immune functions after laparoscopic cholecystectomy. Surgery 115:424–428
140. Schietroma M, et al. (2001) Evaluation of immune response in patients after open or laparoscopic cholecystectomy. Hepatogastroenterology 48:642–646
141. Liang JT, et al. (2002) Prospective evaluation of laparoscopyassisted colectomy versus laparotomy with resection for management of complex polyps of the sigmoid colon. World J Surg 26:377–383
142. Ordemann J, et al. (2001) Cellular and humoral inflammatory response after laparoscopic and conventional colorectal resections. Surg Endosc 15:600–608

143. Eggermont AM, Steller EP, Sugarbaker PH (1987) Laparotomy enhances intraperitoneal tumor growth and abrogates the antitumor effects of interleukin-2 and lymphokine-activated killer cells. Surgery 102:71–78

144. Schwenk W, et al. (2000) Inflammatory response after laparoscopic and conventional colorectal resections–results of a prospective randomized trial. Langenbecks Arch Surg 385:2–9

145. Wu FPK, et al. (2003) Systemic and peritoneal inflammatory response after a laparoscopic or conventional colon resection in cancer patients: a prospective, randomized trial. Dis Colon Rectum 46:147–155

146. Sietses C, et al. (2000) Laparoscopic surgery preserves monocytemediated tumor cell killing in contrast to the conventional approach. Surg Endosc 14:456–460

147. Nishiguchi K, et al. (2001) Comparative evaluation of surgical stress of laparoscopic and open surgeries for colorectal carcinoma. Dis Colon Rectum 44:223–230

148. Kuntz C, et al. (2000) Short- and long-term results after laparoscopic vs conventional colon resection in a tumor-bearing small animal model. Surg Endosc 14:561–567

149. Delgado S, et al. (2001) Acute phase response in laparoscopic and open colectomy in colon cancer: randomized study. Dis Colon Rectum 44:638–646

150. Fukushima R, et al. (1996) Interleukin-6 and stress hormone responses after uncomplicated gasless laparoscopic-assisted and open sigmoid colectomy. Dis Colon Rectum 39(10 Suppl):S29–S34

151. Tang CL, et al. (2001) Randomized clinical trial of the effect of open versus laparoscopically assisted colectomy on systemic immunity in patients with colorectal cancer. Br J Surg 88:801–807

152. Schiedeck TH, et al. (2000) Laparoscopic surgery for the cure of colorectal cancer: results of a German five-center study. Dis Colon Rectum 43:1–8

153. Millikan KW, et al. (1996) Superior mesenteric and portal vein thrombosis following laparoscopic-assisted right hemicolectomy: report of a case. Dis Colon Rectum 39:1171–1175

154. Franklin ME, et al. (2000) Laparoscopic surgery for stage III colon cancer: long-term follow-up. Surg Endosc 14:612–616

155. Poulin EC, et al. (1999) Laparoscopic resection does not adversely affect early survival curves in patients undergoing surgery for colorectal adenocarcinoma. Ann Surg 229:487–492

156. Schwenk W, et al. (1998) Laparoscopic versus conventional colorectal resection: a prospective randomised study of postoperative ileus and early postoperative feeding. Langenbecks Arch Surg 383:49–55

157. Delgado F, et al. (1999) Laparoscopic colorectal cancer resection: initial follow-up results. Surg Laparosc Endosc Percutan Tech 9:91–98

158. Cook TA, Dehn TC (1996) Port-site metastases in patients undergoing laparoscopy for gastrointestinal malignancy. Br J Surg 83:1419–1420

159. Hoffman GC, et al. (1996) Minimally invasive surgery for colorectal cancer: initial follow-up. Ann Surg 223:790–796, discussion 796798

160. Molenaar CB, Bijnen AB, de Ruiter P (1998) Indications for laparoscopic colorectal surgery. results from the Medical Centre Alkmaar, The Netherlands. Surg Endosc 12:42–45

161. Quattlebaum JK Jr, Flanders HD, Usher CH (1993) Laparoscopically assisted colectomy. Surg Laparosc Endosc 3:81–87

162. Ballantyne GH (1995) Laparoscopic-assisted colorectal surgery: review of results in 752 patients. Gastroenterologist 3:75–89

163. Fleshman JW, et al. (1996) Early results of laparoscopic surgery for colorectal cancer: retrospective analysis of 372 patients treated by Clinical Outcomes of Surgical Therapy (COST) Study Group. Dis Colon Rectum 39(10 Suppl):S53–S58

164. Rosato P, et al. (1998) Port-site and wound metastases following laparoscopic resection of colorectal carcinoma: the experience of the Italian registry. Presented at the 33rd Congress of the European Society for Surgical Research (ESSR)

165. Vukasin P, et al. (1996) Wound recurrence following laparoscopic colon cancer resection: results of the American Society of Colon and Rectal Surgeons Laparoscopic Registry. Dis Colon Rectum 39(10 Suppl):S20–S23
166. Gellman L, Salky B, Edye M (1996) Laparoscopic assisted colectomy. Surg Endosc 10:1041–1044
167. Kwok KY, et al. (1996) Laparoscopic-assisted large bowel resection. Ann Acad Med Singapore 25 650–652
168. Guillou PJ, Darzi A, Monson JR (1993) Experience with laparoscopic colorectal surgery for malignant disease. Surg Oncol 2(Suppl 1):43–49
169. Croce E, et al. (1997) Laparoscopic colectomy: the absolute need for a standard operative technique. Jsls 1:217–224
170. Kawamura YJ, et al. (1995) Laparoscopic-assisted colectomy and lymphadenectomy without peritoneal insufflation for sigmoid colon cancer patients. Dis Colon Rectum 38:550–552
171. Alexander RJ, Jaques BC, Mitchell KG (1993) Laparoscopically assisted colectomy and wound recurrence. Lancet 341:249–250
172. O'Rourke N, et al. (1993) Tumor inoculation during laparoscopy. Lancet 342:368
173. Walsh DC, Wattchow DA, Wilson TG (1993) Subcutaneous metastases after laparoscopic resection of malignancy. Aust N Z J Surg 63:563–565
174. Fusco MA, Paluzzi MW (1993) Abdominal wall recurrence after laparoscopic-assisted colectomy for adenocarcinoma of the colon: report of a case. Dis Colon Rectum 36:858–861
175. Cirocco WC, Schwartzman A, Golub RW (1994) Abdominal wall recurrence after laparoscopic colectomy for colon cancer. Surgery 116:842–846
176. Nduka CC, et al. (1994) Abdominal wall metastases following laparoscopy. Br J Surg 81:648–652
177. Champault G, et al. (1994) [Neoplastic colonization of trocart paths: should laparoscopic surgery be stopped for digestive cancers?] Presse Med 23:1313
178. Ramos JM, et al. (1994) Laparoscopy and colon cancer: is the port site at risk? A preliminary report. Arch Surg 129:897–899 discussion 900
179. Cohen SM, Wexner SD (1993) Laparoscopic colorectal resection for cancer: the Cleveland Clinic Florida experience. Surg Oncol 2(Suppl 1):35–42
180. Jacquet P, et al. (1995) Cancer recurrence following laparoscopic colectomy: report of two patients treated with neated intraperitoneal chemotherapy. Dis Colon Rectum 38:1110–1114

Colonic Cancer – Update 2006

Ruben Veldkamp, M. Gholghesaei, H. Jaap Bonjer, Dirk W. Meijer, M. Buunen, J. Jeekel, B. Anderberg, M. A. Cuesta, Alfred Cuschieri, Abe Fingerhut, J. W. Fleshman, P. J. Guillou, E. Haglind, J. Himpens, Christoph A. Jacobi, J. J. Jakimowicz, Ferdinand Koeckerling, Antonio M. Lacy, Emilio Lezoche, John R. T. Monson, Mario Morino, Edmund A. M. Neugebauer, S. D. Wexner, R. L. Whelan

Definition

No new data available.

Epidemiology and Clinical Course

No new data available.

Diagnostics

No new data available.

Operative Versus Conservative Treatment

No new data available.

Choice of Surgical Approach and Procedure

The choice of surgical approach, laparoscopic or open, in colon cancer is dependent on both short- and long-term results. Since publication of the consensus on laparoscopic resection of colon cancer, one single center and three multicenter randomized controlled trials published their results following laparoscopic versus open surgery for colon cancer. The Clinical Outcomes of Surgical Therapy Study Group (COST) trial [1] and the trial by Leung et al. [2] (Hong Kong) reported the long-term outcome. The Conventional Versus Laparoscopic Assisted Surgery in Patients with Colorectal Cancer (CLASICC) trial [3] and the Colon Cancer Laparoscopic or Open Resection (COLOR) trial [4] published the short-term results. In this update, we will discuss these studies.

Intraoperative and Immediate Postoperative Results

In the COLOR trial [4], a European multicenter randomized study, 1,248 patients with colon cancer were included. The duration of surgery was 32 min longer in the laparoscopic group (202 vs. 170 min, $p < 0.0001$), while blood loss was 75 ml less (100 vs. 175 ml, $p < 0.0001$). Similar differences in intraoperative results between laparoscopic and open colon resection were reported in the Hong Kong trial. The laparoscopic procedure took 45 min longer (189 vs. 144 min, $p < 0.001$), but was associated with less blood loss (169 vs. 238 ml, $p = 0.06$).

After surgery, the recovery of patients was faster following laparoscopic surgery in the COLOR trial: 1 day earlier recovery of bowel movements (3.6 vs. 4.6 days, $p < 0.0001$) and fluid intake (2.9 vs. 3.8 days, $p < 0.0001$) and fewer analgesics requirements. This resulted in a shorter hospital stay (8.2 vs. 9.3 days, $p < 0.0001$). The Hong Kong and CLASICC trials also documented faster postoperative recovery of bowel function, less need for analgesics and shorter hospital stay. The COST [1], COLOR [4], CLASICC [3] and Hong Kong [2] trials did not report a difference in postoperative in-hospital morbidity, mortality, resection margins or number of harvested lymph nodes.

The costs of laparoscopic and open surgery for colon cancer were investigated by Janson et al. [5] in a subset of Swedish patients randomized in the COLOR trial. Costs were calculated up to 12 weeks after surgery. All relevant costs to society were included. Two hundred and ten patients were included in the primary analysis, 98 of whom were operated on laparoscopically and 112 with open surgery. The cost of surgery was significantly higher for the laparoscopic group than for the open group (difference in means € 1,171, $p < 0.001$), as was the cost of the first admission (difference in means € 1,556, $p = 0.015$) and the total costs to the healthcare system (difference in means € 2,244, $p = 0.018$). The total costs to society did not differ significantly between groups (difference in means for laparoscopic versus open surgery € 1,846, $p = 0.104$). Janson et al. [5] concluded that within 12 weeks of surgery for colon cancer, there was no difference in the total costs to society; however, the laparoscopic procedure was more costly to the healthcare system.

The results of the aforementioned large randomized trials confirm the conclusions from the original consensus statement regarding intraoperative and immediate postoperative results of laparoscopic resection of colon cancer compared with those for the open procedure. Laparoscopic surgery for colon cancer is a safe and feasible procedure, improving short-term outcome.

Long-Term Results

Since publication of the consensus on laparoscopic versus open surgery for colon cancer, all major randomized controlled trials no longer include patients and two trials published their results. Results of the trial by Lacy et al. [6] have already been discussed in the consensus.

The COST trial is so far the only large multicenter trial to have published long-term outcome results comparing laparoscopic with open surgery for colon cancer. In this study, 3-year overall and cancer-free survival were not different; however, this trial did not achieve its accrual goal and stopped randomization after 872 patients. Tinmouth and Tomlinson [7] stated that "We can conclude with 95 percent certainty that patients who are treated laparoscopically have at most a 16 percent increase in the risk of death and 11 percent increase in the risk of recurrence." The number of patients treated per center was low, which may have led to learning-curve effects in this trial; therefore, this trial did not close the debate on long-term safety of laparoscopic colon cancer surgery.

Leung et al. [2] included 403 patients with rectosigmoid cancer in a single-center randomized trial. Survival after laparoscopic and open colectomy was similar. The long-term outcomes of the CLASICC and COLOR trials have not yet been published.

It can be concluded that patients with colon cancer who are operated on laparoscopically have similar long-term survival to patients operated on with open surgery. However, a meta-analysis of all major randomized trials is to be performed to achieve the highest level of evidence for this subject. Given the advantages of laparoscopic surgery in the immediate postoperative period, laparoscopy should be implemented in the treatment of colon cancer with curative intent.

Technical Aspects of Surgery

No new data available.

Peri- and Postoperative Care

No new data available.

References

1. Clinical Outcomes of Surgical Therapy Study Group (2004) A comparison of laparoscopically assisted and open colectomy for colon cancer. N Engl J Med 350:2050–2059
2. Leung KL, Kwok SP, Lam SC et al (2004) Laparoscopic resection of rectosigmoid carcinoma: prospective randomised trial. Lancet 363:1187–1192
3. Guillou PJ, Quirke P, Thorpe H et al (2005) Short-term endpoints of conventional versus laparoscopic-assisted surgery in patients with colorectal cancer (MRC CLASICC trial): multicentre, randomised controlled trial. Lancet 365:1718–1726
4. Veldkamp R, Kuhry E, Hop WC et al (2005) Laparoscopic surgery versus open surgery for colon cancer: short-term outcomes of a randomised trial. Lancet Oncol 6:477–484
5. Janson M, Bjorholt I, Carlsson P et al (2004) Randomized clinical trial of the costs of open and laparoscopic surgery for colonic cancer. Br J Surg 91:409–417
6. Lacy AM, Garcia-Valdecasas JC, Delgado S, Castells A, Taura P, Pique JM, Visa J (2002) Laparoscopy-assisted colectomy versus open colectomy for treatment of non-metastatic colon cancer: a randomised trial. Lancet 359:2224–2229
7. Tinmouth J, Tomlinson G (2004) Laparoscopically assisted versus open colectomy for colon cancer. N Engl J Med 351:933–934; author reply 933–934

The EAES Clinical Practice Guidelines on Obesity Surgery (2005)

Stefan Sauerland, Luigi Angrisani, Mituku Belachew, J.M. Chevallier,
Franco Favretti, Nicholas Finer, Abe Fingerhut, Manuel García Caballero,
J.A. Guisado Macias, R. Mittermair, Mario Morino, Simon Msika,
Francesco Rubino, Roberto Tacchino, Rudolf Weiner,
Edmund A.M. Neugebauer

Introduction

Obesity is an increasingly serious health problem in nearly all Western countries [76, 108, 320]. Although various preventive and conservative treatment options are available, it has been estimated that obesity-related illnesses, such as diabetes mellitus, knee osteoarthritis, systemic hypertension and heart failure, are responsible for an estimated 3–6% of total health care costs [6, 230, 279]. A recent study on the association between different grades of obesity and the number of life-years lost indicated that life expectancy can be up to 20 years shorter in severe obesity [104]. The consequences of obesity are by far more severe than those of smoking or alcohol [319].

Definition and classification of obesity is based primarily on the body mass index (BMI), calculated as weight divided by the square of height with kilograms per square meter as the unit of measurement [17]. For Caucasians, a BMI of 30–35 is considered as class 1 obesity, 35–40 as class 2, and over 40 as class 3. Morbid obesity is usually defined as a BMI of over 40 or a BMI over 35 in combination with comorbidities [238]. In addition, some surgeons speak of super- and mega-obesity, if a patient's BMI exceeds 50 or 70, respectively. Alternatively, absolute or relative increases in body weight may be used to define obesity.

Given the enormous importance of morbid obesity and the limited efficacy of dietetic and pharmacological treatments, surgical treatment has become increasingly popular. The number of procedures performed has more than doubled within a few years [64, 78, 289]. This dramatic growth can be attributed in part also to the introduction of new surgical techniques, e.g. the adjustable silicone gastric band (AGB), and the rise of laparoscopic surgery. Traditionally, there are two types of operations for morbid obesity: Gastric restrictive operations (where food intake is restricted) and malabsorptive operations (where aliments are diverted from absorption via a gastrointestinal shortcut). Both types of obesity surgery are now being performed laparoscopically [38]. The aim of these guidelines is to systematically review the clinical effectiveness of the various surgical procedures and to support surgeons and other physicians in the provision of high-quality care for morbidly obese patients.

Methods

Selection of Topics and Experts

Considering the current controversy regarding the best surgical treatment for morbid obesity, the Scientific Committee and the Executive Board of the EAES decided to provide the surgical community with evidence-based guidelines. The aim and focus of these guidelines cover key questions regarding effective and efficient surgical treatment of obesity, including patient selection, choice of surgical technique, management of complications and follow-up.

A panel was appointed to develop clinical practice guidelines and consisted of representatives from key disciplines, i.e. surgeons specialized in obesity treatment, general surgeons, nutritionists, and epidemiologists from across Europe. Experts were selected according to scientific and clinical expertise, geographical localisation, and membership in societies pertaining to laparoscopic obesity surgery. The Obesity Management Task Force of the European Association for the Study of Obesity (EASO) was represented at the complete process by one nominated delegate (N.F.).

Guideline development started with a list of key questions, which all experts were asked to answer. In May 2004, the panel convened to review and discuss the range of answers on the basis of the scientific evidence. The nominal group process was used to develop statements that were agreeable for all or at least the majority of panel members. A preliminary position paper was compiled and presented to the audience at the EAES congress in June 2004. All comments from the audience were discussed and a final version of the guidelines was agreed on consensually. The project was funded by the EAES. All panelists had to document and sign their relationships to commercial stakeholders in order to rule out possible conflicts of interest.

Literature Searches and Appraisal

According to the hierarchy of research evidence, we tried to locate randomized controlled trials (RCTs, i.e. level 1b evidence) dealing with the key questions. When RCTs were of low quality or completely lacking, non-randomized controlled clinical trials (CCTs, i.e. level 1b evidence) were included. Whenever level 1 and 2 evidence was scarce, case series with comparison of pre- and postoperative status (i.e. level 4 evidence) were used. However, it should be noted that for some studies our grading of evidence led to different opinions of levels than in other similar assessments [55]. Studies were downgraded whenever the intention-to-treat principle was heavily violated or randomization was obviously unconcealed and biased. For each intervention, we considered the validity and homogeneity of study results, effect sizes, safety, and economic consequences. It should be noted that not all studies can be categorized, since studies presenting epidemiologic incidences or prevalences, or proposing ideas or definitions are not amenable to evidence grading. Furthermore, one study could be assigned different levels of evidence, whenever two or more comparisons were performed within one study, some of which may be randomized while other are not.

To identify relevant studies in all languages [5], the electronic databases of Medline (PubMed) and the Cochrane Library (Issue 2, 2004) were used. Searches in Medline spanned from 1966 to May 2004 and used the following wording: "obesity/surgery" [MeSH] OR "obesity, morbid/surgery" [MeSH] OR "gastric bypass" [MeSH] OR "biliopancreatic diversion" [MeSH] OR "anastomosis, Roux en Y" [MeSH] OR "jejunoileal bypass" [MeSH] OR "biliopancreatic bypass" OR "duodenal switch" OR "'gastroplasty" OR gastric band*. Restricting this search to the publication type "clinical trial" yielded 312 articles. In addition, the references of previous evidence-based guidelines on obesity therapy were screened [42, 117, 153]. Recently published systematic reviews of RCTs, CCTs, or case series (levels of evidence 1a, 2a or 4, respectively) and their reference lists were also studied in detail [55, 61–63, 78, 120, 152, 220, 262]. Of note, we considered three abstracts (by Agren, van Rij, and van Woert) to be insufficient sources of information, although the Cochrane review treated them as independent RCTs [63].

All recommendations were graded according to the quality and quantity of the underlying scientific evidence, the risk-benefit balance, and the values expressed by the panelists. We attempted to respect the views of patients, although no patient directly participated in guideline formulation. The grades of recommendations ranged from A (high-quality evidence, usually from RCTs, demonstrating clear benefits) over B (medium quality evidence and/or a disputable risk-benefit ratio) to C (low quality evidence and/or unclear risks and benefits).

Results

Multidisciplinary Evaluation

Before making a decision for obesity surgery, the patient must be seen by surgeon and anaesthesiologist (GoR A), and should also be seen by an expert in dietary/nutritional support (GoR B). The consultation of further specialities depends on the patient's comorbidity (GoR B).

It is beyond any doubt that all patients must be seen by a surgeon and an anaesthesiologist before surgery. While the anaesthesiologists will usually be consulted only a few days before surgery, the surgeon should see the patient at least twice prior to the decision for surgery. Alternatively, a visit with a bariatric primary care physician has been proposed (EL 5 [94]). Since obesity surgery often introduces a durable change of the gastrointestinal tract, the decision for or against surgery requires a well-informed patient. Therefore, a few weeks' time interval between the first visit and the eventual operation are desirable (EL 4 [367]). The role of other specialities in examining and preparing the patient for surgery has evolved over many years [94].

The association between psychologic health and the success of obesity surgery reinforces the role of a psychiatrist or psychologist in assessing possible candidates for surgery. The patient's preoperative motivation has been found to be a predictor of weight loss after gastric bypass (EL 2b [21, 271]), while other psychological factors have little influence on the long-term effectiveness of surgery in other studies (EL 2b [47, 82]). A few authors suggested the need of psychiatric evaluation of all morbidly obese who seek surgical treatment (EL 5 [56, 121]), because some patients were found postoperatively to develop anorexia-like syndromes, post-traumatic stress disorders, or other psychological problems leading to treatment failure (EL 4 [121, 128, 315]). A recent review by Dixon and O'Brien did recommend routine psychologic assessment, although they noted that such an assessment is common, but not standard, practice in the USA (EL 5 [82, 94]) and Europe (EL 4 [231]). This panel therefore agreed with Brolin's position that psychological evaluation is necessary only for selected patients (EL 5 [38]). It is beyond the scope of these guidelines to differentiate here between psychologists, psychiatrists, and other qualified persons.

Nutrition also is a crucial aspect of obesity, both preand postoperatively. Therefore, most surgeons in the field believe that all patients must be evaluated, instructed, and guided by an expert in nutrition. This person may either be a physician with nutritional medicine qualification or a registered dietitian. Similarly, physical exercise should be initiated preoperatively under the guidance of a physical therapy specialist. Although there are no comparative studies on the impact of nutrition and physical exercise therapy, both are considered standard (EL 5 [94]). In addition to the nutritionist, other groups have reported routine consultation of a pneumologist or an endocrinologist (EL 4 [231, 356]).

Indications for Surgery

Obesity surgery should be considered in adult patients with a documented BMI greater than or equal to 35 and related comorbidity, or a BMI of at least 40 (GoR A). All patients must fully understand and agree with postoperative care (GoR A), and must be free of general contraindications (GoR A). Adults with a BMI between 30 and 35 accompanied by substantial obesity-related co-morbidity or after prolonged medical treatment should undergo obesity surgery only in the context of controlled clinical trials (GoR C). No consensus was reached on the usefulness of obesity surgery in adolescent patients.

Many studies and committees have pointed out that in morbidly obese patients "no current [conservative] treatments appear capable of producing permanent weight loss" (EL 5 [125]). So far, only one randomized trial has compared obesity surgery versus non-surgical therapy: In this trial by Andersen et al. [13, 14] (EL 1b), horizontal gastroplasty produced significantly more weight loss and maintenance of weight loss than very low calorie diet (32 versus 9 kg after 2 years). After more than 5 years, 16% of surgical patients had successfully reduced weight as compared to only 2% of diet patients.

The very large, but non-randomized Swedish Obese Subjects (SOS) study (EL 2b) compared different types of obesity surgery versus conservative treatment in a matched-pair design [158, 159]. Women and men with a BMI greater than 38 or 34, respectively, were studied over 2 years. They lost significantly more weight after surgical than after non-surgical treatment and this weight loss resulted in significant improvements of comorbidities, such as diabetes (from a prevalence at baseline of 19–10% after 2 years), hypertension (from 53 to 31%), sleep apnea (from 23 to 8%), dyspnea when climbing stairs (from 87 to 19%), and chest pain when climbing stairs (from 28 to 4%). The SOS study also found health-related quality-of-life (QoL) to be directly correlated with weight loss [159]. As there was a significant difference in QoL even between women with 30–40-kg weight loss and those with more than 40-kg weight loss, it seems as if obesity surgery should aim at the largest possible excess weight loss (EWL). If long-term EWL is less than 50%, a procedure is generally considered a treatment failure.

Traditionally, obesity surgery is considered appropriate for adult patients with either a BMI of 40 or more, or a BMI between 35 and 40 with obesity-related comorbidity. These selection criteria have been laid down in March 1991 by the National Institutes of Health Consensus Development Panel [236–238] and have subsequently been adopted by all major surgical and non-surgical societies [9, 11, 88, 148, 178, 226, 235, 313]. Even though the BMI threshold values of 40 and 35 were arbitrarily chosen, it appears wise to stick to these criteria, because the majority of surgical experience and scientific evidence relates to patients who were selected by such criteria. Off course, the risk-benefit ratio needs to be assessed critically in each individual patient (EL 2b [260]). As the short-term risks of obesity surgery clearly exceed that of conservative treatment (EL 1c [93]), it is advisable that all patients should have tried other ways of weight loss prior to surgery. In costeffectiveness analyses, all major obesity procedures were found to give better results than conservative treatment in morbidly obese patients (EL 2b [62, 235]).

Recent reports have shown that surgical treatment is similarly effective in patients with a BMI between 25 and 35 (EL 4 [15]). According to Dixon and O'Brien [82], the "cut-off of BMI>35 is due for review" also in the USA, where it is currently been evaluated in a RCT. Although no study so far has compared surgical and non-surgical management in patients with a BMI between 30 and 35, obesity surgery is increasingly being performed in this subgroup. Given the strength of the existing evidence, it seems too early to recommend obesity surgery even in cases with a BMI of at least 30 who suffer from substantial obesity-related comorbidity. The majority of the panel favored surgical treatment in well-selected patients with a BMI between 30 and 35 only in the context of controlled clinical trials.

A complex issue in the NIH selection criteria is the proper definition of comorbidities, which warrant obesity surgery due to their seriousness and potential alleviation through weight loss. Comorbidities may be divided in medical, physical and psychological categories. In this respect, medical conditions such as sleep apnea and other hypoventilation syndromes (EL 4 [57, 114]), type II diabetes mellitus (EL 4 [190, 251, 261, 263, 265, 282, 328]), obesity-related cardiomyopathy and hypertension [31, 53, 103, 273, 318, 328], hyperlipidemia (EL 4 [231, 251]), asthma (EL 4 [251]), pseudotumor cerebri (EL 4 [216, 324]), knee osteoarthritis (EL 4 [114]), low back pain (EL 4 [215]), female urinary incontinence (EL 4 [45, 114]) and infertility (EL 4 [113, 204, 360]) are well-documented indications for obesity surgery, because clinical evidence has convincingly proven that weight-loss allows prevention, relevant improvement, or even remission of these conditions. The metabolic effect of obesity surgery in diabetic patients is especially noteworthy, since it goes beyond weight reduction alone (EL 4 [161, 263, 282]; EL 5 [283]). Gastroesophageal reflux, however, was found unresponsive to obesity surgery in some studies (EL 2b [107, 255]), whereas others found an association (EL 4 [81, 114, 149, 251, 311]). Of course, these results varied with the type of surgery.

Physical, social, and psychological problems are important factors in the quality-of-life of obese persons. Although such problems are difficult to communicate and to quantify, they play a leading role in deciding on conservative or surgical treatment of obesity. Various validated instruments are available to assess quality-of-life (QoL) in obese patients [171], but it should be added that most of these QoL questionnaires were validated by their responsiveness to weight loss, so by definition a procedure that produces weight loss will produce improved QoL. The literature is replete with before-and-after-studies (EL 4) about the positive changes in patients' quality-of-life

(QoL) caused by bariatric surgery [135, 347]. This allows us to focus here exclusively on studies with a non-surgical control group. Arcila et al., for example, demonstrated significant improvements in various QoL domains after VBG and RYGB as compared to conservative therapy (EL 2b [19]). In a recent study from Switzerland (EL 2b), obesity surgery proved better than conservative treatment in patients with and without severe psychosocial stress [43]. It can be concluded that deliberation on obesity treatment options must incorporate an assessment of the patient's current physical, social, and psychological status as well as the expected effects of therapy on this status. Therefore, psychological counseling, even superficial, as a screening tool is desirable in all patients before surgery.

Various contraindications must also be taken into account, although most have not been derived from firm clinical evidence. As patients' non-compliance with follow-up schedules can lead to potentially life-threatening complications [26], all candidates for obesity surgery must hold a realistic view of the operation and the necessity for lifelong aftercare (EL 1c). Severe mental or cognitive retardation and malignant hyperphagia are therefore generally considered absolute contraindications, because such patients will be unable to eat and exercise as required postoperatively (EL 5 [82, 121]). On the other hand, minor arid major mental and personality disorders are highly prevalent in morbidly obese patients, but they were not found to be valid predictors of successful therapy (EL 2b [34, 291]). Eating disorders are no general contraindication, even if they are not amenable to psychological and dietary counseling (EL 4 [203]). Nevertheless, such disorders must be known when selecting the type of surgery.

Psychiatric disorders (psychotic, personality, or affective disorders, alcoholism and/or drug abuse, mental retardation, and eating disorders, especially bulimia nervosa, and binge eating disorder), lack of social support, persistent ambivalence to surgery, and marital dysfunction are factors which must be evaluated in particular before surgery. A substantial percentage of bariatric surgery patients suffer from binge eating disorders or binge eating symptoms. The effect of bariatric surgery on the outcome of binge eating symptoms largely depends on the type of operation. In general, the indication for surgery depends on the severity of the mental disorder and its response to psychopharmacological treatment. Repeated assessment of the patient may end in a postponement or cancelling of the operation. Surgery is contraindicated only in the cases of severe mental disease not responding to treatment (EL 4 [56, 203, 336]).

Women of reproductive age, who wish to have children after surgery, should not be denied an operation, because the course of pregnancy and the health of the baby are usually unaffected by previous obesity surgery (EL 2b [79, 113, 202, 205, 309, 350]). Still, postoperative contraception is recommended for about 12 months, after which weight should usually be stabilized. In patients with LABG (laparoscopic adjustable gastric banding), the band can be deflated in case of pregnancy (EL 4 [344]). Finally, liver cirrhosis should not hinder elegibility for obesity surgery (EL 4 [26, 65]).

Before reaching skeletal maturity children should definitely not be offered obesity surgery, but recent pilot studies (EL 4) on adolescents (12–19 years old) suggested that surgery in this age group is as effective as it is in adults [32, 52, 85, 146, 317, 327]. Since about 80% of obese adolescents will remain obese into adulthood, some surgeons have offered surgery to well selected nonadult patients. However, the total number of patients aged between 12 and 18 is small, thus precluding any recommendation on performing surgery in adolescents. Recently, a threshold BMI of 40 (with severe comorbidities) or 50 (with less severe comorbidities) has been proposed for consideration of obesity surgery in adolescents (EL 5 [147]). In this panel, however, there was no consensus on the selection of adolescents for surgery. The balance of the risks and benefits of surgery must be also considered critically at the other end of the age scale. Findings in patients aged between 55 and 70 documented beneficial effects of surgery on weight and some comorbidities (EL 4 [193, 229]). In patients over 60 or 65 years, however, obesity-related comorbidity has usually become more complicated and less reversible (EL 5 [32, 82, 231]). In consequence, the risks of surgery may be no worthwhile (EL 2b [93, 339]), although a fixed age limit can not be recommended.

Preoperative Diagnostics

As for any other major abdominal surgical procedures, all patients should be evalated for their medical history (GoR A) and undergo laboratory tests (GoR B). Despite the lack of sound evidence in the obese, chest radiography, electrocardiography, spirometry, and abdominal ultrasonography may be recommended for the evaluation of obesity-related comorbidity (GoR C). Polysomnography (GoR C) should be done in patients with high risk of sleep apnea. In centers where psychiatric consultation or psychological assessment is not routine, psychological screening should be performed (GoR C). Upper gastrointestinal endoscopy or upper GI series is advisable for all bariatric procedures (GoR C), but is strongly recommended for gastric bypass patients (GoR B).

In the preoperative work-up, as outlined above, patients with apparent psychosocial problems should be seen also by a psychologist or psychiatrist. In the morbidly obese, psychosocial problems are usually associated with an increased motivation for weight loss, which in turn is predictive of the success of surgery (EL 2b [253, 271, 336]). Socioeconomic problems are also highly prevalent [188]. To assess these connections, all patients should be evaluated for psychologic health, quality-of-life, possible personality disorders, social relationships, motivation, expectations and compliance. Many centers use self-developed questionnaires for this purpose (EL 4 [271, 291, 315]). The psychiatric assessment of morbid obesity should include a brief explanation and description of the assessment process, a clinical interview (ideally at least 3 months before surgery), and psychological testing of eating behaviour, quality of life, psychopathology, and personality (EL 5 [95]). The clinical interview should cover the patient's previous weight loss attempts and treatments, eating patterns, eating disorders symptoms, physical activity, attitudes and expectation regarding treatment, psychiatric history, mental and marital status.

Published evidence on the technical preoperative evaluation of obese patients stems largely from case series and general gastrointestinal surgery standards, which were adopted to obesity surgery. Standard investigations are electrocardiography, chest radiography and laboratory tests (EL5 [94, 312]). According to Naef et al. [231] (EL 4), laboratory testing should include a full blood count, liver, kidney (EL 4 [162]), coagulation and thyroid parameters, thyroid hormone stimulating test, a lipid profile, a oral glucose screening test (only in patients not known to be diabetic), and an analysis of arterial blood gas. Urinalysis is also a standard procedure [94].

Ultrasonography of the abdomen is usually done to detect cholecysto- or choledocholithiasis. Being a noninvasive and cheap procedure, abdominal sonography seems to be advisable as a part of the routine preoperative work-up. Even those centers where intraoperative ultrasound is performed, use preoperative ultrasonography as a screening tool.

Specifically important to obese patients is the evaluation of pulmonary function and obstructive sleep apnea. Sugerman and colleagues first described the high prevalence of pulmonary obstructive diseases in morbidly obese patients (EL 4 [322, 323]). To prevent postoperative hypoventilation, it has been recommended that all patients be assessed spirometrically as part of the preoperative work-up and supplied with the necessary therapy (EL 4 [217, 231]; EL 5 [312]). In multivariate analysis, a forced expiratory volume (FEV1) under 80% and an abnormal electrocardiogram were predictive of postoperative intensive care admission (EL 2b [124]). Hypoventilation syndromes were also found to be predictive of thrombembolic complications and anastomotic leakage (EL 2b [93, 285]). American obesity clinics recently recommended routine polysomnography, because sleep apnea was detected in 77–88% of their patients (EL 4 [109, 252]) and was predictive of postoperative complications in other studies. Other groups use the Epworth sleepiness scale or similar instruments to screen for patients who will require polysomnography (EL 4 [299]). Various studies have found a higher preoperative prevalence of pulmonary problems with increasing BMI (EL 2b [214]). One study, however, failed to confirm the predictive value of both, BMI and Epworth sleepiness scale, in the prediction of obstructive breathing disorders (EL 2b [109]). In summary, the threshold for ordering polysomnography should be low and all superobese patients should probably be tested routinely (EL 5 [94]).

Disputable is the evaluation of the upper gastrointestinal (GI) tract by endoscopy, barium meal, both, or none of the two technologies. In the study by Sharaf et al., routine radiologic assessment of the upper GI tract before bariatric surgery led to clinically important findings in only 5.3% of patients (EL 4 [302]). In only six of 814 patients (0.9%), as reported by Ghassemian et al., X-ray examination of the GI tract demonstrated relevant abnormality, and not a single operation had to be delayed due to the results of the GI tract series (EL 4 [122]). Using esophageal manometry, two recent case series found abnormalities in only 13–20% of patients and being without clinical consequences (EL 4 [169, 186]). Jaffin et al., however, described that esophageal disorders were highly prevalent (61%) and associated with postoperative results (EL 4 [150]). Other groups also have advocated routine upper GI tract series before gastric banding, because hiatal hernia may cause band slippage (EL 4 [115, 127]). Endoscopy, however, offers the advantage of visualizing esophageal and gastric mucosa (EL 4 [115, 337]), thus detecting gastritis, reflux, or ulcerations. This may be of special value before any operation with exclusion of the stomach (EL 5 [312]). To make a compromise, this panel advises to perform either upper GI series or endoscopy in all patients. Given the higher prevalence of reflux after VBG (EL 4 [24, 164, 259, 301]), preoperative GI evaluation seems to be of special importance in VBG patients.

Choice of Procedure

Adjustable gastric banding (AGB), vertical banded gastroplasty (VBG), Roux-en-Y gastric bypass (RYGB) and biliopancreatic diversion (BPD) are all effective in the treatment of morbid obesity (GoR B). All four types of procedures should be explained to the patient (GoR C). In terms of weight loss, BPD is superior to RYGB (GoR B), RYGB is superior to VBG (GoR A), and VBG is superior to AGB (GoR A). There is an increased risk of perioperative complications in procedures requiring stapling and anastomoses (GoR A). The reoperation rate is higher for adjustable gastric banding and Mason (but not MacLean) VBG (GoR A). As positive and negative effects differ among the procedures, the choice of procedure should be tailored to the patient's BMI, perioperative risk, metabolic situation, comorbidities and preference as well as to the surgeon's expertise (GoR C). Intragastric balloon, sleeve gastrectomy, and gastric pacemaker are options (GoR C), which require further evaluation.

Since obesity surgery has various competing aims, such as weight loss, adjustability, reversibility, and safety, it is difficult to draw universally valid conclusions about the optimal bariatric procedure. For all types of surgery, there is overwhelming evidence from case series on safety, efficacy, and effectiveness in terms of weight loss, but much less data are available on the comparative evaluation of different bariatric procedures. Therefore, the decision must be taken with the patient's individual situation and the surgeon's expertise in mind. A profound knowledge of the different malabsorptive and gastric restrictive procedures and their pathophysiologic consequences is indispensable.

Biliopancreatic diversion (BPD) was invented by Scopinaro (EL 5 [294, 296]; EL 4 [295]) and later modified by Marceau et al., who added a duodenal switch (EL 4 [136, 200, 201]). BPD with duodenal switch and sleeve gastrectomy was found to be superior (EL 2b [267]), which allows us to leave the original BPD procedure unmentioned in the following considerations. In the long-term after BPD, patients typically lose between 65 and 75% of their excess body weight (EL 4 [267, 293]).

Roux-en-Y gastric bypass (RYGB) was first described by Mason and Ito [207, 208]. Numerous technical modifications have been proposed relating to gastric pouch construction, gastro-jejunal anastomosis, and length of alimentary and biliopancreatic limbs. RYGB usually results in 60–70% EWL [75, 101, 138, 173, 222, 273], but the procedure is much better accepted in the USA (about 70% of all procedures) as compared to Europe [332].

Gastroplasty was first performed horizontally ("gastric partition"), but in 1982 Mason [206] introduced the vertical banded gastroplasty (VBG), which was quickly adopted by surgeons. In this procedure a gastric pouch of about 10–20 ml is created. By using a mesh band or a silastic ring, the gastric pouch outlet can be calibrated and reinforced. Postoperative weight reductions range between 55 and 65% nadir EWL (EL 4 [199, 224, 232, 277, 325]).

In gastric banding, a ring is placed around the gastric cardia. A small pouch is created, thus limiting food intake. Modern gastric bands have an inflatable reservoir to adjust the size of the remaining passage [30, 175]. With the introduction of laparoscopic adjustable gastric banding (LAGB), the procedure has gained worldwide popularity. Being a gastric restrictive procedure, weight loss is less in gastric banding compared to other procedures and usually reaches only 45–55% (EL 4 [49, 67, 83, 249, 250, 330, 342, 367]). Technical details of all four procedures will be discussed in a separate chapter below.

The randomized studies in this field are summarized in Fig. 10.1. In the following, we will discuss key findings of these studies comparing biliopancreatic diversion, gastric bypass, gastroplasty, and gastric banding.

Several randomized studies have compared gastric bypass versus horizontal or vertical gastroplasties. As horizontal gastroplasty has been abandoned

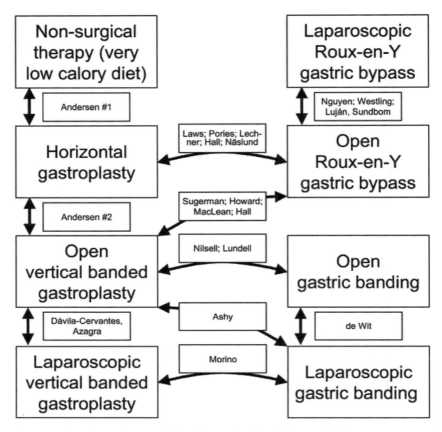

Fig. 10.1. Randomised controlled trials comparing different obesity surgery procedures among each other or versus medical treatment. Please note that the trial by Hall et al. [129] had three arms and therefore appears twice. The trial by Sundbom evaluated hand-assisted laparoscopic Roux-en-Y gastric bypass

since the 1980 s, we will only briefly discuss the four RCTs evaluating this technique. Laws first showed that gastric partitioning produces less weight loss than RYGB (EL 1 b [179]). Other groups (Pories et al. [264], Lechner et al. [181, 182], and Hall et al. [129]) have confirmed this finding (EL 1 b). Finally, Naslund et al. (EL 1 b [233, 234]) found that nearly all of their gastric bypass patients lost more than 25 kg within the first postoperative year, compared to only 18 of 28 gastroplasty patients ($p < 0.01$). The 1987 publication by Andersen et al. [12] (EL 1 b) finally brought horizontal gastroplasty to an end.

Four RCTs compared open RYGB and open vertical banded gastroplasty. In an often-quoted study (EL 1 b), Sugerman et al. [326] compared 3-year results between 20 RYGB and 20 VBG patients. In terms of EWL after 1 year,

RYGB was found to be superior over VBG (68 versus 43%), but postoperative complications, for instance vitamine B_{12} deficiency and vomiting due to stoma stenosis, were more common after RYGB. In the three-armed study from Adelaide, which was already cited above, Hall et al. [129] compared the 3-year success rates defined as more than 50% EWL. Successful treatment was observed in 67% of patients after RYGB, 48% after vertical gastroplasty, and 17% after gastric partition. The RCT by Howard et al. [143] was able to report long-term data. Again, EWL was clearly better in the RYGB than in the VBG cohort. MacLean et al. [196, 198] confirmed these results.

VBG and gastric banding have been compared in three trials (all EL 1 b), but the trials used different surgical approaches (Fig. 10.1). One trial compared both procedures in open access surgery [247], one trial compared open VBG versus LAGB [20], and the third trial compared both procedures in laparoscopic surgery [223]. In the study by Nilsell et al., weight reduction tended to be larger and quicker after VBG, but after 5 years gastric banding patients reached the same level of weight loss. Reoperations were performed more often in the VBG group (11/30 versus 3/29), a finding which contradicts non-randomized data (EL 2 b [29, 333]). In their study of 60 patients, Ashy et al. [20] found greater EWL half a year after VBG as well, but failed to report long-term data. Due to shorter hospital stay, less complications, and adjustability Ashy et al. preferred LAGB over open VBG. In comparing LAGB and laparoscopic VBG, Morino et al. described shorter hospital stay after LAGB, but found fewer complications and reoperations after laparoscopic VBG. Weight loss was also better after VBG. Consequently, this group firmly favored the latter technique and commented that the high complication rates after VBG in the Nilsell study might have been due to not dividing the stomach between the staple lines.

It is difficult to draw summary conclusions from these three trials, because they represent a mixture of surgical procedures and approaches. One common result of the three trials is the better weight reduction after VBG. Data on complication rates, however, are conflicting. A very detailed assessment of comparative and non-comparative studies (EL 2 a) recently concluded that "laparoscopic gastric banding is safer than VBG and RYGB" [55], because short-term mortality and morbidity were found to be lower after LAGB. Still, the ranges of complication rates were wide, thus suggesting a strong effect of surgical expertise. In a large study on laparoscopic RYGB and gastric banding, Biertho et al. concluded that the balance between weight loss and complications favored LAGB in patients with BMI under 40, whereas RYGB might be preferable in case of a BMI between 40 and 50 (EL 3 b, downgraded due to large unadjusted baseline differences [33]).

Of note, no randomized trial so far has compared BPD to other procedures. This is in part a consequence of the 1991 NIH consensus development conference, which simply failed to mention BPD as one of the standard procedures [72]. Two-year follow-up data presented by Rabkin [267] (EL 2b) showed marginally greater EWL after BPD (78%) than after RYGB (74%). In 2004, Deveney et al. [77] confirmed this comparability of EWL after BPD and RYGB (EL 2b). In a small study by Murr et al. [228] (EL 2b), EWL within 4 years was greater after BPD (71%) than after long-limb RYGB (57%), but some cases of liver failure and metabolic bone disease developed in the BPD group. Similarly, EWL after 2 years was 60% following BPD versus 48% following non-adjustable gastric banding (EL 2b [23]), but longer hospital stay and higher major complications rates were also found. In a matched-pair analysis (EL 2b), BPD also resulted in greater EWL (64 versus 48%) when compared to LAGB [86]. In summary, the degree of weight loss caused by BPD is greater, but this is at the expense of other outcomes.

When making a choice between gastric banding, VBG, RYGB and BPD, it is well documented (EL 1b as outlined above, except for BPD) and generally accepted that weight loss is more pronounced after the latter procedures. In fact, weight loss decreased according to the procedures performed in following decreasing order: BPD, RYGB, VBG, and gastric banding. Therefore, in patients with milder degrees of obesity, procedures that produce greater absolute weight loss may not be advantageous, although this can only regarded as a recommendation by rule of thumb. However, the reverse conclusion, that gastric banding and VBG should not be used in massive obesity, does not seem to fully apply, because recent reports showed that LAGB is associated with sufficient EWL also in patients with a BMI of 60–100 (EL 2b [86]; EL 4 [96]).

A remarkable proposal for operative selection among the various procedures was published in 2002 by Buchwald [42], who first reviewed a large number of case series (EL 4) and then constructed a clinical algorithm based on BMI, age, gender, race, body habitus, and comorbidity. For example, according to the algorithm a patient with a BMI of 48 should not receive gastric banding irrespective of other factors. Likewise, a patient with a BMI greater than 55 should receive either BPD or long-limb RYGB. This panel agrees to the relative importance of these parameters for choosing a procedure, but is reluctant to propose any strict criteria. BMI, comorbidity, and age should play a key role in selecting the procedure. Data on other criteria are largely missing, except for psychological parameters as described above.

The concept of selecting the procedure according to eating habits was initially proposed by Sugerman et al. [326]. Although this was a RCT, the study's comparison between sweet eaters and non-sweat eaters was nonrandomized and possibly data-driven (EL 2b). More recent studies have failed to confirm this finding (EL 2b [144]). Notwithstanding, eating habits should influence the choice of the procedure to some degree. Most surgeons require LAGB and VBG patients to accept restrictive dietetic rules, and perform

RYGB or BPD if this criterion is not fulfilled. Comorbidity also plays some role in decision-making. As some, but not all, studies showed that esophageal reflux may get worse after gastric banding (EL 4 [16, 80, 352]), RYGB might be preferable in such cases (EL 4 [24, 36, 110, 164]). The only RCT on this issue, however, failed to find a difference between LAGB and VBG with regard to reflux symptoms (EL 1b [192]).

The intragastric balloon was introduced in 1982 as an as adjunct to non-operative treatment of obesity [116, 246]. A series of small studies compared intragastric balloons against sham control (EL 1b [141, 172, 187, 210, 270, 278]) or no additional intervention (EL 1b [119]). Both, experimental and control groups lost weight due to low-calorie diet, but no additional effect of the balloon was found in five of the seven trials. With newer smooth-surface balloon, mean EWL after 6 months of intragastric balloon treatment was between 20 and 50% (EL 4 [87, 90, 140]) depending on patient compliance and balloon volume (EL 2b [281]). Since the balloon carries a non-negligible risk of prolonged vomiting, pain, gastric ulcers, and spontaneous deflation with intestinal obstruction, the device has not yet become standard (EL 4 [41]; EL 5 [100, 185]). Especially in comparison to obesity surgery, the balloon was found to produce insufficient and non-durable weight loss (EL 2b [166]). Nowadays, however, some centers still use the gastric balloon in selected patients with a BMI between 30 and 35 (EL 4 [281, 335]). It also is being used as a weight-reducing adjuvant therapy before bariatric surgery (EL 4 [87, 209, 345]). Loffredo et al. [189] proposed that the amount of weight reduction obtained with the balloon could serve as a guidance in selecting the type of bariatric procedure (EL 2b) and has started a RCT testing this hypothesis.

Although sleeve (or longitudinal) gastrectomy is a specific step within the BPD operation, some surgeons have used it also as a first-stage procedure in patients with BMI above 60 to reduce surgical risks, followed about a year later either by RYGB or BPD. EWL within the first year after sleeve gastrectomy as the sole procedure has been reported to range between 33 and 45% (EL 4 [7, 272]), but the limited experience with sleeve gastrectomy prohibits any statement about its clinical value. Still, sleeve gastrectomy may be used as an interim procedure in high-risk morbidly obese patients, especially in case of intraoperative hemodynamic instability (EL 4 [7, 272]). Beyond the traditional surgical concepts of gastrorestriction and malabsorption is the gastric pacemaker, a completely new device, which is currently being evaluated in a randomized, placebo-controlled trial [362]. Preliminary data showed an EWL of about 30% after 15 months (EL 4 [69, 217, 219]). Although the technique is minimally invasive with apparently little surgical complications, longer term results are awaited before this device should be used outside trials.

Surgical Access: Open Versus Laparoscopic

All procedures have been proven to be technically feasible via laparoscopy. There is evidence that the laparoscopic approach is advantageous for gastric banding, VBG, and gastric bypass (GoR B). Preliminary data suggest that the laparoscopic approach may be also preferable for BPD, if surgical expertise is available (GoR C), but further studies are needed.

In 1994, laparoscopic Roux-en-Y gastric bypass (RYGB) was described by Wittgrove et al. [357–359] (EL 4), who found it to give superior results as compared to open surgery. Later, laparoscopic Roux-en-Y gastric bypass (RYGB) was compared to open RYGB in three similarly designed RCTs. In the first study by Nguyen et al. [241–243] (EL 1b) EWL was similar after both procedures, whereas reductions in postoperative complications and hospital stay favored the laparoscopic approach. Late anastomotic strictures, however, were seen more frequently after laparoscopic RYGB. Westling and Gustavsson found that weight loss was unaffected by the surgical approach, but postoperative hospital stay was 2 days shorter after laparoscopic surgery (EL 1b [355]). Most recently, laparoscopic and open gastric bypass were compared by Lujan et al. [191] in a well-performed study (EL 1b). The duration of surgery and hospital stay were shorter in the laparoscopic group. Both groups experienced similar degrees of EWL, but the high rate of incisional hernia in the open group (10/51) led to a significant long-term advantage for the laparoscopic technique (0/53). In addition to these three RCTs, a small, but rigidly designed trial by Sundbom and Gustavsson [329] compared hand-assisted laparoscopic versus open RYGB (EL 1b). Weight loss was similar in both groups, as were postoperative complications. DeMaria et al. [74] confirmed these results in a nonrandomised study (EL 2b).

Until now, two RCTs have compared laparoscopic versus open vertical banded gastroplasty. The quality of one trial was good because of properly concealed allocation and blinded outcome assessment (EL 1b [70]), but the second trial should certainly not be classified as level 1 evidence, since all four converted cases were shifted from the laparoscopic into the open group for analysis (EL 2b [22]). Both trials clearly documented a longer duration of surgery in the laparoscopic group. Hospital stay was 4 days in both groups in both trials. Respiratory and physical function was restored quicker after laparoscopic surgery [70]. As EWL was similar, laparoscopic surgery seems to be favorable, although more data are needed.

In adjustable gastric banding, one RCT dealt with the comparative effectiveness of laparoscopic versus open approach in 50 patients (EL 1b [71]). LAGB was found to be advantageous due to a 1-day reduction in hospital stay and fewer readmissions, while reduction of BMI was similar. However, the laparoscopic operation took twice as long as its open counterpart. For non-adjustable gastric banding, level II evidence indicates that laparoscopic surgery produces similar weight loss but quicker reconvalescence as compared to open surgery [112].

As the first laparoscopic biliopancreatic diversion (BPD) was performed only in 1999 (EL 4 [25, 275]), scientific evaluation of this technique has not advanced as for the other procedures. Early results were published by a few centers (EL 4 [25, 256, 275, 297, 346]) and showed promising results in terms of technical feasibility and postoperative morbidity, but long-term data are lacking so far. The only comparative study (performed in superobese patients) found similar weight loss and reconvalescence after laparoscopic and open BPD, but better improvement of comorbidities in the laparoscopic group [165]. This finding, however, should be attributed to different durations of follow-up in the two groups (EL 3b, downgraded accordingly).

In summary, laparoscopic surgery has had a major impact on obesity surgery [55, 287]. According to surveys of American Society of Bariatric Surgery members, the percentage of laparoscopic procedures in relation to all bariatric procedures has increased from about 10% in 1999 to nearly 90% in 2004 [32]. These dramatic changes have been fuelled by affirmative trial data but also commercial interests. A second and equally important effect is the lowered threshold in considering patients for surgery [289].

Training and Qualification

All surgeons performing obesity surgery should have an adequate technical expertise (GoR A). He or she should be a qualified and certified general or gastrointestinal surgeon with additional training in obesity surgery (GoR B). Technical expertise in laparoscopic surgery alone is insufficient to start a bariatric surgery program (GoR B).

According to the Cancun statement of the IFSO (EL 5 [126]), every obesity surgeon should be a "fully trained, qualified, certified general or gastrointestinal surgeon, who has completed a recognized general/gastrointestinal surgery program" with additional training in "bariatric surgery including patient education, support groups, operative techniques, and postoperative follow-up". In addition, the IFSO recommends certain written approvals of expertise, course attendance, membership in an obesity surgery society, continuing medical education, and other criteria. Similar guidelines have been issued for US hospitals (EL 5 [314]), where board-certified training of surgeons and standard hospital infrastructure are formally required. Surgical experience should be documented by "an appropriate volume of cases (open and/or laparoscopic)".

Many published series on different bariatric operations have reported learning curve effects, but there is no clear threshold for the distinction between an unexperienced and an experienced surgeon. Consequently, the

American guidelines recommended that "priviliges should not be granted or denied based on the number of procedures performed". The IFSO statement, however, declared that obesity surgery should be learned from an experienced surgeon, defined as "one who has performed at least 200 bariatric surgical procedures and has 5 or more years experience".

So far, only two clinical studies have explored the volume-outcome relationship in bariatric surgery. Courcoulas et al. found that surgeons with fewer than ten procedures per year had significantly higher morbidity (28 vs 14%) and mortality (5 vs 0.3%) than high-volume surgeons (EL 2b [64]), but this result was partly attributable to better patient selection and overall hospital volume. As medium volume surgeons (with 10–50 cases per year) had also worse results when compared to high-volume surgeons, the authors were unable to recommend a minimum caseload for obesity surgery, although there was a significant trend toward higher mortality among patients in the lower activity group. The second, larger, study looked at hospital volumes and noted a nearly three-fold increase in comorbidityadjusted complication rates in hospitals with less than 100 cases per year. Given the large proportion of lowvolume hospitals and surgeons in Europe, this panel warns against starting a bariatric surgery program without having the necessary prerequisites in terms of staff, infrastructure, and volume requirements.

General Perioperative Aspects

Antibiotic (GoR A) and antithromboembolic (GoR B) prophylaxis should be administered to all obesity surgery patients.

Antibiotic administration was first studied by Pories et al. [266], who gave cefazolin or placebo over two postoperative days to gastric bypass patients (EL 1b). Wound infections were significantly reduced, thus making infection prophylaxis a standard. Antibiotics should always be given in an appropriate dose (EL 1b [105]), but there are no data available to specifically recommend certain groups or dosage regimens of drugs.

Prophylaxis of thromboembolic complications has also been an essential part of bariatric procedures. The incidence of fatal pulmonary embolism has been described to be 0.2% (EL 4 [285, 354]). More recent series, however, have shown that anticoagulation may not be necessary in patients with short operative times, use of postoperative pneumatic compression stockings, and quick mobilisation (EL 4 [123]). The current standard consists of low-dose heparin in combination with intermittent pneumatic compression stockings (EL 5 [363]). Most data in this field have to be extrapolated from other types of surgery, as until today only one small RCT has been performed in obesity surgery (EL 1b [157]). In this study, no difference between daily doses of 5,700 IU vs 9,500 lU nadroparin was detected.

Specific Technical Aspects of the Procedures

Key aspects of surgical technique in LAGB are the pars flaccida approach (GoR B), correct positioning (GoR A) and fixation (GoR A) of the band. In VBG, pouch volume should be less than 30 ml (GoR C) and the staple line should be completely transsected (GoR B). There is variability in many technical aspects of RYGB without clear data to justify clear-cut recommendations. The standard GB includes a pouch volume of about 20 or 30 ml (GoR C), an alimentary limb length of at least 75 cm (GoR C), and a biliary limb of at least 50 cm (GoR C). Long limb distal GB seems to be preferable in superobese patients, as this induces greater weight loss (GoR B). In BPD, the length of common canal should always be greater than 50 cm (GoR C). In BPD with duodenal switch and sleeve gastrectomy, the length should be between 50 and 100 cm (GoR C). There are preliminary data suggesting that closing mesenteric defects may prevent internal hernia (GoR C).

Laparoscopic Adjustable Gastric Banding

Nowadays, adjustable bands are generally preferred to non-adjustable ones, as this avoids postoperative food intolerance, vomiting, and other complications (EL 2b [112]). The selection of banding devices is influenced by clinical but also cost-related data. Most commonly used are the Lap-Band and the Swedish Adjustable Gastric Band [106], which have yielded similar results (EL 2a [111]). All new bands should be compared against these standard devices (EL 4 [366]). One randomized trial showed that the Lap-Band resulted in less complications as compared to the Heliogast band (EL 1b [35]).

The pars flaccida technique is generally preferred in the preparation of the path for the band (EL 2b [68]; EL 4 [274]). In respect to band position, gastric banding was found to be superior over esophagogastric banding (EL 1b [351]). A further study described more dysphagia after esophagogastric banding (EL 2b [177]). Weiner et al. [343], however, favored esophagogastric over retrogastric placement due to a lower risk of band slippage (EL 1b). In a Czech language article, Kasalicky et al. [160] described that cuff fixation is a worthwhile option to prevent band slippage (EL 1b). It is common practice to secure the band by a few non-resorbable gastro-gastric sutures on the anterior gastric wall. Furthermore, fixation of the port to the surface of the anterior rectus sheath is necessary to avoid turning and inaccessibility of the port (EL 2b [348]). The routine use of early postoperative barium swallows to detect gastroin testinal perforations is usually unnecessary (EL 4 [239]). Most authors refrain from inflating the band during the first postoperative weeks (EL 2b [46]).

One interesting study examined whether complete resection of the greater omentum performed together with adjustable gastric banding offers metabolic advantages (EL 1b [334]). Two years after surgery, glucose metabolism (i.e. oral glucose tolerance, fasting plasma glucose, insulin, and insulin sensitivity) was significantly more improved in omentectomized patients, although weight loss was similar in both groups.

Vertical Banded Gastroplasty

There are no randomized trials available to define the technical aspects of the procedure. Nevertheless, the following points are standard in laparoscopic surgery. Dissection at the lesser curvature should preserve vagal nerve branches. A circular stapler (usually 21 mm) should be used to create the transgastric window. The pouch volume should be less than 30 ml, which generally requires calibration with a 34 Fr nasogastric tube.

The pouch outlet should be banded with a polypropylene or polytetrafluoroethylene mesh collar, so that outer circumference and inner lumen are about 5 cm and 1 cm respectively in diameter. In one study, less complications were encountered with polypropylene than with Gore-Tex bands (EL 2b [340]). This panel also discourages the use of silastic rings. According to MacLean et al. [195] (EL 4), the gastric pouch needs to be separated at the vertical staple line and sutured in order to avoid staple line disruption. A small trial by Fobi et al. [102] confirmed a lower complication rate after transsection of the staple line (EL 1b). This holds true also for laparoscopic VBG (EL 4 [137]).

Roux-en-Y Gastric Bypass

Similar to other procedures, pouch volume is believed to be a key aspect in RYGB. Usually, a tube with a balloon is passed into the stomach and inflated with 15–30 ml saline before the gastric pouch is stapled. However, it should be noted that no clinical data so far back up a specific pouch volume. Small staples (3.5 mm) are recommended for creating the pouch, and the dissection at the lesser curvature requires careful management to prevent postoperative distension of the gastric remnant. Measuring pouch size is not the standard (EL 5 [332]).

The Roux limb should be created so that it measures 75–100 cm in patients with BMI under 50, but between 100 and 250 cm in case of a higher BMI. These lengths can be derived from several comparative studies (EL 1b [39, 60]; EL 2b [40, 197]). Brolin et al. [39] compared Roux limb lengths of 75 vs 150 cm in superobese patients and found a difference in BMI of 10 kg/m^2 after 2 years follow-up (EL 1b). Ten years later, Choban and Flancbaum

[60] went even further in their trial when they found greater EWL in those superobese patients, who received a 250 cm as opposed to a 150 cm Roux limb. The length of the biliopancreatic limb was kept similar in all patients. In the second part of this trial, 67 patients with a BMI between 40 and 50 were randomized to Roux limb lengths of either 75 or 150 cm, but here no apparent advantages were noted with one or the other technique [60]. Roux limb length therefore should be adapted to match initial BMI, in patients with BMI over 50. In 2004, a similar recommendation was given by SAGES (Society of American Gastrointestinal Endoscopic Surgeons; EL 4 [152]). The retrocolic-retrogastric, retrocolic-antegastric, and antecolic-antegastric routes all seem acceptable for the Roux limb (EL 4 [4]). Papasavas et al. [257, 258] found slightly less stenoses after retrocolic-retrogastric positioning (EL 2b), while others reported less hernias for the antecolic route (EL 2b [163]).

The creation of the gastrojejunostomy is a further critical aspect of RYGB, because 3–5% of patients may develop stenosis [292]. When reviewing the case series on stenoses (EL 4 [292]), stapled anastomoses appear to give better results than the hand-sewn type. This corresponds well to RCT data in gastric cancer patients (EL 1b [142, 300, 307, 353]). In obese patients there is only a trial with pseudorandomization by alternation (EL 2b [1]), where stenosis occurred in ten of 30 handsewn anastomoses and eight of 60 mechanical anastomoses ($p=0.047$ by Fisher's exact test). Laterolateral anastomoses are currently standard and can be created by circular or linear stapling, although the latter seems perferable. A preliminary comparison between 21 and 25 mm stapled end-to-end anastomoses found no differences (EL 1b [331]). Different devices with similar effectiveness are currently in use (EL 1b [54]). The mesentery defect should be closed in order to avoid internal hernia (EL 4 [97, 154, 258]). A surgical drain should be place at the gastrojejunostomy site (EL 4 [298]), but the nasogastric tube may be removed at the end of the procedure (EL 2b [145]).

Biliopancreatic Diversion

As described above, when speaking of BPD our article refers to biliopancreatic diversion with duodenal switch and sleeve gastrectomy. The vertical subtotal gastrectomy (sleeve gastrectomy) should be performed on a 34–60-Fr bougie along the lesser curvature so that the gastric tube consists of about 10–30% of the original stomach (100–200 ml).

Little data have been published on limb length, but the common limb should measure over 50 cm, but less than 100 cm. Correspondingly, the alimentary canal should be between 200 and 300-cm long. Duodenoileostorny can be created by circular stapling, linear stapling with hand sutures, or a completely hand-sewn technique (EL 2b [346]). The integrity of all staple lines needs to be confirmed by methylene blue testing. To shorten the duration of surgery in high-risk patients, some authors have proposed to perform BPD either as a two-stage procedure with gastrectomy first (EL 4 [7, 272]) or without gastrectomy (EL 4 [276]).

General Aspects

Other simultaneous procedures may be carried out in obesity surgery patients. First, ventral hernia should be repaired by mesh implantation under the same anaesthesia, as this reduces the risk of bowel ischemia (EL 2b [89, 286]). Second, cholecystectomy has been proposed for all patients (with or without gallstones) at the time of surgery (EL 4 [3, 8, 50, 99, 290]), because obesity surgery furthers postoperative gallstone formation and necessitates cholecystectomy in about 10% of patients following RYGB (EL 4 [3, 8, 73, 305, 306]). Other, more recent studies, however, have shown that simultaneous cholecystectomy can be safely restricted to those patients with asymptomatic gallstones detected on intraoperative ultrasound (EL 4 [134, 155, 338]) or with symptomatic cholecystolithiasis (EL 4 [151]). The postoperative use of ursodeoxycholic acid was shown to reduce the risk of subsequent cholecystolithiasis (EL 1b [218, 321, 364]). A daily dose of 500–600 mg of ursodeoxycholic acid for 6 months was shown to be an effective prophylaxis for gallstone formation.

Long-Term Aftercare

A multidisciplinary approach to aftercare is needed in all patients regardless of the operation (GoR B). Patients should be seen three to eight times during the first postoperative year, one to four times during the second year and once or twice a year thereafter (GoR B). Specific procedures may require specific follow-up schedules (GoR B). Further visits and specialist consultation by surgeon, dietician, psychiatrist, psychologist or other specialists should be done whenever required (GoR C). Outcome assessment after surgery should include weight loss and maintainance, nutritional status, comorbidities, and quality-of-life (GoR C).

Obesity is a "chronic disorder that requires a continuous care model of treatment" [125]. Although there are only a few comparative studies on the frequency, intensity or mode of follow-up, close regular follow-up visits have become routine in most centres (EL 4 [217]). Baltasar et al. highlighted several cases of serious complications and even death which were due to metabolic derangement caused by inadequate follow-up (EL 4 [26]). This is why patients who do not understand or comply with strict follow-up schedules should be denied surgery, as recommended above.

Postop. Months	1	2	3	4	5	6	7	8	9	10	11	12	13	14	15	16	17	18	19	20	21	22	23	24	thereafter
LAGB (minimal)	X		X			X						X												X	once a year
LAGB (intensive)	X	X	X	X		X		X		X		X			X			X			X			X	twice a year
VBG (minimal)	X					X						X												X	once a year
VBG (intensive)	X		X			X			X			X						X						X	once a year
RYGB (minimal)	X					X						X												X	once a year
RYGB (intensive)	X	X	X			X			X			X						X						X	once a year
BPD (minimal)	X		X			X						X												X	once a year
BPD (intensive)	X	X	X			X			X			X						X						X	once a year

Fig. 10.2. Suggested timing of postoperative follow-up visits

The frequency of the visits should be adapted to the procedure, the patient's weight loss over time and the overall probability of complications. Therefore, closer follow-up visits are generally required during the first postoperative year. Shen et al. [304] (EL 3b) examined the association between the number of postoperative visits during the first year and EWL. A significant difference favoring more than six visits per year was found for gastric banding but not for gastric bypass patients. In consequence, many obesity surgeons favor closer follow-up visits after LAGB than after VBG or BPD (EL 4 [46, 217]). Based on current practice patterns (EL 4 [92, 217]), this panel unanimously recommended a follow-up protocol as shown in Fig. 10.2. No data are available to indicate that follow-up should be different after open and laparoscopic surgery. It has been recommended to sonographically exclude gallstones at the 6 and 12 months visit. Follow-up should always be continued lifelong, as long as the surgical procedure or device has not been reverted or removed.

For optimal continuity of care, it seems recommendable to have one physician as the primarily responsible person for follow-up. It is therefore usually the surgeon or the nutritionist, who oversees the patient's course, circulates information to other colleagues and coordinates multidisciplinary consultations. Postoperatively, all patients should be seen several times by the dietician and the psychologist (EL 4 [217, 268]). In addition, it may be necessary to consult the gastroenterologist (for upper gastrointestinal endoscopy), the pneumologist (for sleep apnea), the radiologist or other disciplines. Again, communication and collaboration is essential, since many different comorbidities may be affected by weight reduction.

The importance of psychological counseling is difficult to quantify. Comparisons of patients who attended or quitted postoperative group meeting or psychotherapy (EL 3b, downgraded due to noncomparability of groups) found that attenders had slightly more weight loss and better quality-of-life when compared to nonattenders [139, 245, 269]. Although this panels supports the idea of an intensified postoperative counseling, current data does not justify a firm recommendation.

Nutritional treatment aims to ensure that patients consume a diet that meets normally accepted nutritional recommendations for macro-, micro-nutrients and vitamins in-take, but at a reduced energy intake commensurate with maintaining a reduced body weight. Many patients have pre-existing nutritionally inadequate diets [EL 4 [44, 98, 133]), and deficiencies are commoner in the older and more overweight (EL 2b [183, 184]) and may be exacerbated by drugs commonly used to treat obesity comorbidities (EL 4 [180, 280]). Such deficiencies are more likely to be exacerbated rather than improved by bariatric surgery, especially malabsorptive procedures (EL 4 [27, 91, 130, 194, 268]). For this reason individual nutritional (diet) assessment and advice is necessary both pre- and postoperatively in order to ensure that nutritional status is optimised. It is likely that most patients will require nutritional supplements of vitamins and minerals (EL 2b [37, 51, 131, 308, 310]).

Clinical and scientific documentation of patients' postoperative course should not only focus on weight. Additionally, the clinical course of comorbidities should be closely monitored, and all patients should be questioned about their quality-of-life (QoL), as it recommended by the 1991 NIH conference (EL 5 [238]). For the assessment of QoL, validated instruments are freely available and should be used [221, 254, 361]. In 1997, the ASBS issued guidelines on scientific reporting, which ideally should include the course of BMI and EWL over at least two postoperative years (EL 5 [10]).

Band adjustments are a specific part in the follow-up of LAGB patients. First band filling should be performed between 2 and 8 weeks after band implantationusually after 4 weeks (EL 2b [46]). For this first filling, 1–1.5 ml saline are injected. Band adjustments thereafter should be carried out as required in an individualised manner according to weight loss, satiety and eating behaviour, and gastric problems (e.g. vomiting). Four-, six- or eight-week intervals between adjustments are widely accepted. A much simpler approach for band filling was recently found to produce similar EWL, while reducing workload immensely. Twenty patients treated by Kirchmayr et al. [167] received a bolus-filling 4 weeks after surgery thus obviating the need for subsequent stepwise re-calibration (EL 1b). This panel awaits further studies confirming the safety of this or similar concept. The volume of the pouch should be examined radiographically after 12 months and (as an option) also after 6 months.

Dealing with Complications

Surgeons should be aware that postoperative complications may have an atypical presentation in the obese, and early detection and timely management are necessary to prevent deleterious outcomes (GoR C).

Common to all procedures which employ gastrointestinal suture or anastomoses is the possibility of anastomotic leakage and bleeding [48]. Clinical signs, such as fever, tachycardia, and tachypnea, were found to be highly predictive of anastomotic leaks after RYGB (EL 4 [168]). Generally, anastomotic leakage can be treated by drainage with or without oversewing (EL 4 [298]). Revisional surgery for suspected anastomotic leakage can be done via open or laparoscopic approach (EL 5 [346]). Staple line bleeding with minor or major blood loss can often be treated conservatively (EL 4 [212, 244]; EL 5 [275]). Splenectomy is seldomly required.

Laparoscopic Adjustable Gastric Banding

Complications after LAGB include gastric erosion, band slippage, pouch dilation, occlusion of the stoma, and port-related complications. Gastric erosion usually causes mild pain, various types of infections and prevents further weight loss (EL 4 [2]). When gastric erosion is confirmed on gastroscopy, the band needs to be removed urgently, but not immediately. Patients may be converted to RYGB (EL 4 [156, 341]), VBG, or BPD (EL 4 [84]), or rebanding (EL 4 [118]). However, rebanding should be avoided if further weight reduction is the principal aim (EL 2b [341]).

The incidence of band slippage essentially depends on band positioning (EL 2 [68]). Patients usually complain of burning sensations and discontinuation of weight loss. Initial management consists of band deflation. If the pars flaccida technique was not used in the primary operation, therapy consists of laparoscopic revision (EL 4 [59]). Other alternatives are band repositioning, rebanding, or conversion to other procedures (EL 4 [349]).

Pouch dilatation can occur in the early or late followup. Early dilatation is mostly caused by a wrong position of the band (EL 4 [58]). Patients do not get a feeling of satiety, stop to loose weight, and suffer from vomiting. A contrast meal verifies the diagnosis, but minor degrees of dilatation can be considered not clinically relevant (EL 4 [174]). Therapy consists of immediate gastric tube placement and band deflation followed by reinflation after a few months. In case pouch dilatation persists, band repositioning or conversion to other procedures should be tried (EL 4 [248]).

Access ports can twist or become infected. While port rotation can be corrected by revisional surgical fixation (EL 4 [170, 225, 349]), infection requires port removal. First, the tube is placed in the abdominal cavity. When infection has settled down, the tube is reconnected, and a new port is place at a different position. A spontaneous disconnection between tube and port should be suspected in patients who report an acute abdominal pain (EL 4 [365]). Laparoscopic grasping of the tube with reattachment is a feasible treatment option (EL 4 [365]).

Vertical Banded Gastroplasty

After VBG, the range of complications includes stoma stenosis, pouch dilatation, band erosion and staple line disruption. Erosion or infection of the band at the pouch outlet should be treated by band removal (EL 4 [340]). In severe cases, conversion to LAGB or other procedures may be necessary (EL 4 [66, 176]). As described above, staple line disruption should be prevented intraoperatively by the use of MacLean's technique with complete transsection of the vertical staple line with oversewing (EL 1b [102]; EL 2b [195]). The advantage of not transsecting the staple line, however, is that small disruptions can be accepted without major effects on weight loss (EL 4 [213]). Severe cases of esophageal reflux after VBG may require conversion RYGB (EL 4 [24]).

Roux-en-Y Gastric Bypass

Stoma stenosis, gastric distension, anastomotic leakage, gastrojejunal ulcers and nutritional deficiencies may occur after RYGB. Stoma stenosis due to anastomotic strictures usually occurs during the first postoperative months (EL 4 [284, 292]). Most cases of stoma stenosis are amenable to endoscopic dilatation, but some require conversion for persistence of stenosis or perforation caused by dilatation (EL 4 [28, 288, 292]). On the opposite site, an unwanted dilatation of the gastrojejunostomy may respond to sclerotherapy (EL 4 [316]). Stomal ulceration can usually be treated conservatively with an H2 blocker and sucralfacte (EL 4 [284]).

Biliopancreatic Diversion

The spectrum of complications after BPD is similar to RYGB. Complications have been found to be more likely in patients converted from other procedures to BPD (EL 3b [26]). According to the report by Anthone et al. [18], a lengthening of the common canal can be necessary to treat hypalbuminaemia or persistent diarrhea (EL 4). In that study, the initial length of the common canal was 100 cm.

Discussion

During the last years, the rapidly growing and often lucrative field of obesity surgery has attracted many laparoscopic surgeons. As also the prevalence of obesity has increased steadily, the number of bariatric operations has increased dramatically. Although obesity surgery represents the only therapeutic opportunity for strong and long-term weight loss, balancing between treatment benefits and side effects is often difficult, because many morbidly obese patients present with severe comorbidity. Furthermore, also the less than morbidly obese population is seeking help of bariatric surgeons. This led to the decision to summarize the state of the art in the field of obesity surgery. The EAES guidelines developed here were also necessary to update previous guidelines of other societies.

Since the results of this consensus conference have been derived directly from the relevant literature by an interdisciplinary panel, it can be hoped that they find widespread acceptance [132]. However, the recommendations are no "cookbook", because national and local circumstances will often necessitate modifications. This European consensus represents a common ground, which can be transferred to all obesity surgery centres. Still, any scientific recommendation represents a compromise between practically orientated firmness of language and its underlying scientific basis. Often, the scarceness of reliable evidence precluded the panel from formulating important decisions. On the other hand, it would have been of no practical value to come up with only bland generalities. Therefore, some recommendations were agreed upon, although only weak evidence had been found to support them, whereas other crucial points, like the choice of surgical procedure, were left unresolved, although some medium-quality, but not convincing evidence was available.

Among the possible shortcomings of these guidelines is the absence of an anesthesiologist, an internist, and a patient in the panel, since the paragraphs on preoperative and postoperative care cover also important aspects of general medicine. As most of the panel members are working in multidisciplinary teams, it can be expected that the most common non-surgical aspects of obesity surgery have been adequately addressed. The input of the nutritionist and the psychiatrist was very valuable. A patient representative often acts as a safeguard against recommending a procedure with unpleasant non-medical side effects and related problems with compliance. However, due to the difficulties in finding a competent person, patients are usually not participating in clinical guideline development. Furthermore, the inclusion of additional persons would have led to a panel size that makes group discussions difficult to moderate [211, 227, 240].

Owing to the lack of published data on various aspects of obesity surgery these recommendations also highlight the need for future studies. Especially the relative effectiveness of the different laparoscopic procedures is worth a number of controlled trials. Some technical modifications and newer devices also require scientific evaluation. Future studies should pay closer attention to the different subgroups of obese and morbidly obese patients, because different risk-benefit ratios are likely in these heterogeneous groups of patients. Since some ongoing studies were already identified during the guideline development process, it should be noted that the present recommendations need to be updated after about 5 years in order to take advantage of this new knowledge [303].

References

1. Abdel-Galil E, Sabry AA (2002) Laparoscopic Roux-en-Y gastric bypass-evaluation of three different techniques. Obes Surg 12:639–642
2. Abu-Abeid S, Keidar A, Gavert N, Blanc A, Szold A (2003) The clinical spectrum of band erosion following laparoscopic adjustable silicone gastric banding for morbid obesity. Surg Endosc 17:861–863
3. Aidonopoulos AP, Papavramidis ST, Zaraboukas TG, Habib HW, Pothoulakis IG (1994) Gallbladder findings after cholecystectomy in morbidly obese patients. Obes Surg 4:8–12
4. Ali MR, Sugerman HJ, DeMaria EJ (2002) Techniques of laparoscopic Roux-en-Y gastric bypass. Semin Laparosc Surg 9:94–104
5. Allison DB, Faith MS, Gorman BS (1996) Publication bias in obesity treatment trials? Int J Obes Relat Metab Disord 20:931–937
6. Allison DB, Zannolli R, Narayan KM (1999) The direct health care costs of obesity in the United States. Am J Public Health 89:1194–1199
7. Almogy G, Crookes PF, Anthone GJ (2004) Longitudinal gastrectomy as a treatment for the high-risk super-obese patient. Obes Surg 14:492–497
8. Amaral JF, Thompson WR (1985) Gallbladder disease in the morbidly obese. Am J Surg 149:551–557
9. American College of Endocrinology (ACE), American Association of Clinical Endocrinologists (AACE). AACE/ACE position statement on the prevention, diagnosis and treatment of obesity. Jacksonville (FL): American Association of Clinical Endocrinologists, 1998
10. American Society for Bariatric Surgery (1997) Guidelines for reporting results in bariatric surgery. Obes Surg 7:521–522
11. American Society for Bariatric Surgery, Society of American Gastrointestinal Endoscopic Surgeons (2000) Guidelines for laparoscopic and open surgical treatment of morbid obesity. Obes Surg 10:378–379
12. Andersen T, Backer OG, Astrup A, Quaade F (1987) Horizontal or vertical banded gastroplasty after pretreatment with very-low-calorie formula diet: a randomized trial. Int J Obes 11:295–304
13. Andersen T, Backer OG, Stokholm KH, Quaade F (1984) Randomized trial of diet and gastroplasty compared with diet alone in morbid obesity. N Engl J Med 310:352–356
14. Andersen T, Stokholm KH, Backer OG, Quaade F (1988) Longterm (5-year) results after either horizontal gastroplasty or very-low-calorie diet for morbid obesity. Int J Obes 12:277–284
15. Angrisani L, Favretti F, Furbetta F, Iuppa A, Doldi SB, Paganelli M, Basso N, Lucchese M, Zappa M, Lesti G, Capizzi FD, Giardiello C, Di Lorenzo N, Paganini A, Di Cosmo L, Veneziani A, Laci-tignola S, Silecchia G, Alkilani M, Forestieri P, Puglisi F, Gardinazzi A, Toppino M, Campanile F, Marzano B, Bernante P, Perrotta G, Borrelli V, Lorenzo M (2004) Italian Group for Lap-Band System: Results of multicenter study on patients with BMI kg/m^2. Obes Surg 14:415–418
16. Angrisani L, Iovino P, Lorenzo M, Santoro T, Sabbatini F, Claar E, Nicodemi O, Persico G, Te-sauro B (1999) Treatment of morbid obesity and gastroesophageal reflux with hiatal hernia by Lap-Band. Obes Surg 9:396–398
17. Anonymous (2000) Obesity: preventing and managing the global epidemic. Report of a WHO consultation. World Health Organ Tech Rep Ser 894:1–253
18. Anthone GJ, Lord RV, DeMeester TR, Crookes PF (2003) The duodenal switch operation for the treatment of morbid obesity. Ann Surg 238:618–628
19. Arcila D, Velazquez D, Gamino R, Sierra M, Salin-Pascual R, Gonzalez-Barranco J, Herrera MF (2002) Quality of life in bariatric surgery. Obes Surg 12:661–665
20. Ashy ARA, Merdad AA (1998) A prospective study comparing vertical banded gastroplasty versus laparoscopic adjustable gastric banding in the treatment of morbid and super-obesity. Int J Surg 83:108–110
21. Averbukh Y, Heshka S, El-Shoreya H, Flancbaum L, Geliebter A, Kamel S, Pi-Sunyer FX, Laferrere B (2003) Depression score predicts weight loss following Roux-en-Y gastric bypass. Obes Surg 13:833–836

22. Azagra JS, Goergen M, Ansay J, De Simone P, Vanhaverbeek M, Devuyst L, Squelaert J (1999) Laparoscopic gastric reduction surgery. Preliminary results of a randomized, prospective trial of laparoscopic vs open vertical banded gastroplasty. Surg Endosc 13:555–558

23. Bajardi G, Ricevuto G, Mastrandrea G, Branca M, Rinaudo G, Cali F, Diliberti S, Lo Biundo N, Asti V (2000) Surgical treatment of morbid obesity with biliopancreatic diversion and gastric banding: report on an 8-year experience involving 235 cases. Ann Chir 125:155–162

24. Balsiger BM, Murr MM, Mai J, Sarr MG (2000) Gastroesophageal reflux after intact vertical banded gastroplasty: correction by conversion to Roux-en-Y gastric bypass. J Gastrointest Surg 4:276–281

25. Baltasar A, Bou R, Miro J, Bengochea M, Serra C, Perez N (2002) Laparoscopic biliopancreatic diversion with duodenal switch: technique and initial experience. Obes Surg 12:245–248

26. Baltasar A, del Rio J, Escriva C, Arlandis F, Martinez R, Serra C (1997) Preliminary results of the duodenal switch. Obes Surg 7:500–504

27. Baltasar A, Serra C, Perez N, Bou R, Bengochea M (2004) Clinical hepatic impairment after the duodenal switch. Obes Surg 14:77–83

28. Barba CA, Butensky MS, Lorenzo M, Newman R (2003) Endoscopic dilation of gastroesophageal anastomosis stricture after gastric bypass. Surg Endosc 17:416–420

29. Belachew M, Jacqet P, Lardinois F, Karler C (1993) Vertical banded gastroplasty vs adjustable silicone gastric banding in the treatment of morbid obesity: a preliminary report. Obes Surg 3:275–278

30. Belachew M, Legrand MJ, Defechereux TH, Burtheret MP, Jacquet N (1994) Laparoscopic adjustable silicone gastric banding in the treatment of morbid obesity. A preliminary report. Surg Endosc 8:1354–1356

31. Benotti PN, Bistrain B, Benotti JR, Blackburn G, Forse RA (1992) Heart disease and hypertension in severe obesity: the benefits of weight reduction. Am J Clin Nutr 55:586S–590S

32. Benotti PN, Burchard KW, Kelly JJ, Thayer BA (2004) Obesity. Arch Surg 139:406–414

33. Biertho L, Steffen R, Ricklin T, Horber FF, Pomp A, Inabnet WB, Herron D, Gagner M (2003) Laparoscopic gastric bypass versus laparoscopic adjustable gastric banding: a comparative study of 1,200 cases. J Am Coll Surg 197:536–545

34. Black DW, Goldstein RB, Mason EE (2003) Psychiatric diagnosis and weight loss following gastric surgery for obesity. Obes Surg 13:746–751

35. Blanco-Engert R, Weiner S, Pomhoff I, Matkowitz R, Weiner RA (2003) Outcome after laparoscopic adjustable gastric banding, using the Lap-Band® and the Heliogast® band: a prospective randomized study. Obes Surg 13:776–779

36. Bloomberg RD, Urbach DR (2002) Laparoscopic Roux-en-Y gastric bypass for severe gastroesophageal reflux after vertical banded gastroplasty. Obes Surg 12:408–411

37. Boylan LM, Sugerman HJ, Driskell JA (1988) Vitamin E, vitamin B-6, vitamin B-12, and folate status of gastric bypass surgery patients. J Am Diet Assoc 88:579–585

38. Brolin RE (2002) Bariatric surgery and long-term control of morbid obesity. JAMA 288:2793–2796

39. Brolin RE, Kenler HA, German JH, Cody RP (1992) Long-limb gastric bypass in the superobese-a prospective randomized study. Ann Surg 215:387–395

40. Brolin RE, LaMarca LB, Kenler HA, Cody RP (2002) Malabsorptive gastric bypass in patients with superobesity. J Gastrointest Surg 6:195–205

41. Brown TH, Davidson PF, Terrell S, Rayford P, Larson GM (1988) The effect of an intragastric balloon on weight loss, gastric acid secretion, and serum peptide levels. Am Surg 54:109–112

42. Buchwald H (2002) A bariatric surgery algorithm. Obes Surg 12:733–746

43. Buddeberg-Fischer B, Klaghofer R, Sigrist S, Buddeberg C (2004) Impact of psychosocial stress and symptoms on indication for bariatric surgery and outcome in morbidly obese patients. Obes Surg 14:361–369

44. Buffington C, Walker B, Cowan GS Jr, Scruggs D (1993) Vitamin D deficiency in the morbidly obese. Obes Surg 3:421–424
45. Bump RC, Sugerman HJ, Fantl JA, McClish DK (1992) Obesity and lower urinary tract function in women: effect of surgically induced weight loss. Am J Obstet Gynecol 167:392–399
46. Busetto L, Pisent C, Segato G, De Marchi F, Favretti F, Lise M, Enzi G (1997) The influence of a new timing strategy of band adjustment on the vomiting frequency and the food consumption of obese women operated with laparoscopic adjustable silicone gastric banding (LAP-BAND). Obes Surg 7:505–512
47. Busetto L, Segato G, De Marchi F, Foletto M, De Luca M, Caniato D, Favretti F, Lise M, Enzi G (2002) Outcome predictors in morbidly obese recipients of an adjustable gastric band. Obes Surg 12:83–92
48. Byrne TK (2001) Complications of surgery for obesity. Surg Clin North Am 81:1181–1193, vii–viii
49. Cadiere GB, Himpens J, Hainaux B, Gaudissart Q, Favretti S, Segato G (2002) Laparoscopic adjustable gastric banding. Semin Laparosc Surg 9:105–114
50. Calhoun R, Willbanks O (1987) Coexistence of gallbladder disease and morbid obesity. Am J Surg 154:655–658
51. Cannizzo F Jr, Kral JG (1998) Obesity surgery: a model of programmed undernutrition. Curr Opin Clin Nutr Metab Care 1:363–368
52. Capella JF, Capella RF (2003) Bariatric surgery in adolescence, is this the best age to operate? Obes Surg 13:826–832
53. Carson JL, Ruddy ME, Duff AE, Holmes NJ, Cody RP, Brolin RE (1994) The effect of gastric bypass surgery on hypertension in morbidly obese patients. Arch Intern Med 154:193–200
54. Champion JK, Williams MD (2003) Prospective randomized comparison of linear staplers during laparoscopic Roux-en-Y gastric bypass. Obes Surg 13:855–860
55. Chapman AE, Kiroff G, Game P, Foster B, O'Brien P, Ham J, Maddern GJ (2004) Laparoscopic adjustable gastric banding in the treatment of obesity: a systematic literature review. Surgery 135:326–351
56. Charles SC (1987) Psychiatric evaluation of morbidly obese patients. Gastroenterol Clin North Am 16:415–432
57. Charuzi I, Lavie P, Peiser J, Peled R (1992) Bariatric surgery in morbidly obese sleep-apnea patients: short- and long-term follow-up. Am J Clin Nutr 55:594S–596S
58. Chelala E, Cadiere GB, Favretti F, Himpens J, Vertruyen M, Bruyns J, Maroquin L, Lise M (1997) Conversions and complications in 185 laparoscopic adjustable silicone gastric banding cases. Surg Endosc 11:268–271
59. Chevallier JM, Zinzindohoue F, Douard R, Blanche JP, Berta JL, Altman JJ, Cugnenc PH (2004) Complications after laparoscopic adjustable gastric banding for morbid obesity: experience with 1,000 patients over 7 years. Obes Surg 14:407–414
60. Choban PS, Flancbaum L (2002) The effect of Roux limb lengths on outcome after Roux-en-Y gastric bypass: a prospective, randomized clinical trial. Obes Surg 12:540–545
61. Clegg A, Colquitt J, Sidhu M, Royle P, Walker A (2003) Clinical and cost effectiveness of surgery for morbid obesity: a systematic review and economic evaluation. Int J Obes Relat Metab Disord 27:1167–1177
62. Clegg AJ, Colquitt J, Sidhu MK, Royle P, Loveman E, Walker A (2002) The clinical effectiveness and cost-effectiveness of surgery for people with morbid obesity: a systematic review and economic evaluation. Health Technol Assess 6:1–153
63. Colquitt J, Clegg A, Sidhu M, Royle P (2003) Surgery for morbid obesity. Cochrane Database of Systematic Reviews, Issue 2, 2003. Update Software, Oxford:
64. Courcoulas A, Schuchert M, Gatti G, Luketich J (2003) The relationship of surgeon and hospital volume to outcome after gastric bypass surgery in Pennsylvania: a 3-year summary. Surgery 134:613–623

65. Dallal RM, Mattar SG, Lord JL, Watson AR, Cottam DR, Eid GM, Hamad G, Rabinovitz M, Schauer PR (2004) Results of laparoscopic gastric bypass in patients with cirrhosis. Obes Surg 14:47–53

66. Dargent J (1997) Two cases of conversion of vertical ring gastroplasty to adjustable silicone gastric banding. Obes Surg 7:34–38

67. Dargent J (1999) Laparoscopic adjustable gastric banding: lessons from the first 500 patients in a single institution. Obes Surg 9:446–452

68. Dargent J (2003) Pouch dilatation and slippage after adjustable gastric banding: is it still an issue? Obes Surg 13:111–115

69. D'Argent J (2002) Gastric electrical stimulation as therapy of morbid obesity: preliminary results from the French study. Obes Surg 12(Suppl 1):21S–25S

70. Davila-Cervantes A, Borunda D, Dominguez-Cherit G, Gamino R, Vargas-Vorackova F, Gon-zalez-Barranco J, Herrera MF (2002) Open versus laparoscopic vertical banded gastroplasty: a randomized controlled double blind trial. Obes Surg 12:812–818

71. de Wit LT, Mathus-Vliegen L, Hey C, Rademaker B, Gouma DJ, Obertop H (1999) Open versus laparoscopic adjustable silicone gastric banding: a prospective randomized trial for treatment of morbid obesity. Ann Surg 230:800–807

72. Deitel M (1994) The NIH consensus development conference revisited. Obes Surg 4:83–84

73. Delaney AG, Duerson MC, O'Leary JP (1980) The incidence of cholelithiasis after jejunoileal bypass. Int J Obes 4:243–248

74. DeMaria EJ, Schweitzer MA, Kellum JM, Meador J, Wolfe L, Sugerman HJ (2002) Hand-assisted laparoscopic gastric bypass does not improve outcome and increases costs when compared to open gastric bypass for the surgical treatment of obesity. Surg Endosc 16:1452–1455

75. DeMaria EJ, Sugerman HJ, Kellum JM, Meador JG, Wolfe LG (2002) Results of 281 consecutive total laparoscopic Roux-en-Y gastric bypasses to treat morbid obesity. Ann Surg 235:640–647

76. Detournay B, Fagnani F, Phillippo M, Pribil C, Charles MA, Sermet C, Basdevant A, Eschwege E (2000) Obesity morbidity and health care costs in France: an analysis of the 1991–1992 Medical Care Household Survey. Int J Obes Relat Metab Disord 24:151–155

77. Deveney CW, MacCabee D, Marlink K, Welker K, Davis J, McConnell DB (2004) Roux-en-Y divided gastric bypass results in the same weight loss as duodenal switch for morbid obesity. Am J Surg 187:655–659

78. Diez-del Val I, Martinez-Blazquez C (2003) Cirugia de la obesidad morbida: medicina basada en la evidencia. Cir Esp 74:185–192

79. Dixon JB, Dixon ME, O'Brien PE (2001) Pregnancy after Lap-Band surgery: management of the band to achieve healthy weight outcomes. Obes Surg 11:59–65

80. Dixon JB, O'Brien PE (1999) Gastroesophageal reflux in obesity: the effect of lap-band placement. Obes Surg 9: 527–531 81. Dixon JB, O'Brien PE (2002) Changes in comorbidities and improvements in quality of life after LAP-BAND placement. Am J Surg 184:51S–54S

82. Dixon JB, O'Brien PE (2002) Selecting the optimal patient for LAP-BAND placement. Am J Surg 184:17S–20S

83. Doherty C, Maher JW, Heitshusen DS (2002) Long-term data indicate a progressive loss in efficacy of adjustable silicone gastric banding for the surgical treatment of morbid obesity. Surgery 132:724–728

84. Dolan K, Fielding G (2004) Bilio pancreatic diversion following failure of laparoscopic adjustable gastric banding. Surg Endosc 18:60–63

85. Dolan K, Fielding G (2004) A comparison of laparoscopic adjustable gastric banding in adolescents and adults. Surg Endosc 18:45–47

86. Dolan K, Hatzifotis M, Newbury L, Fielding G (2004) A comparison of laparoscopic adjustable gastric banding and biliopancreatic diversion in superobesity. Obes Surg 14:165–169

87. Doldi SB, Micheletto G, Perrini MN, Rapetti R (2004) Intragastric balloon: another option for treatment of obesity and morbid obesity. Hepatogastroenterology 51:294–297
88. Douketis JD, Feightner JW, Attia J, Feldman WF, with the Canadian Task Force on Preventive Health Care (1999) Periodic health examination, 1999 update: 1. Detection, prevention and treatment of obesity. CMAJ 160:513–525
89. Eid GM, Mattar SG, Hamad G, Cottam DR, Lord JL, Watson A, Dallal M, Schauer PR (2004) Repair of ventral hernias in morbidly obese patients undergoing laparoscopic gastric bypass should not be deferred. Surg Endosc 18:207–210
90. Evans JD, Scott MH (2001) Intragastric balloon in the treatment of patients with morbid obesity. Br J Surg 88:1245–1248
91. Faintuch J, Matsuda M, Cruz ME, Silva MM, Teivelis MP, Garrido AB Jr, Gama-Rodrigues JJ (2004) Severe protein-calorie malnutrition after bariatric procedures. Obes Surg 14:175–181
92. Favretti F, O'Brien PE, Dixon JB (2002) Patient management after LAP-BAND placement. Am J Surg 184:38S–41S
93. Fernandez AZ Jr, Demaria EJ, Tichansky DS, Kellum JM, Wolfe LG, Meador J, Sugerman HJ (2004) Multivariate analysis of risk factors for death following gastric bypass for treatment of morbid obesity. Ann Surg 239:698–703
94. Ferraro DR (2004) Preparing patients for bariatric surgery-the clinical considerations. Clinician Reviews 14:57–63
95. Fettes PH, Williams DE (1996) Assessment, and treatment of morbid obesity. In: Thompson JK (ed) Body image, eating disorder, and obesity: An integrative guide for assessment and treatment of morbid obesity. American Psychological Association, Washington, pp 441–461
96. Fielding GA (2003) Laparoscopic adjustable gastric banding for massive superobesity (>60 body mass index kg/m²). Surg Endosc 17:1541–1545
97. Filip JE, Mattar SG, Bowers SP, Smith CD (2002) Internal hernia formation after laparoscopic Roux-en-Y gastric bypass for morbid obesity. Am Surg 68:640–643
98. Fletcher RH, Fairfield KM (2002) Vitamins for chronic disease prevention in adults: clinical applications. JAMA 287:3127–3129
99. Fobi M, Lee H, Igwe D, Felahy B, James E, Stanczyk M, Fobi N (2002) Prophylactic cholecys-tectomy with gastric bypass operation: incidence of gallbladder disease. Obes Surg 12:350–353
100. Fobi MA (1993) Operations that are questionable for control of obesity. Obes Surg 3:197–200
101. Fobi MA, Lee H, Holness R, Cabinda D (1998) Gastric bypass operation for obesity. World J Surg 22:925–935
102. Fobi MA, Lee H, Igwe D Jr, Stanczyk M, Tambi JN (2001) Prospective comparative evaluation of stapled versus transected silastic ring gastric bypass: 6-year follow-up. Obes Surg 11:18–24
103. Foley EF, Benotti PN, Borlase BC, Hollingshead J, Blackburn GL (1992) Impact of gastric restrictive surgery on hypertension in the morbidly obese. Am J Surg 163:294–297
104. Fontaine KR, Redden DT, Wang C, Westfall AO, Allison DB (2003) Years of life lost due to obesity. JAMA 289:187–193
105. Forse RA, Karam B, MacLean LD, Christou NV (1989) Antibiotic prophylaxis for surgery in morbidly obese patients. Surgery 106:750–757
106. Forsell P, Hellers G (1997) The Swedish Adjustable Gastric Banding (SAGB) for morbid obesity: 9 year experience and a 4-year follow-up of patients operated with a new adjustable band. Obes Surg 7:345–351
107. Frederiksen SG, Johansson J, Johnsson F, Hedenbro J (2000) Neither low-calorie diet nor vertical banded gastroplasty influence gastro-oesophageal reflux in morbidly obese patients. Eur J Surg 166:296–300
108. Freedman DS, Khan LK, Serdula MK, Galuska DA, Dietz WH (2002) Trends and correlates of class 3 obesity in the United States from 1990 through 2000. JAMA 288:1758–1761

109. Frey WC, Pilcher J (2003) Obstructive sleep-related breathing disorders in patients evaluated for bariatric surgery. Obes Surg 13:676–683

110. Frezza EE, Ikramuddin S, Gourash W, Rakitt T, Kingston A, Luketich J, Schauer P (2002) Symptomatic improvement in gastroesophageal reflux disease (GERD) following laparoscopic Roux-en-Y gastric bypass. Surg Endosc 16:1027–1031

111. Fried M, Miller K, Kormanova K (2004) Literature review of comparative studies of complications with Swedish band and Lap-Band. Obes Surg 14:256–260

112. Fried M, Peskova M, Kasalicky M (1998) Assessment of the outcome of laparoscopic nonadjustable gastric banding and stoma adjustable gastric banding: surgeon's and patient's view. Obes Surg 8:45–48

113. Friedman D, Cuneo S, Valenzano M, Marinari GM, Adami GF, Gianetta E, Traverse E, Scopinaro N (1995) Pregnancies in an 18-year follow-up after biliopancreatic diversion. Obes Surg 5:308–313

114. Frigg A, Peterli R, Peters T, Ackermann C, Tondelli P (2004) Reduction in co-morbidities 4 years after laparoscopic adjustable gastric banding. Obes Surg 14:216–223

115. Frigg A, Peterli R, Zynamon A, Lang C, Tondelli P (2001) Radiologic and endoscopic evaluation for laparoscopic adjustable gastric banding: preoperative and follow-up. Obes Surg 11:594–599

116. Frimberger E, Kuhner W, Weingart J, Ottenjann R (1982) Intragastraler Appetit-Depressor-Ballon. Munch Med Wochenschr 124:39–40

117. Gandjour A, Westenhofer J, Wirth A, Fuchs C, Lauterbach KW (2001) Development process of an evidence-based guideline for the treatment of obesity. Int J Qual Health Care 13:325–332

118. Gavert N, Szold A, Abu-Abeid S (2004) Safety and feasibility of revisional laparoscopic surgery for morbid obesity: conversion of open silastic vertical banded gastroplasty to laparoscopic adjustable gastric banding. Surg Endosc 18:203–206

119. Geliebter A, Melton PM, McCray RS, Gage D, Heymsfield SB, Abiri M, Hashim SA (1991) Clinical trial of silicone-rubber gastric balloon to treat obesity. Int J Obes 15:259–266

120. Gentileschi P, Kini S, Catarci M, Gagner M (2002) Evidencebased medicine: open and laparoscopic bariatric surgery. Surg Endosc 16:736–744

121. Gertler R, Ramsey-Stewart G (1986) Pre-operative psychiatric assessment of patients presenting for gastric bariatric surgery (surgical control of morbid obesity). Aust N Z J Surg 56:157–161

122. Ghassemian AJ, MacDonald KG, Cunningham PG, Swanson M, Brown BM, Morris PG, Pories WJ (1997) The workup for bariatric surgery does not require a routine upper gastrointestinal series. Obes Surg 7:16–18

123. Gonzalez QH, Tishler DS, Plata-Munoz JJ, Bondora A, Vickers SM, Leath T, Clements RH (2004) Incidence of clinically evident deep venous thrombosis after Laroscopic Roux-en-Y Gastric bypass. Surg Endosc 18:1082–1084

124. Gonzalez R, Bowers SP, Venkatesh KR, Lin E, Smith CD (2003) Preoperative factors predicitve of complicated postoperative management after Roux-en-Y gastric bypass for morbid obesity. Surg Endosc 17:1900–1914

125. Goodrick GK, Poston WS 2nd, Foreyt JP (1996) Methods for voluntary weight loss and control: update 1996. Nutrition 12:672–676

126. Gowan GSM Jr (1998) The Cancun IFSO statement on bariatric surgeon qualifications. Obes Surg 8:86

127. Greenstein RJ, Nissan A, Jaffin B (1998) Esophageal anatomy and function in laparoscopic gastric restrictive bariatric surgery: implications for patient selection. Obes Surg 8:199–206

128. Guisado JA, Vaz FJ, Lopez-Ibor JJ, Lopez-Ibor MI, del Rio J, Rubio MA (2002) Gastric surgery and restraint from food as triggering factors of eating disorders in morbid obesity. Int J Eat Disord 31:97–100

129. Hall JC, Watts JM, O'Brien PE, Dunstan RE, Walsh JF, Slavotinek AH, Elmslie RG (1990) Gastric surgery for morbid obesity. The Adelaide Study. Ann Surg 211:419–427

130. Hamoui N, Anthone G, Crookes PF (2004) Calcium metabolism in the morbidly obese. Obes Surg 14:9–12
131. Hamoui N, Kim K, Anthone G, Crookes PF (2003) The significance of elevated levels of parathyroid hormone in patients with morbid obesity before and after bariatric surgery. Arch Surg 138:891–897
132. Hayward RS, Wilson MC, Tunis SR, Bass EB, Guyatt G (1995) Users' guides to the medical literature. VIII. How to use clinical practice guidelines. A. Are the recommendations valid? The Evidence-Based Medicine Working Group. JAMA 274:570–574
133. Henderson L, Irving K, Gregory J (2003) The National Diet & Nutrition Survey: adults aged 19 to 64 years. Vitamin and mineral intake and urinary analytes. The Stationery Office, London, UK
134. Herbst CA, Mittelstaedt CA, Staab EV, Buckwalter JA (1984) Intraoperative ultrasonography evaluation of the gallbladder in morbidly obese patients. Ann Surg 200:691–692
135. Herpertz S, Kielmann R, Wolf AM, Langkafel M, Senf W, Hebebrand J (2003) Does obesity surgery improve psychosocial functioning? A systematic review. Int J Obes Relat Metab Disord 27:1300–1314
136. Hess DS, Hess DW (1998) Biliopancreatic diversion with a duodenal switch. Obes Surg 8:267–282
137. Hess DW, Hess DS (1994) Laparoscopic vertical banded gastroplasty with complete transection of the staple-line. Obes Surg 4:44–46
138. Higa KD, Boone KB, Ho T, Davies OG (2000) Laparoscopic Roux-en-Y gastric bypass for morbid obesity: technique and preliminary results of our first 400 patients. Arch Surg 135:1029–1034
139. Hildebrandt SE (1998) Effects of participation in bariatric support group after Roux-en-Y gastric bypass. Obes Surg 8:535–542
140. Hodson RM, Zacharoulis D, Goutzamani E, Slee P, Wood S, Wedgwood KR (2001) Management of obesity with the new intragastric balloon. Obes Surg 11:327–329
141. Hogan RB, Johnston JH, Long BW, Sones JQ, Hinton LA, Bunge J, Corrigan SA (1989) A double-blind, randomized, shamcontrolled trial of the gastric bubble for obesity. Gastrointest Endosc 35:381–385
142. Hori S, Ochiai T, Gunji Y, Hayashi H, Suzuki T (2004) A prospective randomized trial of hand-sutured versus mechanically stapled anastomoses for gastroduodenostomy after distal gastrectomy. Gastric Cancer 7:24–30
143. Howard L, Malone M, Michalek A, Carter J, Alger S, Van Woert J (1995) Gastric bypass and vertical banded gastroplasty: a prospective randomized comparison and 5-year follow-up. Obes Surg 5:55–60
144. Hudson SM, Dixon JB, O'Brien PE (2002) Sweet eating is not a predictor of outcome after Lap-Band placement. Can we finally bury the myth? Obes Surg 12:789–794
145. Huerta S, Arteaga JR, Sawicki MP, Liu CD, Livingston EH (2002) Assessment of routine elimination of postoperative nasogastric decompression after Roux-en-Y gastric bypass. Surgery 132:844–848
146. Inge TH, Garcia V, Daniels S, Langford L, Kirk S, Roehrig H, Amin R, Zeller M, Higa K (2004) A multidisciplinary approach to the adolescent bariatric surgical patient. J Pediatr Surg 39:442–447
147. Inge TH, Krebs NF, Garcia VF, Skelton JA, Guice KS, Strauss RS, Albanese CT, Brandt ML, Hammer LD, Harmon CM, Kane TD, Klish WJ, Oldham KT, Rudolph CD, Helmrath MA, Donovan E, Daniels SR (2004) Bariatric surgery for severely overweight adolescents: concerns and recommendations. Pediatrics 114:217–223
148. International Federation for the Surgery of Obesity (1997) Statement on patient selection for bariatric surgery. Obes Surg 7:41
149. Iovino P, Angrisani L, Tremolaterra F, Nirchio E, Ciannella M, Borrelli V, Sabbatini F, Mazzacca G, Ciacci C (2002) Abnormal esophageal acid exposure is common in morbidly obese patients and improves after a successful Lap-band system implantation. Surg Endosc 16:1631–1635

150. Jaffin BW, Knoepflmacher P, Greenstein R (1999) High prevalence of asymptomatic esophageal motility disorders among morbidly obese patients. Obes Surg 9:390–395
151. Jan JC, Hong D, Patterson EJ (2004) Concomitant cholecystectomy is not necessary for laparoscopic gastric bypass or laparoscopic adjustable gastric banding-effective use of ursodeoxycholic acid [abstract]. Surg Endosc 18(Suppl.):S185
152. Jones DB, Provost DA, DeMaria EJ, Smith CD, Morgenstern L, Schirmer B (2004) Optimal management of the morbidly obese patient: SAGES appropriateness conference statement. Surg Endosc: published online (DOI 10.1007/s00464-00004-0813200466)
153. Jones DB, Provost DA, DeMaria EJ, Smith CD, Morgenstern L, Schirmer B (2004) Optimal management of the morbidly obese patient: SAGES appropriateness conference statement. Surg Endosc 18:1029–1037
154. Jones KB (1996) Biliopancreatic limb obstruction in gastric bypass at or proximal to the jejunojejunostomy: a potentially deadly, catastrophic event. Obes Surg 6:485–493
155. Jones KB Jr (1995) Simultaneous cholecystectomy: to be or not to be. Obes Surg 5:52–54
156. Jones KB Jr (2001) Revisional bariatric surgery-safe and effective. Obes Surg 11:183–189
157. Kalfarentzos F, Stavropoulou F, Yarmenitis S, Kenagias I, Karamesini M, Dimitrako-poulos A, Maniati A (2001) Prophylaxis of venous thromboembolism using two different doses of low-molecular-weight heparin (nadroparin) in bariatric surgery: a prospective randomized trial. Obes Surg 11:670–676
158. Karason K, Lindroos AK, Stenlof K, Sjostrom L (2000) Relief of cardiorespiratory symptoms and increased physical activity after surgically induced weight loss: results from the Swedish Obese Subjects study. Arch Intern Med 160:1797–1802
159. Karlsson J, Sjostrom L, Sullivan M (1998) Swedish obese subjects (SOS)-an intervention study of obesity. Two-year follow-up of health-related quality of life (HRQL) and eating behavior after gastric surgery for severe obesity. Int J Obes Relat Metab Disord 22:113–126
160. Kasalicky M, Fried M, Peskova M (2002) [Are complications of gastric banding decreased with cuff fixation?]. Sbornik Lekarsky 103:213–222
161. Khateeb NI, Roslin MS, Chin D, Khan N, Anhalt H (1999) Significant improvement in HbA1c in a morbidly obese type 2 diabetic patient after gastric bypass surgery despite relatively small weight loss. Diabetes Care 22:651
162. Khurana RN, Baudendistel TE, Morgan EF, Rabkin RA, Elkin RB, Aalami OO (2004) Postoperative rhabdomyolysis following laparoscopic gastric bypass in the morbidly obese. Arch Surg 139:73–76
163. Kieran JA, Safadi BY, Morton JM, Hsu G, Curet MJ (2004) Antecolic Roux-Y gastric bypass for morbid obesity is associated with shorter operative times and fewer internal hernias [abstract]. Surg Endosc 18(Suppl.):S198
164. Kim CH, Sarr MG (1992) Severe reflux esophagitis after vertical banded gastroplasty for treatment of morbid obesity. Mayo Clin Proc 67:33–35
165. Kim WW, Gagner M, Kini S, Inabnet WB, Quinn T, Herron D, Pomp A (2003) Laparoscopic vs open biliopancreatic diversion with duodenal switch: a comparative study. J Gastrointest Surg 7:552–557
166. Kirby DF, Wade JB, Mills PR, Sugerman HJ, Kellum JM, Zfass AM, Starkey JV, Birkenhauer R, Hamer RM (1990) A prospective assessment of the Garren-Edwards Gastric Bubble and bariatric surgery in the treatment of morbid obesity. Am Surg 56:575–580
167. Kirchmayr W, Klaus A, Muhlmann G, Mittermair R, Bonatti H, Aigner F, Weiss H (2004) Adjustable gastric banding: assessment of safety and efficacy of bolus-filling during follow-up. Obes Surg 14:387–391
168. Kolakowski S Jr, Kirkland ML, Schuricht AL (2004) Routine postoperative barium swallow evaluation after Roux-en-Y gastric bypass: is it necessary? [abstract]. Surg Endosc 18(Suppl):S185
169. Korenkov M, Köhler L, Yücel N, Grass G, Sauerland S, Lempa M, Troidl H (2002) Esophageal motility and reflux symptoms before and after bariatric surgery. Obes Surg 12:72–76

170. Korenkov M, Sauerland S, Yücel N, Köhler L, Goh P, Schierholz J, Troidl H (2003) Port function after laparoscopic adjustable gastric banding for morbid obesity. Surg Endosc 17:1068–1071

171. Korolija D, Sauerland S, Wood-Dauphinee S, Abbou CC, Eypasch E, Garcia-Caballero M, Lumsden MA, Millat B, Monson JRT, Nilsson G, Pointner R, Schwenk W, Shamiyeh A, Szold A, Targarona E, Ure B, Neugebauer E (2004) Evaluation of quality of life after laparoscopic surgery: evidence-based guidelines of the European Association for Endoscopic Surgery. Surg Endosc 18:879–897

172. Krakamp B, Leidig P, Gehmlich D, Paul A (1997) Der Magenvolumen-Reduzierungsballon zur Gewichtsreduktion: Welche Berechtigung hat diese umstrittene Methode? Zentralbl Chir 122:349–357

173. Kreitz K, Rovito PF (2003) Laparoscopic Roux-en-Y gastric bypass in the "megaobese". Arch Surg 138:707–710

174. Kuzmak LI, Burak E (1993) Pouch enlargement: Myth or reality? Impressions from serial upper gastrointestinal series in silicone gastric banding patients. Obes Surg 3:57–62

175. Kuzmak LI, Yap IS, McGuire L, Dixon JS, Young MP (1990) Surgery for morbid obesity. Using an inflatable gastric band. AORN J 51:1307–1324

176. Kyzer S, Raziel A, Landau O, Matz A, Charuzi I (2001) Use of adjustable silicone gastric banding for revision of failed gastric bariatric operations. Obes Surg 11:66–69

177. Labeck B, Nehoda H, Kuhberger-Peer R, Klocker J, Hourmont K, Aigner F, Weiss HG (2001) Adjustable gastric and esophagogastric banding. Is a pouch compulsory? Surg Endosc 15:1193–1196

178. Lauterbach K, Westenhofer J, Wirth A, Hauner H (1998) Evidenz-basierte Leitlinie zur Behandlung der Adipositas in Deutschland. Hauser, Köln

179. Laws HL, Piantadosi S (1981) Superior gastric reduction procedure for morbid obesity: a prospective, randomized trial. Ann Surg 193:334–340

180. Lawson J (2002) Drug-induced metabolic bone disorders. Semin Musculoskelet Radiol 6:285–297

181. Lechner GW, Callender AK (1981) Subtotal gastric exclusion and gastric partitioning: a randomized prospective comparison of one hundred patients. Surgery 90:637–644

182. Lechner GW, Elliott DW (1983) Comparison of weight loss after gastric exclusion and partitioning. Arch Surg 118:685–692

183. Ledikwe JH, Smiciklas-Wright H, Mitchell DC, Jensen GL, Friedmann JM, Still CD (2003) Nutritional risk assessment and obesity in rural older adults: a sex difference. Am J Clin Nutr 77:551–558

184. Ledikwe JH, Smiciklas-Wright H, Mitchell DC, Miller CK, Jensen GL (2004) Dietary patterns of rural older adults are associated with weight and nutritional status. J Am Geriatr Soc 52:589–595

185. Levine GM (1988) Intragastric balloons: an unfulfilled promise. Ann Intern Med 109:354–356

186. Lew JI, Daud A, DiGorgi F, Davis DG, Bessler M (2004) Routine preoperative esophageal manometry does not affect outcome of laparoscopic adjustable silicone gastric banding [abstract]. Surg Endosc 18(Suppl):S185

187. Lindor KD, Hughes RW Jr, Ilstrup DM, Jensen MD (1987) Intragastric balloons in comparison with standard therapy for obesity-a randomized, double-blind trial. Mayo Clin Proc 62:992–996

188. Livingston EH, Ko CY (2004) Socioeconomic characteristics of the population eligible for obesity surgery. Surgery 135:288–296

189. Loffredo A, Cappuccio M, De Luca M, de Werra C, Galloro G, Naddeo M, Forestieri P (2001) Three years experience with the new intragastric balloon, and a preoperative test for success with restrictive surgery. Obes Surg 11:330–333

190. Long SD, O'Brien K, MacDonald KG Jr, Leggett-Frazier N, Swanson MS, Pories WJ, Caro JF (1994) Weight loss in severely obese subjects prevents the progression of impaired glucose tolerance to type II diabetes. A longitudinal interventional study. Diabetes Care 17:372–375

191. Lujan JA, Frutos MD, Hernandez Q, Liron R, Cuenca JR, Valero G, Parrilla P (2004) Laparoscopic versus open gastric bypass in the treatment of morbid obesity: a randomized prospective study. Ann Surg 239:433–437
192. Lundell L, Ruth M, Olbe L (1997) Vertical banded gastroplasty or gastric banding for morbid obesity: effects on gastro-oesophageal reflux. Eur J Surg 163:525–531
193. Macgregor AM, Rand CS (1993) Gastric surgery in morbid obesity. Outcome in patients aged 55 years and older. Arch Surg 128:1153–1157
194. MacLean LD, Rhode B, Shizgal HM (1987) Nutrition after vertical banded gastroplasty. Ann Surg 206:555–563
195. MacLean LD, Rhode BM, Forse RA (1990) Late results of vertical banded gastroplasty for morbid and super obesity. Surgery 107:20–27
196. MacLean LD, Rhode BM, Forse RA, Nohr R (1995) Surgery for obesity—an update of a randomized trial. Obes Surg 5:145–150
197. MacLean LD, Rhode BM, Nohr CW (2001) Long- or short-limb gastric bypass? J Gastrointest Surg 5:525–530
198. MacLean LD, Rhode BM, Sampalis J, Forse RA (1993) Results of the surgical treatment of obesity. Am J Surg 165:155–162
199. Magnusson M, Freedman J, Jonas E, Stockeld D, Granstrom L, Naslund E (2002) Five-year results of laparoscopic vertical banded gastroplasty in the treatment of massive obesity. Obes Surg 12:826–830
200. Marceau P, Biron S, Bourque RA, Potvin M, Hould FS, Simard S (1993) Biliopancreatic diversion with a new type of gastrectomy. Obes Surg 3:29–35
201. Marceau P, Hould FS, Simard S, Lebel S, Bourque RA, Potvin M, Biron S (1998) Biliopancreatic diversion with duodenal switch. World J Surg 22:947–954
202. Marceau P, Kaufman D, Biron S, Hould FS, Lebel S, Marceau S, Kral JG (2004) Outcome of pregnancies after biliopancreatic diversion. Obes Surg 14:318–324
203. Marinari GM, Camerini G, Novelli GB, Papadia F, Murelli F, Marini P, Adami GF, Scopinaro N (2001) Outcome of biliopancreatic diversion in subjects with Prader-Willi Syndrome. Obes Surg 11:491–495
204. Marinari GM, Murelli F, Camerini G, Papadia F, Carlini F, Stabilini C, Adami GF, Scopinaro N (2004) A 15-year evaluation of biliopancreatic diversion according to the Bariatric Analysis Reporting Outcome System (BAROS). Obes Surg 14:325–328
205. Martin LF, Finigan KM, Nolan TE (2000) Pregnancy after adjustable gastric banding. Obstet Gynecol 95:927–930
206. Mason EE (1982) Vertical banded gastroplasty for obesity. Arch Surg 117:701–706
207. Mason EE, Ito C (1969) Gastric bypass. Ann Surg 170:329–339
208. Mason EE, Ito CC (1967) Gastric bypass in obesity. Surg Clin North Am 47:1345–1354
209. Mathus-Vliegen EM, Tytgat GN (1990) Intragastric balloons for morbid obesity: results, patient tolerance and balloon life span. Br J Surg 77:76–79
210. Mathus-Vliegen EMH, Tytgat GNJ, Veldhuyzen-Offermans EAML (1990) Intragastric balloon in the treatment of supermorbid obesity. Double-blind, sham-controlled, crossover evaluation of 500-milliliter balloon. Gastroenterology 99:362–369
211. McKneally MF, McPeek BM, DS, Spitzer WO, Troidl H (1998) Organizing meetings, panels, seminars, consensus conferences. In: Troidl H, McKneally MF, Mulder DS, Wechsler AS, McPeek B, Spitzer WO (eds) Surgical research. Basic principles and clinical practice, 3rd ed. Springer, Berlin Heidelberg New York, pp 341–355
212. Mehran A, Szomstein S, Zundel N, Rosenthal R (2003) Management of acute bleeding after laparoscopic Roux-en-Y gastric bypass. Obes Surg 13:842–847
213. Melissas J, Christodoulakis M, Schoretsanitis G, Harocopos G, de Bree E, Gramatikakis J, Tsiftsis D (1998) Staple-line disruption following vertical banded gastroplasty. Obes Surg 8:15–20
214. Melissas J, Christodoulakis M, Schoretsanitis G, Sanidas E, Ganotakis E, Michaloudis D, Tsiftsis DD (2001) Obesity-associated disorders before and after weight reduction by vertical banded gastroplasty in morbidly vs super obese individuals. Obes Surg 11:475–481

215. Melissas J, Volakakis E, Hadjipavlou A (2003) Low-back pain in morbidly obese patients and the effect of weight loss following surgery. Obes Surg 13:389–393
216. Michaelides EM, Sismanis A, Sugerman HJ, Felton WL 3rd (2000) Pulsatile tinnitus in patients with morbid obesity: the effectiveness of weight reduction surgery. Am J Otol 21:682–685
217. Miller K, Hell E (2003) Laparoscopic surgical concepts of morbid obesity. Langenbecks Arch Surg 388:375–384
218. Miller K, Hell E, Lang B, Lengauer E (2003) Gallstone formation prophylaxis after gastric restrictive procedures for weight loss: a randomized double-blind placebo-controlled trial. Ann Surg 238:697–702
219. Miller K, Holler E, Hell E (2002) Intragastrale Stimulation als erste nichtrestriktive und nichtmalab-sorptive Behandlungsmethode der morbiden Adipositas. Zentralbl Chir 127:1049–1054
220. Monteforte MJ, Turkelson CM (2000) Meta-analysis: Bariatric surgery for morbid obesity. Obes Surg 10:391–401
221. Moorehead MK, Ardelt-Gattinger E, Lechner H, Oria HE (2003) The validation of the Moorehead-Ardelt Quality of Life Questionnaire II. Obes Surg 13:684–692
222. Moose D, Lourie D, Powell W, Pehrsson B, Martin D, LaMar T, Alexander J (2003) Laparoscopic Roux-en-Y gastric bypass: minimally invasive bariatric surgery for the superobese in the community hospital setting. Am Surg 69:930–932
223. Morino M, Toppino M, Bonnet G, del Genio G (2003) Laparoscopic adjustable silicone gastric banding versus vertical banded gastroplasty in morbidly obese patients: a prospective randomized controlled clinical trial. Ann Surg 238:835–842
224. Morino M, Toppino M, Bonnet G, Rosa R, Garrone C (2002) Laparoscopic vertical banded gastroplasty for morbid obesity. Assessment of efficacy. Surg Endosc 16:1566–1572
225. Mortele KJ, Pattijn P, Mollet P, Berrevoet F, Hesse U, Ceelen W, Ros PR (2001) The Swedish laparoscopic adjustable gastric banding for morbid obesity: radiologic findings in 218 patients. AJR Am J Roentgenol 177:77–84
226. Msika S (2003) [Surgery for morbid obesity: 2. Complications. Results of a Technologic Evaluation by the ANAES]. J Chir (Paris) 140:4–21
227. Murphy MK, Black NA, Lamping DL, McKee CM, Sanderson CFB, Askham J, Marteau T (1998) Consensus development methods, and their use in clinical guideline development. Health Technol Assessment 2:i–iv, 1–88
228. Murr MM, Balsiger BM, Kennedy FP, Mai JL, Sarr MG (1999) Malabsorptive procedures for severe obesity: comparison of pancreaticobiliary bypass and very very long limb Roux-en-Y gastric bypass. J Gastrointest Surg 3:607–612
229. Murr MM, Siadati MR, Sarr MG (1995) Results of bariatric surgery for morbid obesity in patients older than 50 years. Obes Surg 5:399–402
230. Must A, Spadano J, Coakley EH, Field AE, Colditz G, Dietz WH (1999) The disease burden associated with overweight and obesity. JAMA 282:1523–1529
231. Naef M, Sadowski C, de Marco D, Sabbioni M, Balsiger B, Laederach K, Burgi U, Buchler MW (2000) Die vertikale Gastroplastik nach Mason zur Behandlung der morbiden Adipositas: Ergebnisse einer prospektiven klinischen Studie. Chirurg 71:448–455
232. Naslund E, Freedman J, Lagergren J, Stockeld D, Granstrom L (1999) Three-year results of laparoscopic vertical banded gastroplasty. Obes Surg 9:369–373
233. Naslund I, Jarnmark I, Andersson H (1988) Dietary intake before and after gastric bypass and gastroplasty for morbid obesity in women. Int J Obes 12:503–513
234. Naslund I, Wickbom G, Christoffersson E, Agren G (1986) A prospective randomized comparison of gastric bypass and gastroplasty. Complications and early results. Acta Chir Scand 152:681–689
235. National Institute for Clinical Excellence (2002) Guidance on the use of surgery to aid weight reduction for people with morbid obesity (Technology Appraisal No. 46). National Institute for Clinical Excellence, London

236. National Institutes of Health (1998) Clinical guidelines on the identification, evaluation, and treatment of overweight and obesity in adults-the evidence report. Obes Res 6(Suppl 2):51S–209S
237. National Institutes of Health Consensus Development Conference Panel (1991) Gastrointestinal surgery for severe obesity. Ann Intern Med 115:956–961
238. National Institutes of Health Consensus Development Panel (1992) Gastrointestinal surgery for severe obesity. Am J Clin Nutr 55(Suppl 2):615–619
239. Nehoda H, Hourmont K, Mittermair R, Lanthaler M, Sauper T, Peer R, Aigner F, Weiss H (2001) Is a routine liquid contrast swallow following laparoscopic gastric banding mandatory? Obes Surg 11:600–604
240. Neugebauer E, Troidl H (1995) Consensus methods as tools to assess medical technologies. Surg Endosc 9:481–482
241. Nguyen NT, Goldman C, Rosenquist CJ, Arango A, Cole CJ, Lee SJ, Wolfe BM (2001) Laparoscopic versus open gastric bypass: a randomized study of outcomes, quality of life, and costs. Am Surg 234:279–291
242. Nguyen NT, Ho HS, Fleming NW, Moore P, Lee SJ, Goldman CD, Cole CJ, Wolfe BM (2002) Cardiac function during laparoscopic vs open gastric bypass. Surg Endosc 16:78–83
243. Nguyen NT, Ho HS, Palmer LS, Wolfe BM (2000) A comparison study of laparoscopic versus open gastric bypass for morbid obesity. J Am Coll Surg 191:149–157
244. Nguyen NT, Rivers R, Wolfe BM (2003) Early gastrointestinal hemorrhage after laparoscopic gastric bypass. Obes Surg 13:62–65
245. Nicolai A, Ippoliti C, Petrelli MD (2002) Laparoscopic adjustable gastric banding: essential role of psychological support. Obes Surg 12:857–863
246. Nieben OG, Harboe H (1982) Intragastric balloon as an artificial bezoar for treatment of obesity. Lancet 1:198–199
247. Nilsell K, Thorne A, Sjostedt S, Apelman J, Pettersson N (2001) Prospective randomised comparison of adjustable gastric banding and vertical banded gastroplasty for morbid obesity. Eur J Surg 167:504–509
248. Niville E, Dams A (1999) Late pouch dilation after laparoscopic adjustable gastric and esophagogastric banding: incidence, treatment, and outcome. Obes Surg 9:381–384
249. O'Brien PE, Brown WA, Smith A, McMurrick PJ, Stephens M (1999) Prospective study of a laparoscopically placed, adjustable gastric band in the treatment of morbid obesity. Br J Surg 86:113–118
250. O'Brien PE, Dixon JB (2002) Weight loss and early and late complications – the international experience. Am J Surg 184:42S–45S
251. O'Brien PE, Dixon JB, Brown W, Schachter LM, Chapman L, Burn AJ, Dixon ME, Scheinkestel C, Halket C, Sutherland LJ, Korin A, Baquie P (2002) The laparoscopic adjustable gastric band (Lap-Band): a prospective study of medium-term effects on weight, health and quality of life. Obes Surg 12:652–660
252. O'Keeffe T, Patterson EJ (2004) Evidence supporting routine polysomnography before bariatric surgery. Obes Surg 14:23–26
253. Olsson SA, Ryden O, Danielsson A, Nilsson Ehle P (1984) Weight reduction after gastroplasty: the predictive value of sugrical, metabolic, and psychological variables. Int J Obes 8:245–258
254. Oria HE, Moorehead MK (1988) Bariatric Analysis and Reporting Outcome System (BAROS). Obes Surg 8:487–499
255. Ovrebo KK, Hatlebakk JG, Viste A, Bassoe HH, Svanes K (1998) Gastroesophageal reflux in morbidly obese patients treated with gastric banding or vertical banded gastroplasty. Ann Surg 228:51–58
256. Paiva D, Bernardes L, Suretti L (2001) Laparoscopic biliopancreatic diversion for the treatment of morbid obesity: initial experience. Obes Surg 11:619–622
257. Papasavas PK, Caushaj PF, McCormick JT, Quinlin RF, Hayetian FD, Maurer J, Kelly JJ, Gagne DJ (2003) Laparoscopic management of complications following laparoscopic Roux-en-Y gastric bypass for morbid obesity. Surg Endosc 17:610–614

258. Papasavas PK, O'Mara MS, Quinlin RF, Maurer J, Caushaj PF, Gagne DJ (2002) Laparoscopic reoperation for early complications of laparoscopic gastric bypass. Obes Surg 12:559–563
259. Papavramidis ST, Theocharidis AJ, Zaraboukas TG, Christoforidou BP, Kessissoglou II, Aidonopoulos AP (1996) Upper gastrointestinal endoscopic and histologic findings before and after vertical banded gastroplasty. Surg Endosc 10:825–830
260. Patterson EJ, Urbach DR, Swanstrom LL (2003) A comparison of diet and exercise therapy versus laparoscopic Roux-en-Y gastric bypass surgery for morbid obesity: a decision analysis model. J Am Coll Surg 196:379–384
261. Pinkney JH, Sjostrom CD, Gale EAM (2001) Should surgeons treat diabetes in severely obese people? Lancet 357:1357–1359
262. Podnos YD, Jimenez JC, Wilson SE, Stevens CM, Nguyen NT (2003) Complications after laparoscopic gastric bypass: a review of 3464 cases. Arch Surg 138:957–961
263. Polyzogopoulou EV, Kalfarentzos F, Vagenakis AG, Alexandrides TK (2003) Restoration of euglycemia and normal acute insulin response to glucose in obese subjects with type 2 diabetes following bariatric surgery. Diabetes 52:1098–1103
264. Pories WJ, Flickinger EG, Meelheim D, Van Rij AM, Thomas FT (1982) The effectiveness of gastric bypass over gastric partition in morbid obesity: consequence of distal gastric and duodenal exclusion. Ann Surg 196:389–399
265. Pories WJ, Swanson MS, MacDonald KG, Long SB, Morris PG, Brown BM, Barakat HA, deRamon RA, Israel G, Dolezal JM, et al (1995) Who would have thought it? An operation proves to be the most effective therapy for adult-onset diabetes mellitus. Ann Surg 222:339–352
266. Pories WJ, van Rij AM, Burlingham BT, Fulghum RS, Meelheim D (1981) Prophylactic cefazolin in gastric bypass surgery. Surgery 90:426–432
267. Rabkin RA (1998) Distal gastric bypass/duodenal switch procedure, Roux-en-Y gastric bypass and biliopancreatic diversion in a community practice. Obes Surg 8:53–59
268. Rabkin RA, Rabkin JM, Metcalf B, Lazo M, Rossi M, Lehman Becker LB (2004) Nutritional markers following duodenal switch for morbid obesity. Obes Surg 14:84–90
269. Rabner JG, Greenstein RJ (1993) Antiobesity surgery: Is a structured support group desirable? Obes Surg 3:381–390
270. Ramhamadany EM, Fowler J, Baird IM (1989) Effect of the gastric balloon versus sham procedure on weight loss in obese subjects. Gut 30:1054–1057
271. Ray EC, Nickels MW, Sayeed S, Sax HC (2003) Predicting success after gastric bypass: the role of psychosocial and behavioral factors. Surgery 134:555–564
272. Regan JP, Inabnet WB, Gagner M, Pomp A (2003) Early experience with two-stage laparoscopic Roux-en-Y gastric bypass as an alternative in the super-super obese patient. Obes Surg 13:861–864
273. Reinhold RB (1994) Late results of gastric bypass surgery for morbid obesity. J Am Coll Nutr 13:326–331
274. Ren CJ, Fielding GA (2003) Laparoscopic adjustable gastric banding: surgical technique. J Laparoendosc Adv Surg Tech A 13:257–263
275. Ren CJ, Patterson E, Gagner M (2000) Early results of laparoscopic biliopancreatic diversion with duodenal switch: a case series of 40 consecutive patients. Obes Surg 10:514–524
276. Resa JJ, Solano J, Fatas JA, Bias JL, Monzon A, Garcia A, Lagos J, Escartin J (2004) Laparoscopic biliopancreatic diversion: technical aspects and results of our protocol. Obes Surg 14:329–333
277. Ridings P, Sugerman HJ (1994) Vertical banded gastroplasty for the treatment of morbid obesity. Br J Surg 81:776
278. Rigaud D, Trostler N, Rozen R, Vallot T, Apfelbaum M (1995) Gastric distension, hunger and energy intake after balloon implantation in severe obesity. Int J Obes Relat Metab Disord 19:489–495
279. Rissanen AM (1996) The economic and psychosocial consequences of obesity. Ciba Found Symp 201:194–206

280. Roe DA (1985) Drug-food and drug-nutrient interactions. J Environ Pathol Toxicol Oncol 5:115–135
281. Roman S, Napoleon B, Mion F, Bory RM, Guyot P, D'Orazio H, Benchetrit S (2004) Intragastric balloon for "non-morbid" obesity: a retrospective evaluation of tolerance and efficacy. Obes Surg 14:539–544
282. Rubino F, Gagner M (2002) Potential of surgery for curing type 2 diabetes mellitus. Ann Surg 236:554–559
283. Rubino F, Marescaux J (2004) Effect of duodenal-jejunal exclusion in a non-obese animal model of type 2 diabetes: a new perspective for an old disease. Ann Surg 239:1–11
284. Sanyal AJ, Sugerman HJ, Kellum JM, Engle KM, Wolfe L (1992) Stomal complications of gastric bypass: incidence and outcome of therapy. Am J Gastroenterol 87:1165–1169
285. Sapala JA, Wood MH, Schuhknecht MP, Sapala MA (2003) Fatal pulmonary embolism after bariatric operations for morbid obesity: a 24-year retrospective analysis. Obes Surg 13:819–825
286. Sauerland S, Korenkov M, Kleinen T, Arndt M, Paul A (2004) Obesity is a risk factor for recurrence after incisional hernia repair. Hernia 8:42–46
287. Schauer PR (2003) Open and laparoscopic surgical modalities for the management of obesity. J Gastrointest Surg 7:468–475
288. Schauer PR, Ikrammudin S, Gourash W, Ramanathan R, Luketich J (2000) Outcomes after laparoscopic Roux-en-Y gastric bypass for morbid obesity. Ann Surg 232:515–529
289. Schirmer B, Watts SH (2004) Laparoscopic bariatric surgery. Surg Endosc 18:1875–1878
290. Schmidt JH, Hocking MP, Rout WR, Woodward ER (1988) The case for prophylactic cholecystectomy concomitant with gastric restriction for morbid obesity. Am Surg 54:269–272
291. Schrader G, Stefanovic S, Gibbs A, Elmslie R, Higgins B, Slavotinek A (1990) Do psychosocial factors predict weight loss following gastric surgery for obesity? Aust N Z J Psychiatr 24:496–499
292. Schwartz ML, Drew RL, Roiger RW, Ketover SR, Chazin-Caldie M (2004) Stenosis of the gastroenterostomy after laparoscopic gastric bypass. Obes Surg 14:484–491
293. Scopinaro N, Gianetta E, Adami GF, Friedman D, Traverse E, Marinari GM, Cuneo S, Vitale B, Ballari F, Colombini M, Baschieri G, Bachi V (1996) Biliopancreatic diversion for obesity at eighteen years. Surgery 119:261–268
294. Scopinaro N, Gianetta E, Civalleri D, Bonalumi U, Bachi V (1979) Bilio-pancreatic bypass for obesity: I. An experimental study in dogs. Br J Surg 66:613–617
295. Scopinaro N, Gianetta E, Civalleri D, Bonalumi U, Bachi V (1979) Bilio-pancreatic bypass for obesity: II. Initial experience in man. Br J Surg 66:618–620
296. Scopinaro N, Gianetta E, Pandolfo N, Anfossi A, Berretti B, Bachi V (1976) II bypass biliopancreatico. Proposta e studio sperimentale preliminare di un nuovo tipo di intervento per la terapia chirurgica funzionale. Minerva Chir 31:560–566
297. Scopinaro N, Marinari GM, Camerini G (2002) Laparoscopic standard biliopancreatic diversion: technique and preliminary results. Obes Surg 12:362–365
298. Serafini F, Anderson W, Ghassemi P, Poklepovic J, Murr MM (2002) The utility of contrast studies and drains in the management of patients after Roux-en-Y gastric bypass. Obes Surg 12:34–38
299. Serafini FM, MacDowell Anderson W, Rosemurgy AS, Strait T, Murr MM (2001) Clinical predictors of sleep apnea in patients undergoing bariatric surgery. Obes Surg 11:28–31
300. Seufert RM, Schmidt-Matthiesen A, Beyer A (1990) Total gastrectomy and oesophago-jejunostomy-a prospective randomized trial of hand-sutured versus mechanically stapled anastomoses. Br J Surg 77:50–52
301. Seymour K, Mackie A, McCauley E, Stephen JG (1998) Changes in esophageal function after vertical banded gastroplasty as demonstrated by esophageal scintigraphy. Obes Surg 8:429–433
302. Sharaf RN, Weinshel EH, Bini EJ, Rosenberg J, Ren CJ (2004) Radiologic assessment of the upper gastrointestinal tract: does it play an important preoperative role in bariatric surgery? Obes Surg 14:313–317

303. Shekelle PG, Ortiz E, Rhodes S, Morton SC, Eccles MP, Grimshaw JM, Woolf SH (2001) Validity of the Agency for Healthcare Research and Quality clinical practice guidelines: How quickly do guidelines become outdated? JAMA 286:1461–1467
304. Shen R, Dugay G, Rajaram K, Cabrera I, Siegel N, Ren CJ (2004) Impact of patient follow-up on weight loss after bariatric surgery. Obes Surg 14:514–519
305. Shiffman ML, Sugerman HJ, Kellum JH, Brewer WH, Moore EW (1993) Gallstones in patients with morbid obesity. Relationship to body weight, weight loss and gallbladder bile cholesterol solubility. Int J Obes Relat Metab Disord 17:153–158
306. Shiffman ML, Sugerman HJ, Kellum JM, Brewer WH, Moore EW (1991) Gallstone formation after rapid weight loss: a prospective study in patients undergoing gastric bypass surgery for treatment of morbid obesity. Am J Gastroenterol 86:1000–1005
307. Shoji Y, Nihei Z, Hirayama R, Mishima Y (1995) Experiences with the linear cutter technique for performing Roux-en-Y anastomosis following total gastrectomy. Surg Today 25:27–31
308. Skroubis G, Sakellaropoulos G, Pouggouras K, Mead N, Nikiforidis G, Kalfarentzos F (2002) Comparison of nutritional deficiencies after Roux-en-Y gastric bypass and after biliopancreatic diversion with Roux-en-Y gastric bypass. Obes Surg 12:551–558
309. Skull AJ, Slater GH, Duncombe JE, Fielding GA (2004) Laparoscopic adjustable banding in pregnancy: safety, patient tolerance and effect on obesity-related pregnancy outcomes. Obes Surg 14:230–235
310. Slater GH, Ren CJ, Siegel N, Williams T, Barr D, Wolfe B, Dolan K, Fielding GA (2004) Serum fat-soluble vitamin deficiency and abnormal calcium metabolism after malabsorptive bariatric surgery. J Gastrointest Surg 8:48–55
311. Smith SC, Edwards CB, Goodman GN (1997) Symptomatic and clinical improvement in morbidly obese patients with gastroesophagealreflux disease following Roux-en-Y gastric bypass. Obes Surg 7:479–484
312. Sociedad Espanola de Cirugia de la Obesidad (SECO) (2004) Recommendaciones de la SECO para la practica de la cirugia bariatrica (Declaracio'n de Salamanca). Cir Esp 75:312–314
313. Sociedad Espanola para el Estudio de la Obesidad (SEEDO) (2000) Consenso SEEDO'2000 para la evaluacion del sobrepeso y la Obesidad y el establecimiento de criterios de intervencion terapeutica. "Med Clin (Barc)" 115:587–597
314. Society of American Gastrointestinal Endoscopic Surgeons (SAGES) (2003) Guidelines for institutions granting bariatric priviliges utilizing laparoscopic techniques. Surg Endosc 17:2037–2040
315. Sogg S, Mori DL (2004) The Boston interview for gastric bypass: determining the psychological suitability of surgical candidates. Obes Surg 14:370–380
316. Spaulding L (2003) Treatment of dilated gastrojejunostomy with sclerotherapy. Obes Surg 13:254–257
317. Stanford A, Glascock JM, Eid GM, Kane T, Ford HR, Ikramuddin S, Schauer P (2003) Laparoscopic Roux-en-Y gastric bypass in morbidly obese adolescents. J Pediatr Surg 38:430–433
318. Stokholm KH, Nielsen PE, Quaade F (1982) Correlation between initial blood pressure and blood pressure decrease after weight loss: A study in patients with jejunoileal bypass versus medical treatment for morbid obesity. Int J Obes 6:307–312
319. Sturm R (2002) The effects of obesity, smoking, and drinking on medical problems and costs. Obesity outranks both smoking and drinking in its deleterious effects on health and health costs. Health Aff (Millwood) 21:245–253
320. Sturm R (2003) Increases in clinically severe obesity in the United States, 1986–2000. Arch Intern Med 163:2146–2148
321. Sugerman HJ, Brewer WH, Shiffman ML, Brolin RE, Fobi MA, Linner JH, MacDonald KG, MacGregor AM, Martin LF, Oram-Smith JC, Popoola D, Schirmer BD, Vickers FF (1995) A multicenter, placebo-controlled, randomized, double-blind, prospective trial of prophylactic ursodiol for the prevention of gallstone formation following gastric-bypass-induced rapid weight loss. Am J Surg 169:91–97

322. Sugerman HJ, Fairman RP, Baron PL, Kwentus JA (1986) Gastric surgery for respiratory insufficiency of obesity. Chest 90:81–86
323. Sugerman HJ, Fairman RP, Sood RK, Engle K, Wolfe L, Kellum JM (1992) Long-term effects of gastric surgery for treating respiratory insufficiency of obesity. Am J Clin Nutr 55:597S–601S
324. Sugerman HJ, Felton WL 3rd, Sismanis A, Kellum JM, DeMaria EJ, Sugerman EL (1999) Gastric surgery for pseudotumor cerebri associated with severe obesity. Ann Surg 229:634–642
325. Sugerman HJ, Londrey GL, Kellum JM, Wolf L, Liszka T, Engle KM, Birkenhauer R, Starkey JV (1989) Weight loss with vertical banded gastroplasty and Roux-Y gastric bypass for morbid obesity with selective versus random assignment. Am J Surg 157:93–102
326. Sugerman HJ, Starkey JV, Birkenhauer R (1987) A randomized prospective trial of gastric bypass versus vertical banded gastroplasty for morbid obesity and their effects on sweets versus non-sweets eaters. Ann Surg 205:613–624
327. Sugerman HJ, Sugerman EL, DeMaria EJ, Kellum JM, Kennedy C, Mowery Y, Wolfe LG (2003) Bariatric surgery for severely obese adolescents. J Gastrointest Surg 7:102–108
328. Sugerman HJ, Wolfe LG, Sica DA, Clore JN (2003) Diabetes and hypertension in severe obesity and effects of gastric bypass-induced weight loss. Ann Surg 237:751–758
329. Sundbom M, Gustavsson S (2004) Randomized clinical trial of hand-assisted laparoscopic versus open Roux-en-Y gastric bypass for the treatment of morbid obesity. Br J Surg 91:418–423
330. Suter M, Giusti V, Heraief E, Zysset F, Calmes JM (2003) Laparoscopic gastric banding: Beyond the learning curve. Surg Endosc 17:1418–1425
331. Svahn J, Haag B, Wasielwski A, Ballantyne GH, Schmidt H (2003) 21 mm vs 25 mm EEA: Does gastrojejunostomy size make a difference? [abstract]. Surg Endosc 17(Suppl):S228
332. Talieh J, Kirgan D, Fisher BL (1997) Gastric bypass for morbid obesity: a standard surgical technique by consensus. Obes Surg 7:198–202
333. Taskin M, Apaydin BB, Zengin K, Taskin U (1997) Stoma adjustable silicone gastric banding versus vertical banded gastroplasty for the treatment of morbid obesity. Obes Surg 7:424–428
334. Thorne A, Lonnqvist F, Apelman J, Hellers G, Arner P (2002) A pilot study of long-term effects of a novel obesity treatment: omentectomy in connection with adjustable gastric banding. Int J Obes Relat Metab Disord 26:193–199
335. Totte E, Hendrickx L, Pauwels M, Van Hee R (2001) Weight reduction by means of intragastric device: experience with the Bioenterics intragastric balloon. Obes Surg 11:519–523
336. Valley V, Grace DM (1987) Psychosicial risk factors in gastric surgery for obesity: identifying guidelines for screening. Int J Obes 11:105–113
337. Verset D, Houben JJ, Gay F, Elcheroth J, Bourgeois V, Van Gossum A (1997) The place of upper gastrointestinal tract endoscopy before and after vertical banded gastroplasty for morbid obesity. Dig Dis Sci 42:2333–2337
338. Villegas L, Schneider B, Provost D, Chang C, Scott D, Sims T, Hill L, Hynan L, Jones D (2004) Is routine cholecystectomy required during laparoscopic gastric bypass? Obes Surg 14:206–211
339. Vishne TH, Ramadan E, Alper D, Avraham Z, Seror D, Dreznik Z (2004) Long-term follow-up and factors influencing success of silastic ring vertical gastroplasty. Dig Surg 21:134–141
340. Waaddegaard P, Clemmesen T, Jess P (2002) Vertical gastric banding for morbid obesity: a long-term follow-up study. Eur J Surg 168:220–222
341. Weber M, Muller MK, Michel JM, Belal R, Horber F, Hauser R, Clavien PA (2003) Laparoscopic Roux-en-Y gastric bypass, but not rebanding, should be proposed as rescue procedure for patients with failed laparoscopic gastric banding. Ann Surg 238:827–834

342. Weiner R, Blanco-Engert R, Weiner S, Matkowitz R, Schaefer L, Pomhoff I (2003) Outcome after laparoscopic adjustable gastric banding-8 years experience. Obes Surg 13:427–434

343. Weiner R, Bockhorn H, Rosenthal R, Wagner D (2001) A prospective randomized trial of different laparoscopic gastric banding techniques for morbid obesity. Surg Endosc 15: 63–68

344. Weiner R, Emmerlich V, Wagner D, Bockhorn H (1998) Management und Therapie von postoperativen Komplikationen nach "gastric banding" wegen morbider Adipositas. Chirurg 69:1082–1088

345. Weiner R, Gutberlet H, Bockhorn H (1999) Preparation of extremely obese patients for laparoscopic gastric banding by gastricballoon therapy. Obes Surg 9:261–264

346. Weiner RA, Blanco-Engert R, Weiner S, Pomhoff I, Schramm M (2004) Laparoscopic biliopancreatic diversion with duodenal switch: Three different duodeno-ileal anastomotic techniques and initial experience. Obes Surg 14:334–340

347. Weiner S, Weiner R, Pomhoff I (2003) Lebensqualitat nach bariatrischen Eingriffen – ein Überblick. Chir Gastroenterol 19:70–75

348. Weiss H, Nehoda H, Labeck B, Hourmont K, Lanthaler M, Aigner F (2000) Injection port complications after gastric banding: incidence, management and prevention. Obes Surg 10:259–262

349. Weiss HG, Kirchmayr W, Klaus A, Bonatti H, Muhlmann G, Nehoda H, Himpens J, Aigner F (2004) Surgical revision after failure of laparoscopic adjustable gastric banding. Br J Surg 91:235–241

350. Weiss HG, Nehoda H, Labeck B, Hourmont K, Marth C, Aigner F (2001) Pregnancies after adjustable gastric banding. Obes Surg 11:303–306

351. Weiss HG, Nehoda H, Labeck B, Peer-Kuehberger R, Oberwalder M, Aigner F, Wetscher GJ (2002) Adjustable gastric and esophagogastric banding: a randomized clinical trial. Obes Surg 12:573–578

352. Weiss HG, Nehoda H, Labeck B, Peer-Kuhberger MD, Klingler P, Gadenstatter M, Aigner F, Wetscher GJ (2000) Treatment of morbid obesity with laparoscopic adjustable gastric banding affects esophageal motility. Am J Surg 180:479–482

353. West of Scotland, Highland Anastomosis Study Group (1991) Suturing or stapling in gastrointestinal surgery: a prospective randomized study. Br J Surg 78:337–341

354. Westling A, Bergqvist D, Bostrom A, Karacagil S, Gustavsson S (2002) Incidence of deep venous thrombosis in patients undergoing obesity surgery. World J Surg 26:470–473

355. Westling A, Gustavsson S (2001) Laparoscopic vs open Roux-en-Y gastric bypass: a prospective, randomized trial. Obes Surg 11:284–292

356. Wiesner W, Schob O, Hauser RS, Hauser M (2000) Adjustable laparoscopic gastric banding in patients with morbid obesity: radiographic management, results, and postoperative complications. Radiology 216:389–394

357. Wittgrove AC, Clark GW (1996) Laparoscopic gastric bypass, Roux-en-Y: Experience of 27 cases, with 3–18 months follow-up. Obes Surg 6:54–57

358. Wittgrove AC, Clark GW, Schubert KR (1996) Laparoscopic gastric bypass, Roux-en-Y: Technique and results in 75 patients with 3–30 months follow-up. Obes Surg 6:500–504

359. Wittgrove AC, Clark GW, Tremblay LJ (1994) Laparoscopic gastric bypass, Roux-en-Y: Preliminary report of five cases. Obes Surg 4:353–357

360. Wittgrove AC, Jester L, Wittgrove P, Clark GW (1998) Pregnancy following gastric bypass for morbid obesity. Obes Surg 8:461–466

361. Wolf AM, Falcone AR, Kortner B, Kuhlmann HW (2000) BAROS: an effective system to evaluate the results of patients after bariatric surgery. Obes Surg 10:445–450

362. Wolff S, Pross M, Knippig C, Malfertheiner P, Lippert H (2002) Gastric pacing. Eine neue Methode in der Adipositaschirurgie. Chirurg 73:700–703

363. Wu EC, Barba CA (2000) Current practices in the prophylaxis of venous thromboembolism in bariatric surgery. Obes Surg 10:7–14

364. Wudel LJ Jr, Wright JK, Debelak JP, Allos TM, Shyr Y, Chapman WC (2002) Prevention of gallstone formation in morbidly obese patients undergoing rapid weight loss: results of a randomized controlled pilot study. J Surg Res 102:50–56
365. Yoffe B, Sapojnikov S, Lebedev V, Goldblum C (2003) Disconnection of port after laparoscopic gastric banding: causes and solution. Obes Surg 13:784–787
366. Zieren J, Ablassmaier B, Enzweiler C, Muller JM (2000) Disaster with a new type of band for gastric banding. Obes Surg 10:22–25
367. Zinzindohoue F, Chevallier JM, Douard R, Elian N, Ferraz JM, Blanche JP, Berta JL, Altman JJ, Safran D, Cugnenc PH (2003) Laparoscopic gastric banding: a minimally invasive surgical treatment for morbid obesity: prospective study of 500 consecutive patients. Ann Surg 237:1–9

Morbid Obesity – Update 2006

Mario Morino, Gitana Scozzari

Definition, Epidemiology and Clinical Course

No new data available.

Diagnostics

No new data available.

Operative Versus Conservative Treatment

Two important studies comparing bariatric surgery versus conservative treatment were published in 2004 [6, 20].

The 10-year results of the prospective controlled Swedish Obese Subjects Study were reported in the by Sjöström et al. [20] (EL 2b). This trial compared 641 patients who were submitted to surgery (156 bandings, 451 vertical banded gastroplasties, VGBs, and 34 gastric bypasses) with 627 obese patients of the control group. At 10 years, the body weight had increased by 1.6% in the control group and had decreased by 16.1% in the surgery group ($p < 0.001$). The surgery group had lower 2- and 10-year incidence rates of diabetes, hypertryglicerydemia and hyperuricemia than the control group, whereas differences between the two groups in the incidence of hypercholesterolemia and hypertension were undetectable.

Christou et al. [6] (EL 2b) reported an observational study using a combination of hospital and provincial insurance administrative databases to assess the effectiveness of bariatric surgery and to compare the mortality, morbidity and healthcare use in morbidly obese patients treated with bariatric surgery with a cohort of matched morbidly obese patients who were not treated surgically. Bariatric surgery resulted in a significant reduction in the mean percentage excess weight loss (EWL) (67.1%, $p < 0.001$). Bariatric surgery patients had significant risk reductions for developing cardiovascular, cancer, endocrine, infectious, psychiatric and mental disorders compared with controls, with the exception of haematologic (no difference) and digestive diseases (increased rates in the bariatric cohort). The mortality rate in the bariatric surgery cohort was

0.68% compared with 6.17% in controls, which translates to a reduction in the relative risk of death by 89%. This is a significant observation because it not only suggest the role of morbidity as a risk factor for early mortality but also provides evidence that surgical treatment of obesity produces a significant reduction in mortality. It is important to note that weight loss in the series by Christou et al. [6] was significantly higher that in the study by Sjöström et al. [20] (67 vs 25%) presumably as a consequence of the higher percentage of Roux-en-Y gastric bypasses (RYGBs) (80 vs 5%). In the Swedish study, 95% of surgical procedures were VBG and adjustable gastric banding; both procedures are associated with less weight loss compared with RYGB.

Therefore, compared with conventional therapy, bariatric surgery results in better long-term weight loss, improved lifestyle, amelioration of risk factors and decreased overall mortality (EL 2b).

Choice of Surgical Approach and Procedure

The laparoscopic approach is considered the gold standard for bariatric procedures and no papers comparing the laparoscopic with the open approach were published between 2004 and 2005.

Two randomized controlled trials (RCTs) comparing laparoscopic RYGB (LRYGB) and laparoscopic VBG (LVBG) [12, 17] (EL 1b) confirmed the results obtained from similar trials in open surgery: LRYGB is a time-consuming, demanding technique with a higher early complication rate compared with LVBG (17.8 vs 2.5%), but LRYGB results in a higher 2-year EWL (71.4 vs 53.1% in the study by Lee et al. [12] and 84.4 vs 59.8% in the study by Olbers et al. [17]).

A further RCT compared LRYGB with the mini-gastric bypass [13] (EL 1b) and showed similar results for resolution of metabolic syndrome, improvement of quality of life (QOL) and EWL at 2 years; nevertheless, the operative morbidity rate was higher for LRYGB (20 vs 7.5%).

VBG and RYGB were also compared in terms of oesophageal function in a prospective nonrandomized series by Ortega et al. [18]: on the basis of manometric and pH-metric results at 3 and 12 months postoperatively, the authors concluded that RYGB is significantly better than VBG as an antireflux procedure (EL 3).

These data were confirmed by Di Francesco et al. [10], who demonstrated that VBG reduced weight but not gastro-oesophageal reflux in obese patient at 1-year follow-up. The authors concluded that VBG should not be proposed for obese patients with reflux symptoms and positive functional tests (EL 3). It is important to note that no comparative data on long-term results of different bariatric procedures are available.

The results of a new bariatric procedure, the Implantable Gastric Stimulator (IGS), a pacemaker-like device that induces satiety, have been presented in a multicentric prospective series of 69 patients with a mean body mass index (BMI) of 41 [8]. Postoperative morbidity was limited to one case, while the mean EWL was 17% at 6 months and 21% at 10 months. It is not possible to draw any conclusion from this article owing to the reduced number of patients, the limited follow-up and the limited quality of data presented (EL 5). Furthermore, the authors stated that "the exact mechanism of action of electrical stimulation therapy for obesity remains to be defined".

Technical Aspects of Surgery

A review article on the physiologic effects of pneumoperitoneum by Nguyen and Wolfe [14] showed that morbidly obese patients have a higher intra-abdominal pressure of 2–3 times that of nonobese patients. The increased intra-abdominal pressure enhances venous stasis, reduces intraoperative portal venous blood flow, decreases intraoperative urinary output, lowers respiratory compliance, increases airway pressure and impairs cardiac function. Intraoperative management to minimize the adverse changes includes appropriate ventilatory adjustment to avoid hypercapnia and acidosis, the use of sequential compression devices to minimize venous stasis, and optimization of intravascular volume to minimize the effects of increased intra-abdominal pressure on renal and cardiac function.

Laparoscopic adjustable gastric banding is the most frequently applied bariatric technique in Europe and Australia. Different techniques and different bands have been proposed but comparative data are lacking.

O'Brien et al. [16] published a RCT comparing the so-called perigastric with the pars flaccida techniques (EL 1b). Patients operated by the pars flaccida technique had a reduced number of long-term complications (16 vs 42%) and a reduced number of revisional procedures; at 2 years, weight loss, correction of comorbidities and QOL were similar in the two groups.

In a second study, the two more frequently used bands, the LapBand and the Swedish Band, were compared in a RCT by Suter et al. [21] (EL 1b); it is important to note that the LapBand was placed using the perigastric technique, while the Swedish Band was placed using the pars flaccida technique. The two main findings were that early band-related morbidity was higher with the Swedish Band and that weight loss was initially faster with the LapBand. No differences could be found between the two groups regarding late morbidity, late reoperations (10% in each group), and EWL at 2 and 3 years. The two studies present contrasting results concerning the perigastric and the pars flaccida techniques; therefore, existing data are insufficient to define which should be the preferred technique.

The technique of RYGB has not been standardized, a fact which results in a tremendous degree of variation from medical centre to medical centre. It has been shown that increasing the Roux limb length may improve weight loss after RYGB, especially in patients with preoperative BMI > 50 [3, 4].

A RCT by Inabnet et al. [11] addressed this issue comparing 25 RYGBs with a biliopancreatic limb of 50 cm and an alimentary limb of 100 cm with 23 RYGBs with a biliopancreatic limb of 100 cm and an alimentary limb of 150 cm. The BMI decreased equally in both groups with no differences at 3, 6 and 12 months follow-up (EL 1 b).

Different technical devices have been recently proposed to facilitate or improve laparoscopic bariatric surgery, including robot-assisted procedures [1] and different staple-line reinforcement materials [2, 7, 15]. In a short series, Ali et al. [1] (EL 4) showed the feasibility of robot-assisted LRYGB using the Zeus robotic surgical system and addressed the problem of the learning curve defined as "significant but manageable".

Different materials have been tested in order to reduce staple-line bleeding and/or leaks during LRYGB or laparoscopic sleeve gastrectomy. Angrisani et al. [2] using bovine pericardial strips obtained a reduction of intraoperative leaks (methylene blue test) during LRYGB from 12.5 to 0%, but no differences in terms of bleeding or overall complications were found (EL 1 b). Nguyen et al. [15] obtained a significant reduction in staple-line bleeding sites diagnosed intraoperatively (0.4 vs 2.5) and in mean blood loss (84 vs 129 ml) during LRYGB using a glycolic copolymer sleeve to reinforce the staple line (EL 1 b). Furthermore, a significant reduction in peroperative blood loss was found by Consten et al. [7] comparing ten laparoscopic sleeve gastrectomies using a stapled buttressed absorbable polymer membrane to reinforce staple lines with ten cases using a conventional staple line (EL 2 b).

In conclusion, although on a limited number of patients, the use of some form of reinforcement of the staple line during bariatric surgery seems to be effective in improving intraoperative results, but no differences in postoperative complications have been detected by these studies and no data on costs have been reported.

Peri- and Postoperative Care

De Waele et al. [9], in a series of ten patients with a mean BMI of 38 and a mean age of 36 years, showed that laparoscopic adjustable gastric banding may be performed on an ambulatory basis without readmissions or complications (EL 4). The mean time interval between the end of the operation and discharge was 9.6 h (range 8–13 h). A strict selection of patients was advocated.

Factors influencing the outcome of bariatric surgery were evaluated in two different studies.

Poulose [19] reviewed 54,878 patients undergoing bariatric surgery in the USA in 2001 identified using the 2001 Healthcare Cost and Utilization Project

NIS. Risk factors for increased postoperative mortality included male gender, age above 39 years, Medicaid insured, and need for reoperation.

Very similar results were presented in the study by Carbonell et al. [5], who analysed year 2000 data from the Nationwide Inpatient Database for 5,876 RYGBs: male gender and postoperative complications increased mortality; male gender, increasing age and surgery performed in large hospitals were predictors of morbidity (EL 2b).

References

1. Ali MR, Bhaskerrao B, Wolfe BM (2005) Robot-assisted laparoscopic Roux-en-Y gastric bypass. Surg Endosc 19:468–472
2. Angrisani L, Lorenzo M, Borrelli V et al (2004) The use of bovine pericardial strips on linear stapler to reduce extraluminal bleeding during laparoscopic gastric bypass: prospective randomized clinical trial. Obes Surg 14:1198–1202
3. Brolin RE, Kenler HA, Gorman JH et al (1992) Long-limb gastric bypass in the superobese. A prospective randomized study. Ann Surg 215:387–395
4. Bruder SJ, Freeman JB, Brazeau-Gravelle P (1991) Lengthening the Roux-Y limb increases weight loss after gastric bypass: a preliminary report. Obes Surg 1:73–77
5. Carbonell AM, Lincourt AE, Matthews BD et al (2005) National study of the effect of patient and hospital characteristics on bariatric surgery outcomes. Am Surg 71:308–314
6. Christou NV, Sampalis JS, Liberman M et al (2004) Surgery decreases long-term mortality, morbidity, and health care use in morbidly obese patients. Ann Surg 240:416–424
7. Consten EC, Gagner M, Pomp A et al (2004) Decreased bleeding after laparoscopic sleeve gastrectomy with or without duodenal switch for morbid obesity using a stapled buttressed absorbable polymer membrane. Obes Surg 14:1360–1366
8. De Luca M, Segato G, Busetto L et al (2004) Progress in implantable gastric stimulation: summary of results of the European multi-center study. Obes Surg 14:S33–39
9. De Waele B, Lauwers M, Van Nieuwenhove Y et al (2004) Outpatient laparoscopic gastric banding: initial experience. Obes Surg 14:1108–1110
10. Di Francesco V, Baggio E, Mastromauro M et al (2004) Obesity and gastro-esophageal acid reflux: physiopathological mechanisms and role of gastric bariatric surgery. Obes Surg 14:1095–1102
11. Inabnet WB, Quinn T, Gagner M et al (2005) Laparoscopic Roux-en-Y gastric bypass in patients with BMI <50: a prospective randomized trial comparing short and long limb lengths. Obes Surg 15:51–57
12. Lee WJ, Huang MT, Yu PJ et al (2004) Laparoscopic vertical banded gastroplasty and laparoscopic gastric bypass: a comparison. Obes Surg 14:626–634
13. Lee WJ, Yu PJ, Wang W et al (2005) Laparoscopic Roux-en-Y versus mini-gastric bypass for the treatment of morbid obesity: a prospective randomized controlled clinical trial. Ann Surg 242:20–28
14. Nguyen NT, Wolfe BM (2005) The physiologic effects of pneumoperitoneum in the morbidly obese. Ann Surg 241:219–226
15. Nguyen NT, Longoria M, Welbourne S et al (2005) Glycolide copolymer staple-line reinforcement reduces staple site bleeding during laparoscopic gastric bypass: a prospective randomized trial. Arch Surg 140:773–778
16. O'Brien PE, Dixon JB, Laurie C et al (2005) A prospective randomized trial of placement of the laparoscopic adjustable gastric band: comparison of the perigastric and pars flaccida pathways. Obes Surg 15:820–826
17. Olbers T, Fagevik-Olsén M, Maleckas A et al (2005) Randomized clinical trial of laparoscopic Roux-en-Y gastric bypass versus laparoscopic vertical banded gastroplasty for obesity. Br J Surg 92:557–562

18. Ortega J, Escudero MD, Mora F et al (2004) Outcome of esophageal function and 24-hour esophageal pH monitoring after vertical banded gastroplasty and Roux-en-Y gastric bypass. Obes Surg 14:1086–1094
19. Poulose BK, Griffin MR, Moore DE et al (2005) Risk factors for post-operative mortality in bariatric surgery. J Surg Res 127:1–7
20. Sjöström L, Lindroos AK, Peltonen M et al (2004) Lifestyle, diabetes, and cardiovascular risk factors 10 years after bariatric surgery. N Engl J Med 351:2683–2693
21. Suter M, Giusti V, Worreth M et al (2005) Laparoscopic gastric banding. A prospective, randomized study comparing the Lapband and the SAGB: early results. Ann Surg 241:55–62

The EAES Clinical Practice Guidelines on Laparoscopic Cholecystectomy, Appendectomy, and Hernia Repair (1994)

Edmund A.M. Neugebauer, Hans Troidl, C.K. Kum, Ernst Eypasch,
Marc Miserez, Andreas Paul

Introduction

In the history of surgery, probably no other surgical development had such a dramatic and pivotal impact on surgery worldwide as endoscopic surgery. There is indeed no field in surgery which is not affected by endoscopic surgery. However, experience with this "new" tool has shown serious limitations and dangers of endoscopic surgical procedures, especially in less-experienced hands. Furthermore, it is not sufficient to demonstrate that an endoscopic surgical approach is feasible and safe; it must also be ascertained that the specific technique has a real benefit for the patients.

Large international societies such as the European Association for Endoscopic Surgery (EAES) have the responsibility to provide a forum for discussion of new developments and to provide guidelines on the best practice in the different fields based on the current state of knowledge. For this reason, the Educational Committee of the EAES decided to perform consensus development conferences (CDCs) to assess the current status of endoscopic surgical approaches for treatment of cholelithiasis, appendicitis, and inguinal hernia. These topics were chosen because of: (1) importance in terms of prevalence and economy, (2) multidisciplinary interest, (3) scientific controversy, and (4) the existence of sufficient research data for evaluation. The second international European Congress of the EAES, in Madrid, September 15–17, 1994, was chosen as a forum for these consensus development conferences. The method, the same for all three CDCs, and the specific results given as answers to previously posed questions are presented in this comprehensive article.

Methods

At their annual meeting in November 1993, the Educational Committee of the EAES decided to perform three consensus development conferences (CDCs) on the topics mentioned. The second European Congress of the EAES in September in Madrid should be the forum for a public session to discuss the final consensus statements. The Cologne group (chairmen H. Troidl, E.

Neugebauer) was authorized to organize the CDCs according to general guidelines in format and conduct. The procedure chosen was the following: A small group of panelists (10–13 members for each conference) was nominated by the Educational Committee of the E.A.E.S. Criteria for selection were (1) clinical expertise in the field of endoscopic surgery, (2) academic activity, (3) community influence, and (4) geographical location. Two chairpersons were determined and all of them (panelists and chairpersons) were asked to provide written agreements to participate. Four months prior to the conferences, each panelist got (1) a table with guidelines to use to estimate the strength of evidence in the literature for the specific endoscopical procedure, and (2) a table with the description of the levels of technology assessment (TA) according to Mosteller (1985). Each panelist was asked to indicate what level of development, in his opinion, the endoscopic procedure had attained in general and was given (3) a table with specific parameters of TA, relevant to the endoscopic procedure under assessment. In this table, the panelists were asked to indicate the status of the endoscopic procedure in comparison with conventional open procedures. The panelists' view must have been supported by evidence in the literature – a reference list was mandatory for each item in this table (always Table 12.1 in the results section of each CDC). Each panelist was given (4) a list of relevant specific questions pertaining to each procedure (questions on indication, technical aspects, training, etc.). The panelists were asked to provide brief answers with references. Guidelines for response were given and the panelists were asked to send their initial evaluations back to the conference organizers 2 months prior to the conference.

The next step was to compile and to analyze the initial evaluation of the panelists and to prepare provisional consensus statements and tables for each topic by the conference organizers. These drafts were then posted to each panelist prior to the Madrid panel meetings. At this time point, a complete list of the whole panel group was released to each panelist. In a 2-h session of each panel in Madrid, all statements and tables were discussed and modified if necessary under the leadership of the chairperson selected. When full agreement could not be obtained, the consensus was formulated on majority agreement. The consensus results of each panel were presented at the same day to the participants of the second European Congress of the EAES in topic-related plenary sessions by one of the chairpersons. Following discussion final consensus statements were formulated by the panel. The full text of the statements is given below.[1])

---

[1]) Mosteller F (1985) Assessing medical technologies. National Academic Press, Washington, DC

Table 12.1. Evaluation of feasibility and efficacy parameters for laparoscopic cholecystectomy by the panelists before the final discussion

Stages of technology assessment	Definitely better	Probably better	Similar	Probably worse	Definitely worse	Percentage of consensus [a]	Strength evidence 0–III [b]
Feasibility							
Safety (intra-op)			2	5	1	75	II
Operation time			4	4		50	II
Postop complications	1	3	4			50	II
Mortality	1	1	6			75	II
Efficacy							
Postoperative pain	8					100	II
Hospital stay	8					100	III
Return to normal activities	8					100	III
Cosmesis	8					100	II
Overall assessment	5	3				100	II

[a] Percentage of consensus was calculated by dividing the number of panelists who voted better (probably and definitely), similar, or worse (probably and definitely) by the total number of panelists who submitted their evaluation forms (8)

[b] Refer to Table 2 for definitions of the grading system

1. Results of EAES Consensus Development Conference on Laparoscopic Cholecystectomy

Chairmen: J. Perissat, Centre de Chirurgie, Université de Bordeaux, Bordeaux, France; W. Wayand, 2nd Department of Surgery, General Hospital, Linz, Austria.

Panelists: A. Cuschieri, Department of Surgery, University of Dundee, Ninewells Hospital 1 Dundee, UK; T.C. Dupont, Jefe del Opto de Cirugia, Hospital Universitario Virgen del Rocio, Seville, Spain; M. Garcia-Caballero, Department of Surgery, Medical Faculty, Malaga, Spain; J. F. Gigot, Department de Chirurgie Digestive, St. Luc Hospital, Bruxelles, Belgium; H. Glise, Department of Surgery, Norra Alsborgs, Lanssjukhus-NAL, Trollhattan, Sweden; C. Liguory, CMC Alma, Paris, France; M. Morino, Surgical Clinic, University of Torino, Turin, Italy; M. Rothmund, Department of Surgery, University of Marburg, Marburg, Germany.

Literature List with Rating

All literature submitted by the panelists as supportive evidence for their evaluation was compiled and rated (Table 12.2). Only papers of grade I and above were considered. The consensus statements were based on these published results.

Table 12.2. Ratings of published literature on laparoscopic cholecystectomy

Study type	Strength of evidence	References
Clinical randomized controlled studies with power and relevant clinical endpoints	III	[5, 26, 30, 37]
Cohort studies with controls: – Prospective, parallel controls – Prospective, historical controls Case-control studies	II	[6, 16, 19, 23, 25, 27, 29, 34, 36, 43, 44, 49, 53, 54, 57, 59]
Cohort studies with literature controls Analysis of databases Reports of expert committees	I	[1–4, 7–15, 17, 18, 20–22, 24, 28, 31–33, 35, 38–42, 45–48, 50–52, 55, 56, 58, 60–65]
Case series without controls Anecdotal reports Belief	0	Not evaluated

Table 12.3. Evaluation of stage of technology attained and strength of evidence

Stages in technology assessment[a]	Level attained/strength of evidence[b]
1. Feasibility Technical performance, applicability, safety, complications, morbidity, mortality	III
2. Efficacy Benefit for the patient demonstrated in centers of excellence	III
3. Effectiveness Benefit for the patient under normal clinical conditions, i.e., good results reproducible with widespread application	II
4. Costs Benefit in terms of cost-effectiveness	I
5. Gold standard	Yes

[a] Mosteller F (1985) Assessing medical technologies. National Academy Press, Washington, DC
[b] Level attained, and if so the strength of evidence in the literature as agreed upon by the panelists

Question 1. What Stage of Technological Development is Laparoscopic Cholecystectomy (LC) at (in Sept. 1994)?

The definitions for the stages in technological development follow the recommendations of the Committee for Evaluating Medical Technologies in Clinical Use. The panel's evaluation as to the attainment of each technological stage by laparoscopic cholecystectomy, together with the strength of evidence in the literature, is presented in Table 12.3. LC is the procedure of choice for symptomatic uncomplicated cholelithiasis. As it is not possible to conduct randomized trials on LC vs open surgery anymore, it is important for all surgeons to audit continually the results of LC. Results of analyses on its cost effectiveness and cost benefits are dependent on the health-care system. Open cholecystectomy remains the standard for comparison.

Question 2: Who Should Undergo LC?

1. The indications for cholecystectomy remain unchanged. LC is indicated for patients who are able to tolerate general anesthesia without undue risk. It is also indicated in patients with calcified (porcelain) gallbladders.
2. Asymptomatic cholelithiases, in general, do not warrant cholecystectomy. Most of the patients remain asymptomatic. It is also rare for complications to occur without symptoms appearing first. Patients with symptomless gallstones that should be followed up closely include:
   i. Diabetics
   ii. Those with sickle cell disease

iii. Children
iv. Those on long-term somatostatin
v. Those on immunosuppressive drugs
3. In the following conditions, LC is usually contraindicated.
    i. Generalized peritonitis
    ii. Septic shock from cholangitis
    iii. Severe acute pancreatitis
    iv. Cirrhosis with portal hypertension
    v. Severe coagulopathy that is not corrected
    vi. Cholecysto-enteric fistula
4. Extreme caution should be taken in the following groups of patients,
    i. Severe associated cardiorespiratory diseases
    ii. Previous upper abdominal surgery
    iii. Acute cholecystitis
    iv. Symptomatic cholecystitis in the second trimester of pregnancy

These cases should be performed only by an experienced team.

Question 3: Is LC Safe and Feasible?

1. The incidence of common bile duct injury is still slightly higher than open surgery. Vascular injury and bowel injury are specific to LC. This is due to surgeon inexperience, limitations of the two-dimensional view, lack of tactile sensation, and extension of indication to more difficult cases. Adequate training with close supervision and strict accreditation is required.
2. Operation time is similar or longer than the open procedure.
3. Morbidity from wound complications and postoperative recovery period are reduced with LC.
4. Mortality risk is similar.
5. In pregnant women, the risk of CO_2 pneumoperitoneum on the fetus in the first trimester is not fully known. LC in the third trimester should be avoided as it is technically difficult and carries a risk of injuring the uterus. Only in the second trimester is LC relatively safe, but it should only be performed by experienced operators in severely symptomatic or complicated cholelithiasis.
6. For acute cholecystitis, publications of data on small numbers of patients by keen endoscopic surgeons have reported complication rates not more than routine LC, even when performed in the same admission. However, the true safety cannot be known until more data are available. The threshold for conversion should be low. Indications for conversion include:
    i. Unclear anatomy
    ii. Gangrenous, friable gallbladder that is difficult to handle

iii. Bleeding
iv. technical problems
v. Unduly long operation time with no progress

Please refer to Table 12.2 for the definitions of the different grades.

Question 4: Is It Beneficial to the Patients?

1. LC leads to markedly less postoperative pain, shorter hospital stay, earlier return to normal activities, and better cosmesis.
2. In general, LC has a distinct advantage over open cholecystectomy.

Question 5: How Should Common Bile Stones Be Managed?

1. The optimal management of common bile duct stones (CBDS), which are present in 10–15% of patients, is not well defined. The common bile duct should be imaged in patients with a previous or present history of jaundice or pancreatitis, or abnormal liver function tests, or when ultrasonography reveals a dilated CBD. Either preoperative endoscopic retrograde cholangio-pancreatography (ERCP) or preoperative IV cholangiography (IVC) or intraoperative cholangiography (IOC) can be used to image the duct.
2. ERCP is the most reliable modality for confirming the presence of CBDS preoperatively in patients with abnormal biochemical or ultrasound findings. Endoscopic sphincterotomy (ES) and stone clearance is currently the established treatment for these patients, and is followed by LC. Studies are needed to compare the two-stage treatment (ERCP, ES + LC) with the single-stage laparaoscopic intervention (LC+laparoscopic removal of CBDS).
3. CBDS found on IOC can be treated by (1) open exploration, (2) laparoscopic exploration, (3) intra-operative ERCP, (4) postoperative ERCP, (5) careful observation, depending on the expertise available. Open exploration remains the standard technique. Laparoscopic techniques of exploration are under evaluation. Postoperative ERCP has the risk, albeit low, of failure.

Question 6. What Are the Special Technical Aspects to Be Considered During LC?

1. If problems are encountered during CO_2 insufflation with the Veress needle, the open technique should be used.
2. The junction between the cystic duct and the gall-bladder must always be clearly defined. Dissection of the junction between the cystic duct and the CBD is not necessary. Dissection in this area, principally done to identify the CBD, is, however, associated with the risk of inadvertent damage to the CBD itself.

3. Coagulation in Calot's triangle should be kept to aminimum. If needed, either bipolar or soft monopolar (less than 200 mV) coagulation is preferred.
4. Either metal clips (at least two) or locking clips are safe for securing the cystic artery and duct. In event of a large cystic duct, a ligature is safer.
5. The prevention of CBD damage by routine intraoperative cholangiogram (IOC) is not proven. However, IOC allows immediate detection of the injury and thus primary repair with better prognosis. IOC should be done when (1) anatomy is not well seen; (2) duct injury is suspected; (3) common bile duct stones are suspected. All surgeons should be trained to perform IOC.
6. To avoid injury to the CBD, the following principles should be adhered to:
7. Unambiguously identify the structures in Calot's triangle
8. Avoid unnecessary coagulation
9. Dissect starting from the gallbladder-cystic duct junction
10. Perform IOC when the anatomy is not clear
11. Convert to open surgery when in doubt
12. Drainage is usually not required
13. Suturing of trocar sites 10 mm or more is recommended especially when such a site has been dilated or extended for extraction of the gallbladder.

Question 7. What Are the Training Recommendations for LC?

Refer to EAES guidelines published in *Surgical Endoscopy* 1994; 5:721–722

References

(Grading of references is given in Table 12.2)

1. Adams DB, Borowicz MR, Wootton FT III, Cunningham JT (1993) Bile duct complications after laparoscopic cholecystectomy. Surgical Endoscopy 7:79–83
2. Airan M, Appel M, Berci G, Coburg AJ, Cohen M, Cuschieri A, Dent T, Duppler D, Easter D, Greene F, Halevey A, Hammer S, Hunter J, Jenson M, Ko ST, McFadyan B, Perissat J, Ponsky J, Ravindranathan P, Sackier JM, Soper N, Van Stiegmann G, Traverse W, Udwadia T, Unger S, Wahlstrom E, Wolfe B (1992) Retrospective and prospective multi-institutional laparoscopic cholecystectomy study organized by the Society of American Gastrointestinal Endoscopic Surgeons. Surgical Endoscopy 6:169–176
3. Assouline Y, Liguory C, Ink O, Fritsch T, Choury AD, Lefebvre JF, Pelletier G, Ruffet C, Etienne JP (1993) Current results of endoscopic sphincterotomy for lithiasis of the common bile duct. Gastroenterol Clin Biol 17:251–258
4. Baird DR, Wilson JP, Mason EM, Duncan TD, Evans JS, Luke JP, Ruben DM, Lukas GW (1992) An early review of 800 cholecystectomies at university-affiliated community teaching hospital Am Surg 58:206–210
5. Barkun JS, Barkun AN, Sampalis JS, Fried G, Taylor B, Wexler MJ, Goresky CA, Meakins JL (1992) Randomised controlled trial of laparoscopic versus mini cholecystectomy. The McGill Gallstone Treatment Group. Lancet 340:1116–1119
6. Bass EB, Pitt HA, Lillemoe KD (1993) Cost-effectiveness of laparoscopic cholecystectomy versus open cholecystectomy. Am J Surg 165:466–417

7. Collet D, Edye M, Magne F, Perissat J (1992) Laparoscopic cholecystectomy in the obese patient. Surg Endosc 6:186–188
8. Collet D, Edye M, Perissat J (1993) Conversions and complications of laparoscopic cholecystectomy. Results of a survey conducted by the French Society of Endoscopic Surgery and Interventional Radiology. Surg Endosc 7:334–338
9. Cotton PB (1993) Endoscopic retrograde cholangiopancreatography and laparoscopic cholecystectomy. Am J Surg 165:474–478
10. Cuschieri A (1993) Approach to the treatment of acute cholecystitis: open surgical, laparoscopic or endoscopic? (editorial; comment). Endoscopy 25:397–398
11. Cuschieri A, Dubois F, Mouiel J, Mouret P, Becker H, Buess G, Trede M, Troidl H (1991) The European experience with laparoscopic cholecystectomy. Am J Surg 161:385–387
12. Davids PH, Ringers J, Rauws EA, de Wit LT, Huibregtse K, der Heyde MN van, Tytgat GH (1993) Bile duct injury after laparoscopic cholecystectomy: the value of endoscopic retrograde cholangiopancreatography (see comments). Gut 34:1250–1254
13. Deziel DJ, Millikan KW, Economou SG, Doolas A, Ko ST, Airan MC (1993) Complications of laparoscopic cholecystectomy: a national survey of 4,292 hospitals and an analysis of 77,604 cases. Am J Surg 165:9–14
14. Eypasch E, Troidl H, Wood-Dauphinee S, Williams JI, Spangenberger W, Ure BM, Neugebauer E (1993) Immediate improval in quality of life after laparoscopic cholecystectomy. Minimally Invasive Ther 2:139–146
15. Feretis C, Apostolidis N, Mallas E, Manouras A, Papadimitriou J (1993) Endoscopic drainage of acute obstructive cholecystitis in patients with increased operative risk. Endoscopy 25:392–395
16. Fisher KS, Reddick EJ, Olsen DO (1991) Laparoscopic cholecystectomy: cost analysis. Surg Laparosc Endosc 1:77–81
17. Fletcher DR, Jones RM, O'Riordan R, Hardy KT (1992) Laparoscopic cholecystectomy for complicated gallstone disease. Surg Endosc 6:179–182
18. Fried CM, Barkun JS, Sigman HH, Joseph L, Clas D, Garzon J, Hinchey EJ, Meakins JL (1994) Factors determining conversion to laparotomy in patients undergoing laparoscopic cholecystectomy. Am J Surg 167:35–39; discussion 39–41
19. Fullarton GM, Darling K, Williams J, MacMillan R, Bell G (1994) Evaluation of the cost of laparoscopic and open cholecystectomy. Br J Surg 81:124–126
20. Gadacz TR, Talamini MA, Lillemoe KD, Yeo CJ (1990) Laparoscopic cholecystectomy. Surg Clin North Am 70:1249–1262
21. Go PM, Schol F, Gouma DJ (1993) Laparoscopic cholecystectomy in The Netherlands. Br J Surg 80:1180–1183
22. Gouma DJ, Go PM (1994) Bile duct injury during laparoscopic and conventional cholecystectomy. J Am Coll Surg 178:229–232
23. Grace PA, Quereshi A, Coleman J, Keane R, McEntee G, Broe P, Osbome H, Bouchier-Hayes D (1991) Reduced postoperative hospitalization after laparoscopic cholecystectomy. Br J Surg 78:160–162
24. Habicht S, Schlumpt R, Ruchmann P, Frick T, Weder W, Largiader F (1992) Is routine intraoperative cholangiography in laparoscopic cholecystectomy truly unnecessary. Helv Chir Acta 58:977–982
25. Hardy KJ, Miller H, Fletcher DR, Jones RM, Shulkes A, Mc-Neil JJ (1994) An evaluation of laparoscopic versus open cholecystectomy. Med J Aust 160:58–62
26. Hauer-Jensen M, Karesen R, Nygaard K, Solheim K, Amlie EJB, Havig O, Rosseland AR (1993) Propective randomised study of routine intraoperative cholangiography during open cholecystectomy: long-term follow-up and multivariate analysis of predictors of choledocholithiasis. Surgery 113:318–323
27. Heintz A, Menke H, Bottger T, Klupp J, Junginger T (1992) Laparoskopische Cholezystektomie: Ergebnisse einer "Matched-Pairs-Analyse". Acta Chirurg Aust 24:182–185
28. Hunter JG (1992) Laparoscopic transcystic common bile duct exploration. Am J Surg 163:53–58

29. Kelley JE, Burrus RG, Burns RP, Graham LD, Chandler KE (1993) Safety, efficacy, cost, and morbidity of laparoscopic versus open cholecystectomy: a prospective analysis of 228 consecutive patients. Am Surg 59:23–27

30. Kunz R, Orth K, Vogel J, Steinacker JM, Meitinger A, Bruckner U, Beger HG (1992) Laparoskopische Cholezystektomie versus Mini-Lap-Cholezystektomie. Ergebnisse einer prospektiven, randomisierten Studie. Chirurg 63:291–295

31. Larsen GM, Vitale GC, Casey J, Evans JS, Gilliam G, Heuser L, McGee G, Rao M, Scherm MJ, Voyles CR (1992) Multipractice analysis of laparoscopic cholecystectomy in 1983 patients. Am J Surg 163:221–226

32. Lauri A, Horton RC, Davidson BR, Burroughs AK, Dooley JS (1993) Endoscopic extraction of bile duct stones: management related to stone size. Gut 34:1718–1721

33. Lefering R, Troidl H, Ure BM (1994) Entscheiden die Kosten? Einweg- oder wiederverwendbare Instrumente bei der laparoskopischen Cholecystektomie? (Do costs decide? Disposable or reusable instruments in laparoscopic cholecystectomy?) Chirurg 65:317–325

34. Lill H, Sitter H, Klotter HJ, Nies C, Guentert-Goemann K, Rothmund M (1992) Was kostet die laparoskopische Cholecystektomie? (What is the cost of laparoscopic cholecystectomy?) Chirurg 63:1041–1044

35. MacMathuna P, White P, Clarke E, Lennon J, Crowe J (1994) Endoscopic sphincterotomy: a novel and safe alternative to papillotomy in the management of bile duct stones. Gut 35:127–129

36. McIntyre RC, Zoeter MA, Weil KC, Cohen MM (1992) A comparison of outcome and cost of open vs laparoscopic cholecystectomy. J Laparoendosc Surg 2:143–149

37. McMahon AJ, Russell IT, Baxter JN, Ross S, Anderson JR, Morran CG, Sunderland G, Galloway D, Ramsey G, O'Dwyer PJ (1994) Laparoscopic versus minilaparotomy cholecystectomy: a randomised trial (see comments). Lancet 343:135–138

38. Miller RE, Kimmelstiel FM (1993) Laparoscopic cholecystectomy for acute cholecystitis. Surg Endosc 7:296–299

39. National Institute of Health (1993) Gallstones and laparoscopic cholecystectomy. NIH Consensus Development Panel on Gallstones and Laparoscopic Cholecystectomy. Surg Endosc 7:271–279

40. Perissat J (1993) Laparoscopic cholecystectomy: the European experience Am J Surg 165:444–449

41. Perissat J, Collet D, Belliard R, Desplantez J, Magne E (1992) Laparoscopic cholecystectomy: the state of the art. A report on 700 consecutive cases. World J Surg 16:1074–1082

42. Petelin JB (1993) Laparoscopic approach to common duct pathology. Am J Surg 165:487–491

43. Peters JH, Ellison EC, Innes JT, Liss JL, Nichols KE, Lomano JM, Roby SR, Front ME, Carey LC (1991) Safety and efficacy of laparoscopic cholecystectomy. Ann Surg 213:3–12

44. Phillips EH, Carroll BJ, Pearlstein AR, Daykhovsky L, Fallas MJ (1993) Laparoscopic choledochoscopy and extraction odcommon bile duct stones. World J Surg 17:22–28

45. Phillips EH, Carroll RT, Rello JM, Fallas MT, Daykhovsky L (1992) Laparoscopic cholecystectomy in acute cholecystitis. Am Surg 58:273–276

46. Pitt HA (1993) Role of open choledochotomy in the treatment of choledocholithiasis. Am J Surg 165:483–486

47. Roselyn JJ, Birnus GS, Hughes EF, Saunders-Kirkwork, Zinner MJ, Gates JA (1993) Open cholecystectomy: a contemporary analysis of 42 474 patients. Am J Surg 218:129–137

48. Salky B, Bauer J (1994) Intravenous cholangiography, ERCP, and selective operative cholangiography in the performance of laparoscopic cholecystectomy. Surg Endosc 8:289–291

49. Schirmer BD, Dix J (1992) Cost effectiveness of laparoscopic cholecystectomy. J Laparoendosc Surg 2:145–150

50. Schlumpf R, Klotz HP, Wehrli H, Herzog U (1994) A nation's experience in laparoscopic cholecystectomy. Prospective multicenter analysis of 3722 cases. Surg Endosc 8:35–41

51. Seifert RE (1988) Long-term follow up after endoscopic sphincterotomy. Endoscopy 20:232–235

52. Soper NJ, Flye MW, Brunt LM, Stockmann PT, Sicard GA, Picus D, Edmundowicz SA, Aliperti G (1993) Diagnosis and management of biliary complications of laparoscopic cholecystectomy. Am J Surg 165:663–669
53. Soper NJ, Barteau JA, Dayman RV, Ashley SW, Dunnegan DL (1992) Comparison of early postoperative results for laparoscopic versus standard open cholecystectomy. Surg Gynecol Obstet 174:114–118
54. Stoker ME, Vose J, O'Mara P, Maini BS (1992) Laparoscopic cholecystectomy. A clinical and financial analysis of 280 operations. Arch Surg 127:589–595
55. Strasberg SM, Clavien PA (1993) Overview of therapeutic modalities for the treatment of gallstone diseases. Am J Surg 165:420–426
56. The Southern Surgeons Club (1991) A prospective analysis of 1518 laparoscopic cholecystectomies. N Engl J Med 324:1073–1078
57. Troidl H, Spangenberger W, Langen R, Al-Jaziri A, Eypasch E, Neugebauer E, Dietrich J (1992) Laparoscopic cholecystectomy. Technical performance, safety, and patient benefits. Endoscopy 24:252–261
58. Ure BM, Troidl H, Spangenberger W, Dietrich A, Lefering R, Neugebauer E (1994) Pain after laparoscopic cholecystectomy. Intensity and localization of pain and analysis of predictors in preoperative symptoms and intraoperative events. Surg Endosc 8:90–96
59. Vander Velpen GC, Shimi SM, Cuschieri A (1993) Outcome after cholecystectomy for symptomatic gall stone disease and effect of surgical access: laparoscopic vs open approach. Gut 34:1448–1451
60. Vincent-Hamelin E, Pallares AC, Felipe JAR, Rosello EL, Caperochipi JA, Cantero JLB, Gomis FD, Corvinos FF, Sanchez SP, Lesquereux JP, Puig OP (1994) National survey on laparoscopic cholecystectomy in Spain. Results of a multi-institutional study conducted by the Committee for Endoscopic Surgery. Surg Endosc 8:770–776
61. Voyles CR, Petro AB, Meena AL, Haick AJ, Koury AM (1991) A practical approach to laparoscopic cholecystectomy. Am J Surg 161:365–370
62. Wilson RG, Macintyre IM, Nixon SJ, Saunders JH, Varma JS, King PM (1992) Laparoscopic cholecystectomy as a safe and effective treatment for severe acute cholecystitis. BMJ 305:394–396
63. Wolfe BM, Gardiner BN, Leary BF, Frey CF (1991) Endoscopic cholecystectomy. An analysis of complications. Arch Surg 126:1192–1198
64. Woods MS, Traverso LW, Kozarek RA, Tsao J, Rossi RL, Cough D, Donohue JH (1994) Characteristics of biliary tract complications during laparoscopic cholecystectomy: a multi-institutional study. Am J Surg 167:27–33
65. Zucker KA, Flowers JL, Bailey RW, Graham SM, Buell J, Imbembo AL (1993) Laparoscopic management of acute cholecystitis. Am J Surg 165:508–514

2. Results of EAES Consensus Development Conference on Laparoscopic Appendectomy

Chairman: E. Eypasch, 2nd Department of Surgery, University of Cologne, Germany; C.K. Kum, Department of Surgery, National University Hospital, Singapore.
Panelists: O.J. McAnenna, Surgical Unit, University College Hospital, Galway, Ireland; M. McMahon, Leeds Institute for Minimally Invasive Therapy, The General Infirmary, Leeds, UK; S. Attwood, Meath Hospital, Dublin, Ireland; E. Schippers, Department of Surgery, Clinic RWTH, Aachen, Germany; J. Jakimowicz, Department of Surgery, Catharina Hospital, Eindhoven, The Netherlands; W. van Erp, Department of Surgery, Diaconessenhuis, Eindho-

Table 12.4. Evaluation of feasibility and efficacy parameters for laparoscopic appendectomy by the panelists before the final discussion

Stages of technology assessment	Definitely better	Probably better	Similar	Probably worse	Definitely worse	Percentage of consensus a)	Strength of evidence 0–III b)
Feasibility							
Safety		1	8	2		73	II
Operation time			3	7	1	73	III
Postop complications		6	4			64	III
Mortality	1		9	1 c)		82	I
Efficacy							
Diagnostic accuracy	7	4				100	II
Wound infection	8	3				100	III
Postoperative pain	4	6	1			91	II
Hospital stay	2	6	3			73	II
Return to normal activities	5	5	1			91	III
Postoperative adhesions	1	7	2 c)			73	I
Cosmesis	4	4	2 c)			73	0
Overall assessment	3	6	1	1		7	II

a) Percentage of consensus was calculated by dividing the number of panelists who voted better (probably and definitely), similar, or worse (probably and definitely) by the total number of panelists [11]

b) Refer to Table 2 for definitions of the grading system

c) One panelist wrote "unknown" or left it blank. He is presumed to have voted with this minority group when the percentage of agreement was calculated.

Table 12.5. Ratings of published literature on laparoscopic appendectomy

Study type	Strength of evidence	References
Clinical randomized controlled studies with power, and relevant clinical end points	III	[2, 6, 10, 12, 23, 33]
Cohort studies with controls – Prospective, parallel controls – Prospective, historical controls Case-control studies	II	[3, 4, 8, 13, 18, 19, 25, 27, 29, 32, 34, 36, 38]
Cohort studies with literature controls Analysis of databases Reports of expert committees	I	[1, 5, 7, 9, 14, 16, 20–22, 24, 26, 30, 37]
Case series without controls Anecdotal reports Belief	0	[15, 17, 28, 31, 35, 39]

ven, The Netherlands. P. Testas, Service de Chirurgie Generate, Centre Hospitalier Bicetre, Le Kremlin-Bicetre Cedex, France; J. A. Lujan Mompean, Department of General Surgery, University Hospital "Virgen de la Arrixac", El Palmar, Murcia, Spain; J. S. Valla, Hopital pour Enfants, Nice, France.

Literature List with Rating

All literature submitted by the panelists as supportive evidence for their evaluation was compiled and rated (Table 12.5). The consensus statements were based on these published results.

Question 1. What Stage of Technological Development is Laparoscopic Appendectomy (LA) at (in Sept. 1994)?

The definitions for the stages in technological development follow the recommendations of the Committee for Evaluating Medical Technologies in Clinical Use. The panel's evaluation as to the attainment of each technological stage by laparoscopic appendectomy, together with the strength of evidence in the literature, is presented in Table 12.6. LA is presently at the efficacy stage of development because most of the data on feasibility and safety originate from centers with a special interest in endoscopic surgery. More data on its use in general and district hospitals are needed to ascertain its effectiveness. Detailed analysis on its cost-effectiveness and cost benefits is also lacking. Although a very promising procedure, it is not yet the gold standard for acute appendicitis.

Table 12.6. Evaluation of stage of technology attained and strength of evidence

Stages in technology assessment[a]	Level attained/strength of evidence[b]
1. Feasibility Technical performance, applicability, safety, complications, morbidity, mortality	III
2. Efficacy Benefit for the patient demonstrated in centers of excellence	III
3. Effectiveness Benefit for the patient under normal clinical conditions, i.e., good results reproducible with widespread application	I
4. Costs Benefit in terms of cost-effectiveness	Unknown
5. Gold standard	No

[a] Mosteller F (1985) Assessing Medical Technologies. National Academy Press, Washington, DC

[b] Level attained, and if so, the strength of evidence in the literature as agreed upon by the panelists. Please refer to Table 12.5 for the definitions of the different grades

Question 2: Is LA Safe and Feasible?

1. There is no evidence in published literature that LA is any less safe than open appendectomy (OA).
2. Operation time, depending on the experience of the surgeon, is similar or longer than the open procedure.
3. Postoperative complications – e.g., bleeding, intraabdominal abscess, re-operation – are not more frequent than OA in the published literature. However, the morbidity associated with widespread application is not yet known.
4. LA is not contraindicated for perforated appendicitis. However, more data for this subgroup of patients is needed.
5. LA may be attempted for an appendiceal abscess by an experienced surgeon if the abscess is to be treated early. Conversion to open surgery should be undertaken when difficulties are encountered. Alternatively, delayed elective LA can be performed after resolution of the abscess with antibiotic therapy.
6. LA can be used in children. It should be performed only by surgeons with ample experience in adult LA. Smaller instruments should be available to improve safety and ergonomy.
7. The safety of LA during pregnancy is not established.
8. The indication for elective LA is the same as for open elective appendectomy.

Question 3: Is It Beneficial to the Patients?

1. Laparascopy improves the diagnostic accuracy of acute right iliac fossa pain, especially in children and young women.
2. LA reduces wound infection rate.
3. There is less postoperative pain in adults. There are no data in children.
4. Hospital stay is similar or less than OA.
5. LA allows earlier return to normal activities.
6. The laparoscopic approach may lead to less post-operative adhesions.
7. Cosmesis may be better than OA.
8. All in all, LA has advantages over OA. However, the potential for serious injuries must be appreciated and avoided in order to make the postoperative advantages worthwhile.

Question 4. What Are the Special Technical Aspects to Be Considered During LA?

The statements here are meant to be guidelines. The surgeon at the operating table has to be the ultimate judge as to what is safe to do.
1. Convert to open surgery if the appendix cannot be found.
2. At diagnostic laparoscopy, there is no obligation to remove the appendix.
3. Bipolar coagulation is a perferred mode of coagulating the artery. Monopolar diathermy may be safe if the appropriate precautions are taken. Use of clips alone or in combination with coagulation is the alternative. Suture ligation of the artery is usually unnecessary. Lasers and staples are not cost-effective.
4. When the base of the appendix is healthy and un-inflamed, one properly applied preformed ligature is probably enough. If in doubt, use two loops. Metal clips alone are not recommended; staples are too expensive and not required in most cases.
5. The appendix should be transected at about 5 mm from the last preformed ligature. It is unnecessary to bury the stump.
6. To avoid wound infection, the appendix should be removed through the port or if too big, within a pouch.
7. Peritoneal toilet is recommended in cases of intraabdominal contamination.
8. The antibiotic policy should be the same as for open appendectomy.

Question 5. What Are the Training Recommendations for LA?

1. LA should be part of the resident's curriculum.
2. At least 20 cases of LA are needed for accredition in general surgery.

Summary

Laparoscopic appendectomy is an efficacious new technology. Its safety and feasibility have been shown in the published literature, mainly from centers with a special interest in endoscopic surgery. However, a few cases of serious complications have been reported. Surgeons should be aware of the potential dangers.

Benefits for the patients, especially in terms of more accurate diagnosis, reduction of wound infection, and earlier return to work, have also been shown in controlled trials, albeit with small numbers of patients. Its effectiveness, compared to open appendectomy, when applied generally to all grades of hospitals, remains to be seen. The cost-effectiveness of LA is not known. Although promising, it is not yet the gold standard for acute appendicitis.

References

(Grading of references is given in Table 12.5)

1. Apelgren KN, Molnar RG, Kisala JM (1992) Is laparoscopic better than open appendectomy? Surg Endosc 6:298–301
2. Attwood SEA, Hill ADK, Murphy PC, Thornton J, Stephens RB (1992) A prospective randomised trial of laparoscopic versus open appendectomy. Surgery 112:497–501
3. Baigrie RJ, Scott-Coombes D, Saidin Z, Vipond MN, Paterson-Brown S, Thompson JN (1992) The selective use of fine catheter peritoneal cytology and laparoscopy reduces the unnecessary appendectomy rate. Br J Clin Pract 46:173
4. De Wilde RL (1991) Goodbye to late bowel obstruction after appendicectomy. Lancet 338:1012
5. El Ghoneimi A, Valla JS, Limonne B, Valla V, Montupet P, Grinda A (1994) Laparoscopic appendectomy in children: report of 1379 cases. J Paediatr Surg 29:786–789
6. Frazee RC, Roberts JW, Symmonds RE, Snyder SK, Hendricks JC, Smith RW, Custer MD 3rd, Harrison JB (1994) A prospective randomised trial comparing open versus laparoscopic appendectomy. Ann Surg 219:725–731
7. Frittz LL, Orlando R (1994) Laparoscopic appendectomy. A safety and cost analysis. Arch Surg 128:521–525
8. Gilchrist BF, Lobe TE, Schropp KP, Kay GA, Hixson SD, Wrenn EL, Philippe PG, Hollabaugh RS (1992) Is there a role for laparoscopic appendectomy in paediatric surgery? J Paediatr Surg 27:209–214
9. Grunewald B, Keating J (1993) Should the 'normal' appendix be removed at operation for appendicitis? J R Coll Surg Edinb 38:158
10. Hebebrand D, Troidl H, Spangenberger W, Neugebauer E, Schwalm T, Gunther MW (1994) Laparoscopic or conventional appendectomy? A prospective randomised trial. Chirurg 65:112–120
11. Hill ADK, Attwood SEA, Stephens RB (1991) Laparoscopic appendectomy for acute appendicitis is safe and effective. Ir J Med Sci 160:268
12. Kum CK, Ngoi SS, Goh PMY, Tekant Y, Isaac JR (1993) Randomized controlled trial comparing laparoscopic appendectomy to open appendectomy. Br J Surg 80:1599–1600
13. Kum CK, Sim EKW, Goh PMY, Ngoi SS, Rauff A (1993) Diagnostic laparoscopy–reducing the number of normal appendectomies. Dis Colon Rectum 36:763–766
14. Lau WY, Fan ST, Yiu TF, Chu KW, Suen HC, Wong KK (1986) The clinical significance of routine histopathological study of the resected appendix and safety of appendiceal inversion. Surg Gynecol Obstet 162:256–258

15. Leahy PF (1989) Technique of laparoscopic appendectomy. Br J Surg 76:616
16. Leape LL, Ramenofsky ML (1980) Laparoscopy for questionable appendicitis: can it reduce the negative appendectomy rate? Am Surg 191:410–413
17. Loh A, Taylor RS (1992) Laparoscopic appendectomy. Br J Surg 79:289–290
18. Lujan JA, Robles R, Parilla P, Soria V, Garcia-Ayllon J (1994) Acute appendicitis. Assessment of laparoscopic appendectomy versus open appendectomy. A prospective trial. Br J Surg 81:133–135
19. McAnena OJ, Austin O, Hederman WP, Gorey TF, Fitzpatrick J, O'Connell PR (1991) Laparoscopic versus open appendicectomy. Lancet 338:693
20. Meinke AK, Kossuth T (1994) What is the learning curve for laparoscopic appendectomy? Surg Endosc 8:371–375
21. Nouailles JM (1990) Technique resultats et limites de l'appen-dicectomie par voie coeliescopique. A propos de 360 malades. Chirugie 116:834–837
22. Nowzaradan Y, Westmorland J, McCarver CT, Harris RJ (1991) Laparoscopic appendectomy for acute appendicitis: indications and current use. J Laparoendosc Surg 1:247–257
23. Olsen JB, Myren CJ, Haahr PE (1993) Randomised study of the value of laparoscopy before appendectomy. Br J Surg 80:922–923
24. Pier A, Gotz F, Bacher C (1991) Laparoscopic appendectomy in 625 cases: from innovation to routine. Surg Endosc Laparosc 1:8–13
25. Reiertsen O, Bakka A, Anderson OK, Larsen S, Rosseland AR (1994) Prospective non-randomised study of conventional versus laparoscopic appendectomy. World J Surg 18:441–446
26. Saye WB, Rives DA, Cochran EB (1992) Laparoscopic appendectomy: three years' experience. Surg Endosc Laparosc 2:109–115
27. Schirmer BC, Schmieg RE, Dix J, Edge SB, Hanks JB (1993) Laparoscopic versus traditional appendectomy for suspected appendicitis. Am J Surg 165:670–675
28. Schreiber JH (1987) Early experience with laparoscopic appendectomy in women. Surg Endosc 1:211–216
29. Schroder DM, Lathrop JC, Lloyd LR, Boccacio JE, Hawasli A (1993) Laparoscopic appendectomy for acute appendicitis: is there a real benefit? Am Surg 59:541–548
30. Scott-Corner CE, Hall TJ, Anglin BL. Muakkassa FF (1992) Laparoscopic appendectomy. Initial experience in teaching program. Ann Surg 215:660–668
31. Semm K (1983) Endoscopic appendectomy. Endoscopy 15:59–63
32. Sosa JL, Sleeman D, McKenny MG, Dygert J, Yarish D, Martin L (1993) A comparison of laparoscopic and conventional appendectomy. J Laparosc Endosc Surg 3:129
33. Tate JJT, Dawson J, Chung SCS, Lau WY, Li AKC (1993) Laparoscopic versus open appendectomy: prospective randomised trial. Lancet 342:633–637
34. Tate JJT, Chung SCS, Dawson J, Leong HT, Chan A, Lau WY, Li AKC (1993) Conventional versus laparoscopic surgery for acute appendicitis. Br J Surg 80:761–764
35. Troidl H, Gaitzsch A, Winkler-Wilfurth A, Mueller W (1993) Fehler und Gefahren bei der laparoskopischen Appendektomie. Chining 64:212–220
36. Ure BM, Spangenberger W, Hebebrand D, Eypasch E, Troidl H (1992) Laparoscopic surgery in children and adolescents with suspected appendicitis. Eur J Paediatr Surg 2:336–340
37. Valla JS, Limonne B, Valla V, Montupet P, Daoud N, Grinda A, Chavrier Y (1991) Laparoscopic appendectomy in children: report of 465 cases. Surg Laparosc Endosc 1:166–172
38. Vallina VL, Velsaco JM, Me Cullough CS (1993) Laparoscopic versus conventional appendectomy. Ann Surg 218:685–692
39. Welch NT, Hinder RA, Fitzgibbons RJ (1991) Incidental appendectomy. Surg Laparosc Endosc 1:116–118

3. Results of EAES Consensus Development Conference on Laparoscopic Hernia Repair

Chairmen: A. Fingerhut, Department de Chirurgie, Centre Hospitaller Intercommunale, Poissy, France; A. Paul, 2nd Department of Surgery, University of Cologne, Germany

Panelists: J.-H. Alexandre, Department de Chirurgie, Hopital Broussais, Paris, France; M. Biichler, University Hospital for Visceral and Transplantation Surgery, Bern, Switzerland; J.L. Dulucq, Department de Chirurgie, M.S.P. Bagatelle, Talence-Bordeaux, France; P. Go, Department of Surgery, University Hospital Maastricht, Maastricht, The Netherlands; J. Himpens Hopital Universitaire St. Pierre, Department de Chirurgie, Bruxelles, Belgium: C. Klaiber, Department of Surgery, General Hospital, Aarberg, Switzerland; E. Laporte, Department of Surgery, Policlinica Teknon, Barcelona, Spain; B. Millat, Department de Chirurgie, Centre Hospitalier Universitaire, Montpellier, France; J. Mouiel, Department de Chirurgie Digestive, Hopital Saint Roche, Nice, France; L. Nyhus, Department of Surgery, College of Medicine, The University of Illinois at Chicago, Chicago, USA; V. Schumpelick, Department of Surgery, Clinic RWTH, Aachen, Germany

Literature List with Rating

All literature submitted by the panelists as supportive evidence for their evaluation was compiled and rated (Table 12.8). The consensus statements were based on these published results.

Question 1. Is There a Need for the Classification of Groin Hernias, and If So, Which Classification Should Be Used?

Several classifications for groin hernias have been proposed (Alexandre, Bendavid, Gilbert, Nyhus, Schumpelick). The majority of the panelists refer to Nyhus's classification (Table 12.9). It is suggested that this classification be applied in future trials. However, the accuracy and reproducibility of any classification in laparoscopic hernia repair still must be demonstrated.

In any case, the minimal requirements for future studies are classifications which accurately describe the defects:
- The type: direct, indirect, femoral or combined
- State of the internal ring (dilated or not)
- Presence and size of the posterior wall defect
- Size and contents of the sac
- Whether primary or recurrent

Table 12.7. Evaluation of feasibility and efficacy for laparoscopic herniorrhaphy by the panelists before the final discussion

Stages of technology assessment	Definitely better	Probably better	Similar	Probably worse	Definitely worse	Strength of evidence 0–III[b]
Feasibility						
Safety of intraabdominal techniques			6	5	1	I
Safety of extraabdominal techniques (54%)[a]	1	4	7	1		I
Operation time (77%)		2	1	8	2	II
Adverse events						
Spermatic cord injury (54%)	1	4	7	1		I
Testicular vessel injury (62%)	1	7	4	1		I
Nerve injury (50%)		3	6	3		I
Ileus (intraabdominal methods) (70%)		1	2	4	3	I
Bleeding (73%)	1	7	2	1		I
Wound infection (70%)	1	6	3			I
Reoperation (50%)	1	4	3	2		I
Disability (75%)	1	8	2	1		I
Mortality (92%)			11		1	I
Efficacy						
Postoperative pain (85%)	4	7		1	1	II
Hospital stay (58%)	3	4	4		1	II
Return to normal activities (75%)	4	5	2		1	II
Cosmesis	2	3	4			I
Recurrence	1	4	5		1	I
Overall assessment (64%)		7	2	2		II

[a] Percentage of agreement calculated by dividing the number of panelists who voted better (probably and definitely), similar, or worse (probably and definitely) by the total number of panelists [9]
[b] Refer to Table 12.8 for definitions of the grading system

Question 2. In What Stage of Technological Development is Endoscopic Hernia Repair (in Sept. 1994)?

Endoscopic hernia repair is presently a feasible alternative for conventional hernia repair if performed by experienced endoscopic surgeons. It appears to be efficacious in the short term. It has not yet reached the effectiveness stage in general practice. Detailed analysis on cost-effectiveness and cost benefits are lacking. Although some aspects of endoscopic hernia repair are

Table 12.8. Ratings of published literature on laparoscopic hernia repair

Study type	Strength of evidence	References
Clinical randomized controlled studies with power and relevant clinical endpoints	III	[42, 43,54]
Cohort studies with controls – Prospective, parallel controls – Prospective, historical controls Case-control studies	II	[7, 15, 36]
Cohort studies with literature controls Analysis of databases Reports of expert committees	I	[2, 3, 5, 6, 8–10, 13, 14, 16–21, 23–35, 38–41, 44–51, 55–61]
Case series without controls Anecdotal reports Belief	0	[1, 4, 11, 12, 22, 37, 52, 53]

Table 12.9. Nyhus classification for groin hernia

Type of hernia	Anatomical defect
I	Indirect hernia-normal internal ring
II	Indirect hernia-dilated internal ring
III A	Direct hernia-posterior wall defect
III B	Large indirect hernia-posterior wall defect
III C	Femoral hernia
IV	Recurrent hernia

See [40]

very promising (e.g., recurrence and bilateral hernia), it cannot be considered the standard treatment. (Table 12.10.)

Question 3. Is Endoscopic Hernia Repair Safe?

Endoscopic hernia repair may be as safe as the open procedure. However, up until now, safety aspects have not been sufficiently evaluated. Most panellists agreed that it has the same potential for serious complications as in open surgery–such as postoperative ileus, nerve injury, and injuries to large vessels. Reporting all complications, fatal or not, is encouraged and necessary for further evaluation.

Table 12.10. Stages of technology assessment in endoscopic hernia repair

Stages in technology assessment[a]	Level attained/strength of evidence[b]
1. Feasibility Technical performance, applicability, safety, complications, morbidity, mortality	I
2. Efficacy Benefit for the patient demonstrated in centers of excellence	II
3. Effectiveness Benefit for the patient under normal clinical conditions, i.e., good results reproducible with widespread application	0
4. Costs Benefit in terms of cost-effectiveness	0
5. Gold standard	No

[a] Mosteller F (1985) Assessing medical technologies. National Academy Press, Washington, DC
[b] Level attained, and if so the strength of evidence in the literature as agreed upon the panelists. Refer to Table 2 for the definitions of the different grades.

Question 4. Is Endoscopic Hernia Repair Beneficial to the Patient?

The potential reduction in the incidence of hematoma and clinically relevant wound infections has yet to be proven. Postoperative pain seems to be diminished. Although it seems to allow earlier return to normal activities, postoperative disability and hospital stay are highly dependent on activity, motivation, and social status of the patient as well as the structure of the health-care system.

Objective measurement (e.g., standardized exercise tests) should be developed and used to evaluate return to normal activity.

As in other endoscopic procedures, there is a potential for better cosmetic results. The long-term recurrence rate for endoscopic hernia repair is not known.

Question 5. Who Is a Potential Candidate for Endoscopic Hernia Repair?

Candidates:
- Type III A–C
- Recurrences (type IV), bilateral hernia
- Type II?

Contraindications:
Absolute:
- High-risk patients for general anesthesia or conventional surgery
- Unconnected bleeding disorders

- Proven adverse reaction to foreign material
- Major intraabdominal disease (e.g., ascites)

Relative:
- Incarcerated or scrotal (sliding) hernia
- Young age (sac resection only)
- Prior major abdominal operations

Question 6. What Concepts Should Be Used in the Future Evaluation of Endoscopic Hernia Repair?

There is a definite need for classification and randomized controlled (multicenter) trials with clear end points:

- Complication and recurrence rates (over 5 years, with less than 5% lost to follow-up)
- Pain and physical activity resumption
- Size, type, and route of mesh placement

Endoscopic techniques should be compared to conventional hernia or open preperitoneal prosthetic mesh repair techniques vs laparoscopic transabdominal preperitoneal (TAPP) and/or extraperitoneal or totally preperitoneal repair (TPP).

Question 7. Should Endoscopic Hernia Repair Be Performed Outside Clinical Trials?

In 1994, we recommend that endoscopic hernia repair should only be performed after appropriate training and with some sort of quality control.

References

(Grading of references is given in Table 12.8)

1. Andrew DR, Gregory RP, Richardson DR (1994) Meralgia paresthetica following laparoscopic inguinal erniorraphy. Br J Surg 81:715
2. Arregui ME, Davis CJ, Yucel O, Nagan RF (1992) Laparoscopic mesh repair of inguinal hernia using a preperitoneal approach: a preliminary report. Surg Laparosc Endosc 2:53–58
3. Arregui ME, Navarrete J, Davis CJ, Castro D, Nagan RF (1993) Laparoscopic inguinal hemiorrhaphy. Techniques and controversies. Surg Clin North Am 73:513–527
4. Barnes FE (1993) Cost-effective hernia repair. Arch Surg 128:600
5. Begin GF (1993) Laparoscopic extraperitoneal treatment of inguinal hernias in adults. A series of 200 cases. Endosc Surg 1:204–206
6. Berliner SD (1989) Biomaterials in hernia repair. In: Nyhus LM, Condon RE (eds). Hernia, 3rd ed. Lippincott, Philadelphia, pp 541–558
7. Brooks DC (1994) A prospective comparison of laparoscopic and tension-free open hemiorrhaphy. Arch Surg 129:361–366

8. Corbitt JD (1993) Transabdominal preperitoneal hemiorrhaphy. Surg Laparosc Endosc 3:328–332
9. Corbitt JD (1994) Transabdominal preperitoneal laparoscopic hemiorrhaphy. In: Arregui ME, Nagan RF (eds) Inguinal hernia: advances or controversies? Radcliffe Medical Press, Oxford, pp 283–287
10. Dulucq JL (1992) Traitement des hernies de l'aine par mise en place d'un patch prothetique sous-peritoneal en pre-peritoneoscopie. Chirurgie 118:83–85
11. Editorial (1993) Surgical innovation under scrutiny. Lancet 342:187–188
12. Eubanks St, Newmann III L, Goehring L, Lucas GW, Adams Ch P, Mason E, Duncan T (1993) Meralgia paresthetica: a complication of laparoscopic hemiorrhaphy. Surg Laparosc Endosc 3:381–385
13. Fiennes A, Taylor R (1994) Learning laparoscopic hernia repair: pitfalls and complications among 178 repairs. In: Arregui ME, Nagan RF (eds) Inguinal hernia: advances or controversies? Radcliffe Medical Press, Oxford, pp 270–274, 407–410
14. Filipi Ch J, Fitzgibbons RJ Jr, Salerno GM. Hart RO (1992) Laparoscopic hemiorrhaphy. Surg Clin North Am 72:1109–1124
15. Fitzgibbons R Jr, Annibali R, Litke B, Filipi C, Salerno G, Comet D (1993) A multicentered clinical trial on laparoscopic inguinal hernia repair: preliminary results. Surg Endosc 7:115
16. Fromont G, Leroy J (1993) Laparoskopischer Leistenhemienverschluss durch subperitoneale Prostheseneinlage (Operation nach Stoppa). Chirurg 64:338–340
17. Geis WP, Crafton WB, Novak MJ, Malago M (1993) Laparoscopic hemiorrhaphy: results and technical aspects in 450 consecutive procedures. Surgery 114:765–774
18. Go PMNYH (1994) Prospective comparison studies on laparoscopic inguinal hernia repair. Surg Endosc 8:719–720
19. Graciac C, Estakhri M, Patching S (1994) Lateral-slit laparoscopic hemiorrhaphy. Surg Endosc 8:592
20. Guillen J, Aldrete JA (1970) Anesthetic factors influencing morbidity and mortality of elderly patients undergoing inguinal hemiorrhaphy. Am J Surg 120:760–763
21. Harrop-Griffiths W (1994) General, regional or local anesthesia for hernia repair. In: Arregui ME, Nagan RF (eds) Inguinal hernia: advances or controversies? Radcliffe Medical Press, Oxford, pp 297–299
22. Hendrickse CW, Evans DS (1993) Intestinal obstruction following laparoscopic inguinal hernia repair. Br J Surg 80:1432
23. Himpens JM (1992) Laparoscopic hernioplasty using a self-expandable (umbrella-like) prosthetic patch. Surg Laparosc Endosc 2:312–316
24. Hoffman HC, Vinton Traverso AL (1993) Preperitoneal prosthetic herniorrhaphy. One surgeon's successful technique. Arch Surg 128:964–970
25. Katkhouda N (1994) Complications of laparoscopic hernia repair. In: Arregui ME, Nagan RF(eds) Inguinal hernia: advances or controversies? Radcliffe Medical Press, Oxford, p 277
26. Kavic MS (1993) Laparoscopic hernia repair. Surg Endosc 7:163–167
27. Kraus MA (1994) Laparoscopic identification of preperitoneal nerve anatomy in the inguinal area. Surg Endosc 8:377–381
28. Lichtenstein IL, Shulman AG, Amid PK, Montllor MM (1989) The tension-free hernioplasty. Am J Surg 157:188–193
29. Lichtenstein IL, Shulman AG, Amid PK (1991) Laparoscopic hernioplasty. Arch Surg 126:1449
30. MacFadyen BV Jr, Arregui ME, Corbitt JD Jr, Filipi Ch J, Fitzgibbons RJ Jr, Franklin ME, Me Keman JB, Olsen DO, Phillips EH, Rosenthal D, Schultz LS, Sewell RW, Smoot RT, Spaw AT, Toy FK, Waddell RL, Zucker KA (1993) Complications of laparoscopic herniorrhaphy. Surg Endosc 7:155–158
31. MacFadyen BV Jr (1994) Laparoscopic inguinal herniorrhaphy: complications and pitfalls. In: Arregui ME, Nagan RF (eds) Inguinal hemia: advances or controversies? Radcliffe Medical Press, Oxford, p 289

32. Macintyre IMC (1992) Laparoscopic herniorrhaphy. Br J Surg 79:1123–1124
33. McKernan JB, Laws HL (1993) Laparoscopic repair of inguinal hernias using a totally extraperitoneal prosthetic approach. Surg Endosc 7:26–28
34. McMahon AJ, Baxter JN, O'Dwyer PJ (1993) Preventing complications of laparoscopy. Br J Surg 80:1593–1594
35. Millat B, Fingerhut A, Gignoux M, Hay J-M, the French Association for Surgical Research (1993) Factors associated with early discharge after inguinal hernia repair in 500 consecutive unselected patients. Br J Surg 80:1158–1160
36. Millikan KW, Kosik ML, Doolas A (1994) A prospective comparison of transabdominal preperitoneal laparoscopic hemia repair versus traditional open hernia repair in a university setting. Surg Laparosc Endosc 4:247–253
37. Notaras MJ (1994) No benefit in hernia repair. BMJ 308:199
38. Nyhus LM, Pollak R, Bombeck CT, Donahue PE (1988) The preperitoneal approach and prosthetic buttress repair for recurrent hemia. Ann Surg 208:733–737
39. Nyhus LM (1992) Laparoscopic hemia repair: a point of view. Arch Surg 127:137
40. Nyhus LM (1993) Individualization of hemia repair: a new era. Surgery 114:1–2
41. Panton ONM, Panton RJ (1994) Laparoscopic hernia repair. Am J Surg 167:535–537
42. Payne JH Jr, Grininger LM, Izawa M, Lindahl PJ, Podoll EF (1994) A randomized prospective comparison between an open and a laparoscopic repair of inguinal hernias. Surg Endosc 8:478
43. Payne JH Jr, Grininger LM, Izawa MT, Podoll EF, Lindahl PJ, Balfour J (1994) Laparoscopic or open inguinal herniorrhaphy?–A randomized prospective trial. Arch Surg (in press)
44. Phillips EH, Carroll BJ, Fallas MJ (1993) Laparoscopic preperitoneal inguinal hernia repair without peritoneal incision. Technique and early clinical results. Surg Endosc 7:159–162
45. Phillips EH, Carroll BJ, Fallas MJ, Arregui ME, Colbit J, Fitzgibbons R, Pietrafita J, Sewell R, Seid A, Shulte R, Toy F, Waddell R (1994) Reasons for recurrence following laparoscopic hernioplasty. In: Arregui ME, Nagan RF (eds) Inguinal hernia: advances or controversies? Radcliffe Medical Press, Oxford, pp 297–299
46. Phillips EH, Carroll BJ (1994) Laparoscopic inguinal hernia repair. Gastrointest Endosc Clin North Am (in press)
47. Rutkow IM (1992) Laparoscopic hernia repair: the socioeconomic tyranny of surgical technology. Arch Surg 127:1271
48. Rutkow IM, Robbins AW (1993) Demographic, classificatory, and socioeconomic aspects of hernia repair in the United States. Surg Clin North Am 73:413–426
49. Rutkow IM, Robbins AW (1993) "Tension-free" inguinal herniorrhaphy: a preliminary report on the "mesh plug" technique. Surgery 114:3–8
50. Schumpelick V, Treutner KH, Arlt G (1994) Inguinal hernia repair in adults. Lancet 344:375–379
51. Sewell R, Waddell R (1994) Complications of laparoscopic inguinal hemia repair. In: Arregui ME, Nagan RF (eds) Inguinal hernia: advances or controversies? Radcliffe Medical Press, Oxford, pp 401–405
52. Spier LN, Lazzaro RS, Procaccino A, Geiss A (1993) Entrapment of small bowel after laparoscopic herniorrhaphy. Surg Endosc 7:535–536
53. Stoker DL, Wellwood JM (1993) Return to work after inguinal hemia repair. Br J Surg 80:1354–1355
54. Stoker DL, Spiegelhalter DJ, Singh R, Wellwood JM (1994) Laparoscopic versus open inguinal hernia repair: randomised prospective trial. Lancet 343:1243–1245
55. Stoppa RE, Warlaumont ChR (1989) The preperitoneal approach and prosthetic repair of groin hernia. In: Nyhus LM, Condon RE (eds) Hernia, 3rd ed. Lippincott, Philadelphia, pp 199–225
56. Stoppa RE, Rives JL, Warlaumont ChR, Palot JP, Verhaeghe PJ, Delattre JF (1984) The use of Dacron in the repair of hernias of the groin. Surg Clin North Am 64:269–285

57. Stoppa R (1987) Hernia of the abdominal wall. In: Chevrel JP (ed) Surgery of the abdominal wall. Springer, Berlin Heidelberg New York, p 155
58. Stuart AE (1994) Taking the tension out of hernia repair. Lancet 343:748
59. Taylor RS, Leopold PW, Loh A (1994) Improved patient well-being following laparoscopic inguinal hernia repair – the St.George's experience. In: Arregui ME, Nagan RF (eds) Inguinal hernia: advances or controversies? Radcliffe Medical Press, Oxford, p 407
60. Testik C, Arregui M, Castro D, Davis C, Dulucq JL, Fitzgibbons R, Franklin M, Hammond J, Me Kernan J, Rosin R, Schultz L, Toy F (1994) Complications and recurrences associated with laparoscopic repair of groin hernias: a multiinstitutional retrospective analysis. In: Arregui ME, Nagan RF (eds) Inguinal hernia: advances or controversies? Radcliffe Medical Press, Oxford, pp 495–500
61. Winchester DJ, Dawes LG, Modelski DD, Nahrwold DL, Pomerantz RA, Prystowsky JB, Rege RV, Joehl RJ (1993) Laparoscopic inguinal hernia repair. A preliminary experience. Arch Surg 128: 781–786

Cholecystolithiasis – Update 2006

Jörg Zehetner, Andreas Shamiyeh, Wolfgang Wayand

Definition, Epidemiology and Clinical Course

Cholecystolithiasis is gallstone formation in the gallbladder. Gallstone disease has a great impact on a surgeon's daily routine. The prevalence of cholecystolithiasis is 10–12% in the western world and about 3–4% in Asian populations [10]. The costs for the treatment of biliary stone disease in the prelaparoscopic aera were estimated at US $ 16 billion in the USA in 1987 [34], about one million people are newly diagnosed annually in the USA, and approximately 600,000 operations are performed a year.

Diagnostics

Abdominal ultrasound is the primary tool for the diagnosis of cholecystolithiasis. In combination with laboratory findings and patient history, the correct diagnosis should be made. In the first years of laparoscopic cholecystectomy (LC), intravenous cholangiography (IVC) was used as a valuable tool for the imaging of the bile duct's anatomy in order to prevent common bile duct injuries and to diagnose possible bile duct stones. IVC is entailed with possible adverse reactions [19] and after initial experience of LC, IVC was considered not to be used as a routine screening modality preoperatively [3]. Spiral CT cholangiography is not suitable for routine diagnosis before LC [28] as well as endoscopic retrograde cholangiopancreatography [18]. Details on the management of common bile duct stones can be found in the appropriate chapter of this book.

Routine gastroscopy prior to LC is still discussed controversially. While some authors claim it as a standard examination before LC, others do not [27, 30, 32]. Endoscopy prior to cholecystectomy should be performed only in patients with a history of upper abdominal pain or discomfort [1, 5, 33].

Operative Versus Conservative Treatment

Operative treatment is indicated for symptomatic gallstones. Conservative treatment is appropriate for asymptomatic gallstones as well as in patients with high operative risk according to the EAES Consensus statements (1994), and this still holds true.

Choice of Surgical Approach and Procedure

The 1994 EAES statement remained unchanged in the updating comments (2000) as well as in 2006: LC is the procedure of choice for symptomatic uncomplicated cholecystolithiasis. The overall rate of cholecystectomy by laparoscopy is about 75% in the western world: In the USA the rate of LC for chronic cholecystitis is 78% with a conversion rate of 6.1% [13]. In Germany, the overall rate is 72% [14] and in Australia 75% [6].

Excluding the randomised controlled trials (RCTs) on acute cholecystitis, timing of surgery or ambulatory surgery, over 40 RCTs are available comparing LC versus open cholecystectomy or minicholecystectomy (MC). MC is defined as open cholecystectomy through a laparotomy smaller than 8 cm [15]. In the first years of LC, the longer operation time was the most significant disadvantage of the minimally invasive approach. Most of the trials found shorter hospital stay, less pain and faster return to normal activity, resulting in less postoperative risk for pulmonary complications not only in healthy patients but also in patients with cirrhotic portal hypertension [7, 9, 21]. However, the main advantages can only be detected during the first days postoperatively. McMahon et al. [17] demonstrated that the benefits of LC diminish beginning after the first week to an equal state 3 months postoperatively.

Majeed et al. [15, 31] concluded in a blinded RCT that LC takes longer to do than small-incision cholecystectomy and does not have any advantages in terms of hospital stay, analgesic consumption or postoperative recovery. Finally there is a blinded multicenter RCT from Sweden comparing LC with MC including 724 randomised patients [24, 25]. The conclusion was shorter sick leave and faster return to work after LC, an equal postoperative complication rate and fewer intraoperative complications in the MC group. The operation time was longer for LC.

Technical Aspects of Surgery

For patient positioning, two possibilities are established: The "French technique", with the surgeon between the patient's legs [4], or the "American technique", with the patient in a supine position with the surgeon standing on the left side. One RCT found better pulmonary function with the French technique [11]. LC is performed by creating a CO_2 pneumoperitoneum. The technical aspects of the pneumoperitoneum (access technique, insufflation gas, etc.) are described in a separate chapter of this book.

The dissection in Callot's triangle should be performed using the "critical view" technique: the two identified structures entering the gallbladder (the duct and the artery) have to be identified clearly before cutting them. These structures might be secured either by metallic or by resorbable clips [23]. Bipolar electrocautery is not safe in the closure of the cystic duct as shown by experimental studies [16, 29]. The dissection is usually done retrograde from the infundibulum to the fundus. In difficult situations, the "fundus" first technique seems to be safe [8, 22, 26].

There is no evidence recommending drainage routinely [12]. One RCT could not prove any advantage of a subphrenic-placed drain in order to evacuate the residual CO_2 gas [20]. Similarly, there is no need for routine antibiotics [2].

Peri- and Postoperative Care

There are no new data available to update the comments from 2000.

References

1. Beyermann K, Stinner B, Hasselmann U, Rothmund M (1992) [Consequences of routine gastroscopy before cholecystectomy]. Langenbecks Arch Chir 377:314–316
2. Catarci M, Mancini S, Gentileschi P, Camplone C, Sileri P, Grassi GB (2004) Antibiotic prophylaxis in elective laparoscopic cholecystectomy. Lack of need or lack of evidence? Surg Endosc 18:638–641
3. Dawson P, Adam A, Benjamin IS (1993) Intravenous cholangiography revisited. Clin Radiol 47:223–225
4. Dubois F, Berthelot G, Levard H (1995) Coelioscopic cholecystectomy: experience with 2006 cases. World J Surg 19:748–752
5. Fahlke J, Ridwelski K, Manger T, Grote R, Lippert H (2001) Diagnostic workup before laparoscopic cholecystectomy—which diagnostic tools should be used? Hepatogastroenterology 48:59–65
6. Fletcher DR, Hobbs MS, Tan P, Valinsky LJ, Hockey RL, Pikora TJ, Knuiman MW, Sheiner HJ, Edis A (1999) Complications of cholecystectomy: risks of the laparoscopic approach and protective effects of operative cholangiography: a population-based study. Ann Surg 229:449–457
7. Harju J, Juvonen P, Eskelinen M, Miettinen P, Pääkkönen M (2006) Minilaparotomy cholecystectomy versus laparoscopic cholecystectomy: a randomized study with special reference to obesity. Surg Endosc 20:583–586
8. Ichihara T, Takada M, Ajiki T, Fukumoto S, Urakawa T, Nagahata Y, Kuroda Y (2004) Tape ligature of cystic duct and fundus-down approach for safety laparoscopic cholecystectomy: outcome of 500 patients. Hepatogastroenterology 51:362–364
9. Ji W, Li LT, Wang ZM, Quan ZF, Chen XR, Li JS (2005) A randomized controlled trial of laparoscopic versus open cholecystectomy in patients with cirrhotic portal hypertension. World J Gastroenterol 11:2513–2517
10. Kratzer W, Mason RA, Kachele V (1999) Prevalence of gallstones in sonographic surveys worldwide. J Clin Ultrasound 27:1–7

11. Kum CK, Eypasch E, Aljaziri A, Troidl H (1996) Randomized comparison of pulmonary function after the 'French' and 'American' techniques of laparoscopic cholecystectomy. Br J Surg 83:938–941
12. Launay-Savary MV, Slim K (2005) [Evidence-based analysis of prophylactic abdominal drainage]. Ann Chir (in press). Epub 2005 Dec 5
13. Livingston EH, Rege RV (2004) A nationwide study of conversion from laparoscopic to open cholecystectomy. Am J Surg 188:205–211
14. Ludwig K, Lorenz D, Koeckerling F (2002) Surgical strategies in the laparoscopic therapy of cholecystolithiasis and common duct stones. ANZ J Surg 72:547–552
15. Majeed AW, Troy G, Nicholl JP, Smythe A, Reed MW, Stoddard CJ, Peacock J, Johnson AG (1996) Randomised, prospective, single-blind comparison of laparoscopic versus small-incision cholecystectomy. Lancet 347:989–994
16. Matthews BD, Pratt BL, Backus CL, Kercher KW, Mostafa G, Lentzner A, Lipford EH, Sing RF, Heniford BT (2001) Effectiveness of the ultrasonic coagulating shears, LigaSure vessel sealer, and surgical clip application in biliary surgery: a comparative analysis. Am Surg 67:901–906
17. McMahon AJ, Russell IT, Baxter JN, Ross S, Anderson JR, Morran CG, Sunderland G, Galloway J, Ramsay G, O'Dwyer PJ (1994) Laparoscopic versus minilaparotomy cholecystectomy: a randomised trial. Lancet 343:135–138
18. Neuhaus H, Ungeheuer A, Feussner H, Classen M, Siewert JR (1992) [Laparoscopic cholecystectomy: ERCP as standard preoperative diagnostic technique]. Dtsch Med Wochenschr 117:1863–1867
19. Nilsson U (1987) Adverse reactions to iotroxate at intravenous cholangiography. A prospective clinical investigation and review of the literature. Acta Radiol 28:571–575
20. Nursal TZ, Yildirim S, Tarim A, Noyan T, Poyraz P, Tuna N, Haberal M (2003) Effect of drainage on postoperative nausea, vomiting, and pain after laparoscopic cholecystectomy. Langenbecks Arch Surg 388:95–100
21. Puggioni A, Wong LL (2003) A metaanalysis of laparoscopic cholecystectomy in patients with cirrhosis. J Am Coll Surg 197:921–926
22. Raj PK, Castillo G, Urban L (2001) Laparoscopic cholecystectomy: fundus-down approach. J Laparoendosc Adv Surg Tech A 11:95–100
23. Rohr S, De Manzini N, Vix J, Tiberio G, Wantz C, Meyer C (1997) [Value of absorbable clips in laparoscopic cholecystectomy. A randomized prospective study]. J Chir (Paris) 134:180–184
24. Ros A, Nilsson E (2004) Abdominal pain and patient overall and cosmetic satisfaction one year after cholecystectomy: outcome of a randomized trial comparing laparoscopic and minilaparotomy cholecystectomy. Scand J Gastroenterol 39:773–777
25. Ros A, Gustafsson L, Krook H, Nordgren CE, Thorell A, Wallin G, Nilsson E (2001) Laparoscopic cholecystectomy versus mini-laparotomy cholecystectomy: a prospective, randomized, single-blind study. Ann Surg 234:741–749
26. Rosenberg J, Leinskold T (2004) Dome down laparosonic cholecystectomy. Scand J Surg 93:48–51
27. Schwenk W, Böhm B, Badke A, Zarras K, Stock W (1992) [Preoperative esophagogastroduodenoscopy before elective surgical therapy of symptomatic cholelithiasis]. Leber Magen Darm 22:225–229
28. Shamiyeh A, Rieger R, Schrenk P, Lindner E, Wayand W (2001) [Spiral CT cholangiography is not suitable for routine diagnosis before laparoscopic cholecystectomy]. Chirurg 72:159–163
29. Shamiyeh A, Vattay P, Tulipan L, Schrenk P, Bogner S, Danis J, Wayand W (2004) Closure of the cystic duct during laparoscopic cholecystectomy with a new feedback-controlled bipolar sealing system in case of biliary obstruction – an experimental study in pigs. Hepatogastroenterology 51:931–933
30. Sosada K, Zurawinski W, Piecuch J, Stepien T, Makarska J (2005) Gastroduodenoscopy: a routine examination of 2,800 patients before laparoscopic cholecystectomy. Surg Endosc 19:1103–1108

31. Squirrell DM, Majeed AW, Troy G, Peacock JE, Nicholl JP, Johnson AG (1998) A randomized, prospective, blinded comparison of postoperative pain, metabolic response, and perceived health after laparoscopic and small incision cholecystectomy. Surgery 123:485–495

32. Thybusch A, Schaube H, Schweizer E, Gollnick D, Grimm H (1996) [Significant value and therapeutic implications of routine gastroscopy before cholecystectomy]. J Chir (Paris) 133:171–174

33. Ure BM, Troidl H, Spangenberger W, Lefering R, Dietrich A, Sommer H (1992) Evaluation of routine upper digestive tract endoscopy before laparoscopic cholecystectomy. Br J Surg 79:1174–1177

34. Zacks SL, Sandler RS, Rutledge R, Brown RS Jr (2002) A population-based cohort study comparing laparoscopic cholecystectomy and open cholecystectomy. Am J Gastroenterol 97:334–340

Inguinal Hernia Repair – Update 2006

Abe Fingerhut, Bertrand Millat, Nicolas Veyrie, Elie Chouillard, Chadli Dziri

Introduction

An update on laparoscopic inguinal hernia repair leads one to realize that while approximately 60 controlled randomized trials have already been performed in this arena, and that at least 15 systematic reviews and meta-analyses [1–15] have analytically summed up these results, there is still controversy as to whether laparoscopic inguinal hernia should be performed or not [16]. The conclusions of all these studies, however, as already alluded to in our previous update [17], have been that laparoscopic mesh repair has similar recurrence rates to open mesh repair (both being better than rraphy techniques), costs more (in operative time and in direct costs) than open mesh or nonmesh repair, with clinically marginal benefits as concerns immediate postoperative pain. After a brief summary of these issues, further discussion will be centered on (1) the practical consequences that arise from the results of these studies and (2) the future directions that must be sought.

Material and Methods

A systematic research of the electronic literature was made using the Cochrane and Medline databases to gain access to all controlled randomized trials, systematic reviews, and meta-analyses involving laparoscopic versus open inguinal hernia repair. The search strategy was that described by Dickersin et al. [18, 19] with the appropriate specific search terms for inguinal hernia repair and controlled trials [clinical trial (PT) and randomized controlled trial (PT), and controlled clinical trial (PT)]. More recent individual studies, either not included in the meta-analyses, or outstanding or highly controversial, were also analyzed.

Results

Of over 60 studies found, our analysis concerns 41.

Overall recurrence rates were 2.3% in meta-analyses [6] and 3% in individual studies; rates were as high as 10.1% [20] for laparoscopic and 3.1–4.9% [20]

for open repairs in multicenter studies. In the study by Schmedt et al. [13] comparing the Lichtenstein technique with laparoscopic hernia repair, recurrence was twice as likely to occur after laparoscopic repair (odds ratio, OR, 2.00; 95% confidence interval, CI, [1.46, 2.74]). The duration of the operation was consistently and statistically significantly longer for laparoscopic repair (approximately 16 min whether in individual studies or in the meta-analyses [6, 10]. Complication rates varied in individual studies from 25 to 39% [20] for laparoscopic repair and from 30 to 33% [20] for the open repair, whereas in one meta-analysis [13] the laparoscopic technique was better than the Lichtenstein technique as concerned the incidence of wound infection (0.39 [0.26, 0.61]), hematoma formation (0.69 [0.54, 0.90]), and chronic pain syndrome (0.56 [0.44, 0.70]). The Lichtenstein technique was associated with less seroma (1.42 [1.13, 1.79]). Control of pain, as expressed either as visual analog scores or as analgesic consumption, was marginally in favor of the laparoscopic repair, but these differences were no longer significant 2 weeks after operation [6].

No difference was found in total morbidity or in the incidence of iatrogenic intestinal lesions, urinary bladder lesions, major vascular lesions, urinary retention, and testicular problems.

Discussion

We will not discuss the feasibility of the techniques nor the classic end points for which, in our opinion, discussion is no longer needed and is somewhat futile.

Mesh or Rraphy?

The results of several meta-analyses suggest that mesh, whether inserted laparoscopically or through a traditional, open incision, is associated with less recurrence than the techniques of rrhaphy [4, 6–9, 12]. Slight variations in outcomes have been noted, however, but these are related to the studies included or not included in the different meta-analyses rather than to the type of approach. Stengel et al. [21] recently abstracted all publications of randomized trials of laparoscopic versus open inguinal hernia repair included in the EU Hernia Trialists meta-analyses. Applying meta-regression to identify variables that were likely to alter the relative risk of hernia recurrence with either route, the authors analyzed 41 randomized trials (7,446 patients). They noted significant statistical heterogeneity across studies (χ^2 test, $P=0.029$), scarce information provided in the original papers, and small sample sizes. The results varied internationally, with trials from the UK, southern Europe, and Australia favoring open hernioplasty (analysis of variance, $P=0.0047$). The number of surgeons participating in each arm influenced outcomes as large numbers of surgeons contributing to the open hernioplasty group predicted better results with endoscopic hernia repair [risk ratio 0.99 with any additional surgeon, 95% CI 0.98–1.00, $P=0.005$]. Because of the diversity in the size of the effect, however, it is doubtful whether data from the available hernia trials should be compiled into a single summary measure. As well, efficacy estimates in hernia surgery are susceptible to technical issues, which need further scientific appraisal on a larger scale.

Laparoscopic or Traditional Open

There has been and continues to be much debate about the benefits of laparoscopic repair of inguinal hernia. The results of laparoscopic hernia repair in large controlled studies [20] reported in the UK [22], and more recently in the USA, although severely criticized by some [16], have clearly shown that laparoscopic hernia repair is not an operation that can be integrated into the general surgeon's armamentarium without raising several important issues. Unquestionably, the results from expert surgeons and centers [23] continue to demonstrate that excellent short-term and long-term outcomes can be achieved, even in the teaching arena. However, the learning curve (i.e., the time necessary to stabilize the duration of operation or reach a stable level or recurrence) for laparoscopic hernia repair has not yet been described in detail [24]. The number of operations to obtain this has been reported to range from 200 to 250 [20, 24] in the overall general population of surgeons who are not claimed experts. The average-to-poor results observed during this long learning curve for all the young surgeons eager to add this technique to their armamentarium require further discussion, concerning ethical and economics issues which will be dealt with later.

Recurrence Rates

Recurrence has been the main end point for several studies and should continue to be the principal criterion for hernia repair [25]. The reasons are several: (1) a bulge in the groin is usually the principal cause for seeking medical advice (far more frequently than any complication); (2) a recurrence is the main reason for reoperation.

The true recurrence rate is very difficult to evaluate in most series and above all in the meta-analyses, essentially because of the variable case-mix in these studies [21]. Moreover, recurrence can be difficult to ascertain, especially when the patient is not seen or examined by a specialist [25]. Moreover, correct evaluation can be plagued by the absence of follow-up, sometimes related to the death of the patient, otherwise to the fact that, not satisfied with the initial attending surgeon, the patient consults another surgeon

[25]. This may explain why the percentage of recurrent hernias operated on in most series is much higher than the actual outcome of the same series, as concerns the recurrence rate.

Complication Rates

Complications rates have been the center of several studies; however, it is important to distinguish between the types of complication rates reported in the literature (overall morbidity, wound complications, deep or intraabdominal complications) and their severity, (i.e., a hematoma at the trocar site insertion resulting from the puncture of the epigastric artery is not comparable with puncture of the iliac artery or vein by a Veress needle or a trocar). Several meta-analyses [3–6, 8, 9] have stated that while there were fewer overall complications with the laparoscopic technique, their severity was greater.

Pain

While it is generally admitted that laparoscopic hernia repair results in less postoperative pain [8, 9], the differences are often minimal and the benefits marginal in terms of analgesic consumption [26, 27]. One reason might be that procedures for measuring pain magnitude, timing of the evaluation of pain, and definitions differ from one study to another, making comparison difficult or even senseless [28]. In any case, these differences hardly exist longer than 2 weeks, usually less than the normal layoff from work, so the criterion of less pain can hardly be expected to contribute to a quicker return to normal activities or to work.

Persistent pain has been reported in up to 54% of patients undergoing operation for hernia repair [28]. Here again, the definition of persistent pain varies greatly across studies for inguinal hernia repair. The presence of foreign material has been suggested to play a major role (plug ?).

Before any reasonable conclusions can be drawn as concerns the question of chronic pain, this issue should now be addressed prospectively using standard definitions and allowing for assessment of the degree of pain [29, 30]. The use of lightweight meshes has recently been advanced to potentially decrease this side effect of mesh [31]. More evidence is required on the loss of utility caused by persisting pain and numbness.

Costs

Costs are a matter of great concern in our budget-constrained health care systems, wherever we look.

Even if the use of reusable instruments (trocars and the associated laparoscopic instruments) has been said to reduce costs [32], sterilization costs, maintenance, and setup times have a price, which has not yet been calculated with precision.

The meshes used for laparoscopic hernia repair are, on average, more expensive than those inserted through a classic inguinal incision.

The question of fixation of the mesh has been debated ever since the start of the laparoscopic hernia repair era. While several authors have said that fixation is necessary and reduces the risk of slippage of the mesh, and consequently, the risk of recurrence, others [32] maintain that fixation is not necessary: at least four controlled trials have found that there was no difference in the recurrence rate when the mesh was not fixated with staples [33–36]. The costs of staples and the firing machine can then be subtracted from the overall costs.

To overcome the purported disadvantages of fixation (costs, chronic neuralgia), the initial study by Katkhouda et al. [37] has led several authors who still believe that fixation is necessary to now use fibrin glue as a method of fixation [38]. More studies are necessary, however, before any coherent policy can be set.

With the goal of determining whether laparoscopic methods are more effective and cost-effective than open mesh methods of inguinal hernia repair, and then whether laparoscopic transabdominal preperitoneal (TAPP) or laparoscopic totally extraperitoneal (TEP) repair is more effective and cost-effective, a review of economic evaluations undertaken by NICE in 2001 [39] was updated and an economic evaluation was performed in 2005 [9]. Laparoscopic repair was more costly to the health service than open repair (extra cost of about £ 300–350 per patient). From the review of economic evaluations, the estimates of incremental cost per additional day at usual activities were between £ 86 and £ 130. When productivity costs were included, they eliminated the cost differential between laparoscopic and open repair. Additional analysis incorporating new trial evidence suggested that TEP repair was associated with significantly more recurrences than open mesh repair, but these data did not greatly influence cost-effectiveness. The authors concluded that for the management of unilateral hernias, the base-case analysis and most of the sensitivity analysis suggest that open flat mesh repair is the least costly option but provides fewer quality-adjusted life years (QALYs) than TEP or TAPP repair. TEP repair is likely to dominate TAPP repair (on average TEP repair is estimated to be less costly and more effective). McCormack et al. [9] and Vale et al. [40] added that laparoscopic repair would be more cost-effective for management of symptomatic bilateral hernias, and possibly also for contralateral occult hernias (see later). The increased adoption of laparoscopic techniques may allow patients to return to usual activities faster. This may, for some people, reduce any loss of income. On the other hand, for the NHS, increased use of laparoscopic repair would lead to an increased requirement for training and the risk of serious complications may be higher.

According to the utility analysis of Vale et al. [40], laparoscopic hernia repair with mesh is not cost-effective compared with open mesh repair in terms of cost per recurrence avoided. As well, it appears unlikely that the extra costs will be offset by the short-term benefits (reduced pain and earlier return to normal activities) [40].

Duration of Operation

The consequences of this time difference, while seemingly minimal, are in fact enormous: if every laparoscopic operation took an average of 16 min longer than the traditional repair, this means that overall all hernia repairs in the USA and France would take an average of 1,792,000 and 600,000 min longer, i.e., 29,867 and 10,000 h longer, respectively. The corresponding costs amount to an average increased cost of US $ 29,867,000 [41] and 7,200,000 (Straetmans, personal communication, EAES 2005), respectively for the year 2003. The increased time necessary to assist a younger colleague with inguinal hernia repair has not been evaluated with precision, but is also important to consider. However, when performed by a resident in training [42] a laparoscopic hernia repair takes on average 120 min compared with 75 min for open repair: a difference of 45 min. Kingsnorth [43] has said that the time that should be allocated to perform a hernia repair by a junior is probably twofold. When compared with those of senior surgeons, incremental costs for the hospital provider were US $ 153 and 106 per open hernia repair when carried out by junior consultants and residents, respectively. The overall incremental costs per year for these procedures were € 8,370 for residents and € 22,922 for junior consultants [42]. Evaluated according to whether the operating surgeon was a junior or a senior resident [44], the extra costs were € 2,907 and 1,855.

The reasons why laparoscopic hernia repair requires more time to perform than open repair, on average, warrant discussion.

Possible reasons might include the time necessary for the peroperative preparation and setup for laparoscopic surgery, frustration because of the small space within which the surgeon has to work, unfamiliarity with (laparoscopic) anatomy, and difficulties arising from a suboptimal trocar setup [45, 46].

The solutions to overcome these time differences may be obtained by several routes: one such direction is to increase operating room efficiency by changing patient flow rather than simply working to streamline existing steps [47]. Another is to have a dedicated laparoscopic surgery suite [48], leading to large and statistically significant differences in setup and put-away times for laparoscopic procedures.

Frustration is a frequently encountered feeling that characterizes many surgeons battling with laparoscopic techniques. Hernia repair is certainly no exception, and at least one article recently dealt with this specific problem [49]. In that paper, frustration, as rated on a scale from 1 (no frustration) to 5 (very frustrated), was reported less often by the surgeons performing the open hernia repair than with the laparoscopic technique ($P = 0.0001$) and was associated with a higher rate of hernia recurrence at 2 years (adjusted OR 2.01, 95% CI 1.15–3.51) in open repair: the level of surgeon frustration correlated with hernia recurrence. However, no such association was found in the laparoscopic group. Frustration level was associated with a higher rate of postoperative complications in both the laparoscopic and the open groups. Procedures in which surgeons expressed frustration were 2.9 times more likely to be accompanied by an intraoperative complication than those in which the surgeon experienced no frustration [49].

Time may also be gained by optimizing the trocar setup in such a way that minimizes the efforts and the stress of laparoscopic surgery, including strict ergonomic principles [46, 50].

Unanswered Questions and Future Directions

When finally even the stoutest proponent admits that the benefits of laparoscopic surgery may not be as thought, the following argument arises: laparoscopic treatment of hernia is best for recurrent hernia and for bilateral hernia – this was the conclusion of a very influential paper published in 2003 [51].

Recurrent Hernia

The argument put forth is that hernia repair would be easier if the incision and dissection of tissues did not have to traverse cicatricial or scarred tissues. The idea behind such a recommendation is that recurrence after a traditional hernia repair by rrhaphy or the Liechtenstein technique would be easier if approached through the transperitoneal or the extraperitoneal routes. If this were true, the Stoppa or Rives operation performed through a midline incision should have allowed the same performance: however, nothing has ever been published to support this. Recurrence after a mesh interposition, whether inserted through a previous Stoppa or Rives operation, or the laparoscopic extraperitoneal or transperitoneal routes, all consisting of a preperitoneal mesh interposition, has been thought to due to too small a mesh, nonfixation, or technical errors.

What about the hernia repair that has already been operated on through both the laparoscopic and the anterior route?

Bilateral Hernia

At a time when the question is arising of whether asymptomatic hernia should be dealt with prophylactly [52], the principle of looking for and then repairing an asymptomatic bilateral hernia warrants serious reflection. Few data, once again, exist in favor of doing so, or not. In a meta-analysis of all published pediatric series (hernia repair from birth to 16 years) of unilateral inguinal hernia repair [11], the incidence of metachronous hernia was 1,062 in 15,310 patients (7%). Gender and age were not risk factors. The risk of metachronous inguinal hernia was 50% greater when the initial hernia was on the left side. Of patients who developed a metachronous hernia, 90% did so within 5 years. The complication rate of metachronous hernia was 0.5%. These authors concluded that there is no role for routine contralateral groin exploration in a patient under 16 years old, except perhaps for left inguinal herniorrhaphy. Patients who do not undergo contralateral groin exploration should be followed up for 5 years.

In a prospective nationwide analysis of laparoscopic versus Lichtenstein repair of inguinal hernia in Denmark, Wara et al. [53] looked at results of hernia repair when nonspecialist surgeons were involved, as recorded in a nationwide registry between 1998 and 2003. The outcome measure was the reoperation rates after laparoscopic ($n=3,606$) and Lichtenstein ($n=39,537$) repair, adjusting for factors predisposing to recurrence. The overall reoperation rates after laparoscopic and Lichtenstein repair of unilateral primary indirect hernia (0 vs 1.0%), primary direct hernia (1.1 vs 3.1%), unilateral recurrent hernia (4.6 vs 4.8%), and bilateral recurrent hernia (2.6 vs 7.6%) did not differ significantly. On the other hand, laparoscopic repair of a bilateral primary hernia was associated with a higher reoperation rate than Lichtenstein repair ($4\cdot8$ vs $3\cdot0$%) ($P=0\cdot017$).

When economic considerations are concerned, McCormack et al. [9] and Vale et al. [40] stated that for management of symptomatic bilateral hernias, laparoscopic repair would be more cost-effective as differences in operation time (a key cost driver) may be reduced and differences in convalescence time are more marked (hence QALYs will increase) for laparoscopic compared with (double) open mesh repair. When possible repair of contralateral occult hernias is taken into account, TEP repair is most likely to be considered cost-effective at threshold values for the cost per additional QALY above £ 20,000. Further research relating to whether the balance of advantages and disadvantages changes when hernias are recurrent or bilateral is also required as current data are limited.

Prosthetic Repair and Other Surgery in the Bogros Space

The consequences of prosthetic hernia repair relative to future surgery for prostate cancer and/or vascular surgery in the Bogros space have been the subject of several publications [54–56]. In summary, there seems to be concern that prosthetic inguinal hernia repair may induce fibrotic changes that make ulterior surgery very difficult, dangerous, or impossible [54]. For the moment, however, there are only case or small-series reports on this subject, the results are contradictory [55], and no formal guidelines have emerged.

Learning Curve and Consequences

The influence of surgeon age and other factors on proficiency in laparoscopic or open hernia repair was studied from data originating in a multicenter, randomized trial comparing open and laparoscopic herniorrhaphies, conducted in Veterans Administration hospitals (CSP 456) [24]. Significant differences in recurrence rates for the laparoscopic procedure as well as for the open procedure related to resident postgraduate year (PGY) level were reported according to the surgeons' experience. On the basis of 1,629 unilateral laparoscopic and open herniorrhaphies in this study, the surgeon's experience (experienced 250 procedures or more; inexperienced fewer than 250 procedures) and the surgeon's age (45 years old or older vs younger than 45) were significant predictors of recurrence in laparoscopic herniorrhaphy. The odds of recurrence for an inexperienced surgeon aged 45 years or older were 1.72 times that of a younger, inexperienced surgeon. For open repairs, although surgeon age and operation time appeared to be related to recurrence, only a median PGY level of less than 3 was a significant independent predictor [24].

As stated in several papers, the learning curve for laparoscopic hernia (i.e., the time necessary to stabilize the duration of operation or to reach a stable level of recurrence) has been reported to be long. For recurrence, the learning curve has been estimated at 200–250 [20, 24]. One must not forget that every surgeon has and will have a learning curve during which the patients operated on will have a greater risk of complications, including recurrence, and the operations will take longer to perform and will have inherent increased costs. Prospective population-based registries of new surgical procedures may be the best way to address this, as a complement to randomized trials assessing effectiveness. Methodologically sound randomized controlled trials are needed to consider the relative merits and risks of TAPP and TEP repair in this respect. Further methodological research is required into the complexity of laparoscopic groin hernia repair and the improvement of performance that accompanies experience.

On the other hand, it is of note that the same learning curve can be as short as five operations for the Lichtenstein technique [57]. While the authors are aware of the necessity to allow time and leniency regarding the question of teaching and learning, especially as concerns laparoscopic technique, the reader has to realize that the line has to be drawn somewhere and sometime to know whether, for laparoscopic hernia repair, the debate on the learning curve should not now be ended.

Conclusions

If good, reproducible, short- and long-term results can be proven, and there are no or few cost-containment arguments, certainly those surgeons who are proficient may want to continue to perform inguinal hernia repair laparoscopically. However, what is in the black zone are the unacceptable complication rates, including a higher recurrence rate, while on the learning curve, when satisfactory results can be obtained easily, quickly, and with few complications [57] using time-proven techniques such as the Lichtenstein and plug methods. Moreover, the time necessary to teach the younger generation might be better used to instruct incoming surgeons to learn easier techniques, that will provide equally efficacious outcomes. In accordance with O'Dwyer [22], for patients with a primary inguinal hernia, laparoscopic repair can no longer be recommended as the repair of choice unless it is undertaken in an expert center in minimal access surgery. As to the role of laparoscopy in recurrent and bilateral inguinal hernia, further clinical trials are needed.

References

1. Bittner R, Sauerland S, Schmedt CG (2005) Comparison of endoscopic techniques vs Shouldice and other open nonmesh techniques for inguinal hernia repair: a meta-analysis of randomized cofntrolled trials. Surg Endosc 19:605–615
2. Chung RS, Rowland DY (1999) Meta-analyses of randomized controlled trials of laparoscopic vs conventional inguinal hernia repairs. Surg Endosc 13:689–694
3. EU Hernia Trialists Collaboration (2000) Laparoscopic compared with open methods of groin hernia repair: systematic review of randomized controlled trials. Br J Surg 87:860–867
4. EU Hernia Trialists Collaboration (2000) Mesh compared with non-mesh methods of open groin hernia repair: systematic review of randomized controlled trials. Br J Surg 87:854–859
5. EU Hernia Trialists Collaboration (2002) Repair of groin hernia with synthetic mesh: meta-analysis of randomized controlled trials. Ann Surg 235:322–332
6. Grant AM (2002) Laparoscopic versus open groin hernia repair: meta-analysis of randomised trials based on individual patient data. Hernia 6:2–10
7. Lau H, Patil NG, Chan-Wing Lee F (2003) Systematic review and meta-analysis of clinical trials comparing endoscopic totally extraperitoneal inguinal hernioplasty with open repair of inguinal hernia repair. Ann Coll Surg 7:2–10

8. McCormack K, Scott NW (2003) Laparoscopic techniques versus open techniques for inguinal hernia repair. Cochrane Database Syst Rev 1:CD001785
9. McCormack K, Wake B, Perez J, Fraser C, Cook J, McIntosh E, Vale L (2005) Laparoscopic surgery for inguinal hernia repair: systematic review of effectiveness and economic evaluation. Health Technol Assess 9:1–203, iii–iv
10. Memon MA, Cooper NJ, Memon B, Memon MI, Abrams KR (2003) Meta-analysis of randomized clinical trials comparing open and laparoscopic inguinal hernia repair. Br J Surg 90:1479–1492
11. Miltenburg DM, Nuchtern JG, Jaksic T, Kozinetz CA, Brandt ML (1997) Meta-analysis of the risk of metachronous hernia in infants and children. Am J Surg 174:741–744
12. Schmedt CG, Leibl BJ, Bittner R (2002) Endoscopic inguinal hernia repair in comparison with Shouldice and Lichtenstein repair. A systematic review of randomized trials. Dig Surg 19:511–517
13. Schmedt CG, Sauerland S, Bittner R (2005) Comparison of endoscopic procedures vs Lichtenstein and other open mesh techniques for inguinal hernia repair: a meta-analysis of randomized controlled trials. Surg Endosc 19:188–199
14. Scott NW, McCormack K, Graham P, Go PM, Ross SJ, Grant AM (2002) Open mesh versus non-mesh for repair of femoral and inguinal hernia. Cochrane Database Rev CD002197
15. Voyles CR, Hamilton BJ, Johnson WD, Kano N (2002) Meta-analysis of laparoscopic inguinal hernia trials favors open hernia repair with preperitoneal mesh prosthesis. Am J Surg 184:6–10
16. Grunwaldt LLJ, Schwaitzberg SD, Rattner DW, Jones DB (2005) Is laparoscopic inguinal hernia repair an operation of the past? J Am Coll Surg 200:616–620
17. Fingerhut A, Millat B, Bataille N, Yachouchi E, Dziri C, Boudet MJ, Paul A (2001) Laparoscopic hernia repair in 2000. Update of the European Association for Endoscopic Surgery (EAES) Consensus Conference in Madrid, June 1994. Surg Endosc 15:1061–1065
18. Dickersin K, Scherer R, Lefebvre C (1994) Identifying relevant studies for systematic reviews. BMJ 309:1286–1291
19. Tumber M, Dickersin K (2004) Publication of clinical trials: accountability and accessibility J Intern Med 256:271–283
20. Neumayer L, Giobbe-Hurder A, Johansson O, Fitzgibbons R Jr, Dunlop D, Gibbs J, Reda D, Henderson W (2004) Open mesh versus laparoscopic mesh repair of inguinal hernia. N Eng J Med 350:1819–1827
21. Stengel D, Bauwens K, Ekkernkamp A (2004) Recurrence risks in randomized trials of laparoscopic versus open inguinal hernia repair: to pool or not to pool (this is not the question). Langenbecks Arch Surg 389:492–498
22. MRC Laparoscopic Groin Hernia Trial Group (1999) Laparoscopic versus open repair of groin hernia: a randomised comparison. Lancet 354:185–190
23. DeTurris SV, Cacchione RN, Mungara A, Pecoraro A, Ferzli GS (2002) Laparoscopic herniorrhaphy: beyond the learning curve. J Am Coll Surg 194:65–73
24. Neumayer LA, Gawande AA, Wang J, Giobbie-Hurder A, Itani KM, Fitzgibbons RJ, Reda D, Jonasson O (2005) Proficiency of surgeons in inguinal hernia repair: effect of experience and age. Ann Surg 242:344–348
25. Hay JM, Boudet MJ, Fingerhut A, Poucher J, Hennet H, Habib E, Veyrieres M, Flamant Y (1995) Shouldice inguinal hernia repair in the male adult: the gold standard? A multicenter controlled trial in 1578 patients. Ann Surg 222:719–727
26. Bringman S, Ramel Heikkinen TJ, Englund T, Westman B, Anderberg B (2003) Tension-free inguinal hernia repair. TEP versus mesh-plug versus Lichtenstein (a prospective randomized trial). Ann Surg 237:142–147
27. Page B, Paterson D, Young D, O'Dwyer PJ (2002) Pain from primary inguinal hernia and the effect of repair on pain. Br J Surg 89:1315–1318
28. Poobalan AS, Bruce J, Smith WC, King PM, Krukowski ZH, Chambers WA (2003) A review of chronic pain after inguinal herniorrhaphy Clin J Pain 19:48–54

29. Kehlet H, Bay-Nielsen M, Kingsnorth A (2002) Chronic postherniorrhaphy pain — a call for uniform assessment. Hernia 6:178–181
30. McCarthy M, Chang CH, Pickard AS, Giobbie-Hurder A, Price DD, Jonasson O, Gibbs J, Fitzgibbons R, Neumayer L (2005) Visual analog scales for assessing surgical pain. J Am Coll Surg 201:245–252
31. O'Dwyer PJ, Alani A, McConnachie A (2005) Groin hernia repair: postherniorrhaphy pain. World J Surg 20:1062–1065
32. Arregui ME, Young SB (2005) Groin hernia repair by laparoscopic techniques: current status and controversies World J Surg 29:1052–1057
33. Ferzli GS, Frezza EE, Pecoraro AM Jr, Ahern KD (1999) Prospective randomized study of stapled versus unstapled mesh in a laparoscopic preperitoneal inguinal hernia repair. J Am Coll Surg 188:461–465
34. Moreno-Egea A, Torralba Martinez JA, Morales Cuenca G, Aguayo Albasini JL (2004) Randomized clinical trial of fixation vs nonfixation of mesh in total extraperitoneal inguinal hernioplasty. Arch Surg 139:1376–1379
35. Parshad R, Kumar R, Hazrah P, Bal S (2005) A randomized comparison of the early outcome of stapled and unstapled techniques of laparoscopic total extraperitoneal inguinal hernia repair. JSLS 9:403–407
36. Smith AI, Royston CM, Sedman PC (1999) Stapled and nonstapled laparoscopic transabdominal preperitoneal (TAPP) inguinal hernia repair. A prospective randomized trial. Surg Endosc 13:804–806
37. Katkhouda N, Mavor E, Friedlander MH, Mason RJ, Kiyabu M, Grant SW, Achanta K, Kirkman EL, Narayanan K, Essani R (2001) Use of fibrin sealant for prosthetic mesh fixation in laparoscopic extraperitoneal inguinal hernia repair. Ann Surg 233:18–25
38. Novik B, Hagedorn S, Mork UB, Dahlin K, Skullman S, Dalenback J (2006) Fibrin glue for securing the mesh in laparoscopic totally extraperitoneal inguinal hernia repair: a study with a 40-month prospective follow-up period. Surg Endosc 20:462–467
39. Motson RW (2002) Why does NICE not recommend laparoscopic herniorraphy? BMJ 324:1092–1094
40. Vale L, Grant A, McCormack K, Scott NW (2004) Cost-effectiveness of alternative methods of surgical repair of inguinal hernia. Int J Technol Assess Health Care 17:192–200
41. Rutkow IM (2003) Demographic and socioeconomic aspects of hernia repair in the United States in 2003. Surg Clin North Am 83:1045–1051
42. Chung RS (2005) How much time do surgical residents need to learn operative surgery? Am J Surg 190:351–353
43. Kingsnorth A (2005) Introduction to current practice of adult hernia repair. World J Surg 29:1044–1045
44. Koperna T (2004) How long do we need teaching in the operating room? The true costs of achieving surgical routine. Langenbecks Arch Surg 389:204–208
45. Reyes DAG, Tang B, Cuschieri A (2006) Minimal access surgery (MAS)-related surgeon morbidity syndromes. Surg Endosc 20:1–13
46. Ferzli GS, Fingerhut A (2004) Trocar placement for laparoscopic abdominal procedures: a simple standardized method. J Am Coll Surg 198:163–173
47. Friedman DM, Sokal SM, Chang Y, Berger DL (2006) Increasing operating room efficiency through parallel processing. Ann Surg 243:10–14
48. Kenyon TA, Urbach DR, Speer JB, Waterman-Hukari B, Foraker GF, Hansen PD, Swanstrom LL (2001) Dedicated minimally invasive surgery suites increase operating room efficiency. Surg Endosc 15:1140–1143
49. Kaafarani HMA, Itani KMF, Giobbie-Hurder A, Gleysteen JJ, McCarthy M, Gibbs J, Neumayer L (2005) Does surgeon frustration and satisfaction with the operation predict outcomes of open or laparoscopic inguinal hernia repair? J Am Coll Surg 200:677–683
50. Fingerhut A, Chouillard E (2005) Ergonomic and technical aspects of laparoscopy for trauma and non trauma emergencies. J Eur Surg 37:8–14

51. Bloor K, Freemantle N, Khadjesari Z, Maynard A (2003) Impact of NICE guidelines on laparoscopic surgery for inguinal hernias: analysis of interrupted time series. Br Med J 326:578–580
52. Fitzgibbons RJ Jr, Giobbie-Hurder A, Gibbs JO, Dunlop DD, Reda DJ, McCarthy M Jr, Neumayer LA, Barkun JS, Hoehn JL, Murphy JT, Sarosi GA Jr, Syme WC, Thompson JS, Wang J, Jonasson O (2006) Watchful waiting vs repair of inguinal hernia in minimally symptomatic men: a randomized clinical trial. JAMA 295:285–292
53. Wara P, Bay-Nielsen M, Juul P, Bendix J, Kehlet H (2005) Prospective nationwide analysis of laparoscopic versus Lichtenstein repair of inguinal hernia. Br J Surg 92:1277–1281
54. Amid PK (2005) Groin hernia repair: open techniques. World J Surg 29:1046–1051
55. Erdogru T, Teber D, Frede T, Marrero R, Hammady A, Rassweiler J (2005) The effect of previous transperitoneal laparoscopic inguinal herniorrhaphy on transperitoneal laparoscopic radical prostatectomy. J Urol 173:769–772
56. Stolzenburg JU, Anderson C, Rabenalt R, Do M, Ho K, Truss MC (2005) Endoscopic extraperitoneal radical prostatectomy in patients with prostate cancer and previous laparoscopic inguinal mesh placement for hernia repair. World J Urol 23:295–299
57. Tocchi A, Liotta G, Mazzoni G, Lepre L, Costa G, Maggiolini F, Miccini M (1998) [Learning curve for "tension-free" reparation of inguinal hernia]. G Chir 19:199–203

The EAES Clinical Practice Guidelines on Diagnosis and Treatment of Common Bile Duct Stones (1998)

Andreas Paul, Bertrand Millat, Ulla Holthausen, Stefan Sauerland, Edmund A.M. Neugebauer, J.C. Berthou, H.-J. Brambs, J.E. Dominguez-Muñoz, P. Goh, L.E. Hammerström, E. Lezoche, J. Périssat, P. Rossi, M.A. Röthlin, R.C.G. Russell, P. Spinelli, Y. Tekant

Introduction

During the last decade, laparoscopic techniques for abdominal surgery have changed the options for the diagnosis and treatment of many abdominal pathologies. Laparoscopic cholecystectomy has now become the standard procedure for removing symptomatic gallbladder stones. New techniques have also been developed for the removal of common bile duct stones (CBDS), which accompany symptomatic gallbladder stones in 10–15% of patients.

A number of different strategies have emerged that combine laparoscopic cholecystectomy with bile duct clearance. There has been a proliferation of publications in this search for a superior or ideal technique. The European Association for Endoscopic Surgery (EAES) recognizes the need to discuss and summarize these controversial developments and to provide practical guidelines based on the current state of knowledge. Bearing in mind the experience of previous consensus development conferences, we decided to use the joint meeting of the EAES and the ELSA (Endoscopic and Laparoscopic Surgeons of Asia) to bring together an international panel of experts in Istanbul.

Methods

In 1996 the EAES decided to hold a consensus development conference (CDC) on CBDS. The Cologne group was authorized by the EAES to organize the CDC according to general guidelines. Twelve internationally known experts were nominated by the Scientific Committee of the EAES. The criteria for selection were clinical and scientific expertise and activity in the diagnosis and/or treatment of CBDS. In order to balance the interests of experts in the areas of surgery, internal medicine, and radiology, panelists from all three specialities were selected.

Prior to the conference, all panelists were asked to survey the literature, list all relevant articles, and estimate the strength of evidence for every article cited. Referring to these articles, the panelists were asked to address the major open questions concerning the management of CBDS. For the five most relevant therapeutic options, they were also asked to comment on the status of each therapy. In regard to the question of laparoscopic common bile duct revision versus endoscopic retrograde cholangiopancreaticography (ERCP) with stone extraction, each panel member was instructed to indicate which technique is superior for several specific situations. All panelists received detailed information on how to answer each section, including a basic description of the CDC process, a scale for ranking the strength of the evidence of medical articles, and a description of levels of technology according to Mosteller [105] and Troidl [164].

In Cologne, all answers were analyzed and subsequently combined into a provisional preconsensus statement. This text was mailed to all panelists a month prior to the Istanbul meeting. The panel members were also informed about the identity of the other members, which had not been previously disclosed.

In Istanbul, all panel members convened for a first meeting on June 18, 1997. Here the provisional statement was scrutinized word by word. The following day, the modified statement was presented to the conference audience for public discussion. During a postconference meeting on the same day, all suggestions made by the audience were discussed by the panelists. Because not all of these questions could be resolved at this time, the chairmen were asked to provide additional literature that would address some of the critical issues. When these points had been cleared and altered in the text, the whole statement was mailed to all the panelists for agreement (Delphi process). In October 1997, the following statement was finalized.

Consensus Statement on the Diagnosis and Treatment of Common Bile Duct Stones

General Comment

Options for the management of common bile duct stones (CBDS) are increasing with the development of new technologies for diagnosis and treatment. While intraoperative cholangiography and open CBD exploration have comprised the applied technology for decades, the introduction of ERCP with endoscopic stone extraction in the 1970s and the more recent introduction of laparoscopic cholecystectomy led to a reappraisal of the situation. For each management policy, numerous publications – from case reports to prospective controlled clinical trials – are available, but evidence-based conclusions an rarely be achieved yet.

In terms of predictors for CBDS, the crucial issue is perhaps not which indicators should best be applied to detect CBDS, but whether we should favor a high rate of negative examinations or a high rate of retained stones, with all their sequelae. The consequences of either strategy are currently not well understood and are often dependent on the local medical and nonmedical conditions.

Nowadays, new imaging techniques in medicine (e.g., magnetic resonance cholangiopancreaticography, MRCP) have opened up new options for the diagnosis of CBDS. Furthermore, any debate about procedure and timing of diagnosis of CBDS leads to this question: Should they all be diagnosed?

Any discussion of an optimal therapy for common bile duct stones must take into account the rare but grave complications that each treatment option, may entail.

In general, the optimal diagnostic and therapeutic strategy seems to be dependent on local circumstances and the experience and expertise of the medical team, since there is still no evidence-based gold standard. In addition, ethical and socioeconomic considerations have an important impact on the controversy. For example, the costs of several techniques are prohibitive in some parts of the world.

Question 1. The Diagnosis of CBDS

What are Good Indicators or Predictive Symptoms/Signs for CBDS?

At the time of cholecystectomy for symptomatic cholelithiasis, 8–15% of patients under the age of 60 years and 15–60% of patients over the age of 60 years have CBDS. This prevalence reflects the prior probability of any patient harboring CBDS before any discriminating test. The prevalence of CBDS has a decisive influence on the predictive value of any indicator. The prevalence of CBDS and the threshold for investigating CBDS vary among individual clinicians.

Among the many parameters investigated, no single indicator is completely accurate in predicting CBDS before cholecystectomy. The indicators can be grouped as follows: symptoms and signs, biochemical parameters, and imaging techniques. Although acute pancreatitis or cholecystitis are associated with a higher prevalence of CBDS, there is no good evidence that a history of pancreatitis is an indicator for CBDS.

Table 15.1 lists the predictive values for the main indicators of CBDS. These data were combined from several primary studies with a meta-analysis [1]. For each individual indicator, the lowest abnormal value is considered to be the threshold. Within a hypothetical population with symptomatic cholelithiasis, a 10% probability (prevalence) of harboring CBDS is assumed. As shown in the example in the table footnote, an individual patient's risk factors can be established by multiplying the relevant positive or negative likelihood ratios.

Table 15.1. Predictive values of preoperative indicators of common bile duct stones (*CBDS*)

Indicator	Sensitivity (95% CI)	Specificity (95% CI)	LR+	LR−
Cholangitis	0.11 (0.02–0.19)	0.99 (0.99–1.00)	18.3	0.93
Preop jaundice	0.36 (0.26–0.45)	0.97 (0.95–0.99)	10.1	0.69
Cholecystitis	0.50 (0.11–0.89)	0.76 (0.45–1.00)	1.6	0.94
Bilirubine ↑	0.69 (0.48–0.90)	0.88 (0.84–0.92)	4.8	0.54
Alkaline phosph ↑	0.57 (0.46–0.69)	0.86 (0.78–0.94)	2.6	0.65
Amylase ↑	0.11 (0.02–0.20)	0.95 (0.93–0.98)	1.5	0.99
CBDS on US	0.38 (0.27–0.49)	1.00 (0.99–1.00)	13.6	0.70
Dilated CBD on US	0.42 (0.28–0.56)	0.96 (0.94–0.98)	6.9	0.77

Data from Abboud et al. [1], reprinted with permission. Data can be read as follows (line 1, cholangitis): from 2 to 19% of patients *with* CBDS have cholangitis (defined as the triad pain–fever–jaundice). Nearly all patients who do *not* have CBDS also do *not* have cholangitis (column 2). A patient with CBDS is 18.3 times more likely to have cholangitis. If we assume prior odds to be 1:9 (i.e., 10% prevalence), we multiply 1/9 by 18.3 to get 2.03. So the posttest odds are about 2:1, which is a 66% probability. However, on the other hand, in a patient without CBDS (column 5), cholangitis is still not unlikely. We receive 1:9.67 posterior odds, or a 9.4% probability.
CI confidence interval, *LR+* positive likelihood ratio, *LR−* negative likelihood ratio, *US* ultrasonography

A cystic duct found to have a diameter of more than 4–5 mm at operation was associated with an increased probability of CBDS (sensitivity, 0.34; PPV, 0.52) in a population of 319 patients with a CBDS prevalence of 12% [59, 61].

In the clinical setting, several groups of patients can be identified, as follows: (a) a *high-risk* group, which fulfills a series of predictive factors resulting in a global probability of CBDS of more than 90% based on the data in Table 15.1; (b) a *medium-risk* group, or group of uncertainty, which fulfills one or several prognostic factors listed in Table 15.1 but for whom the resulting posttest probability (although higher than the pretest probability of 10%) does not reach 90%; (c) a *low-risk* group, which has no signs or symptoms. Although their probability of harboring CBDS is below average, in clinical practice unsuspected CBDS are found in 5% of patients of fewer with symptomatic gallbladder stones.

Question 2. Diagnostic Procedures

Which Diagnostic Tools are Useful in the Detection of CBDS? In What Order Should They Be Applied?

Preoperative ultrasonography (US) misses two of three patients with common bile duct stones. However, it is a useful screening tool for the diagnosis of CBDS because of its noninvasiveness, easy availability, and low costs. Of all tools it should be applied as first. It has a reasonable predictive value if the CBD diameter is dilated as an indirect sign for CBDS. According to the literature, the sensitivity of preoperative US is 0.14–0.40, depending on the investigator's experience, the defined threshold value, and the general prevalence. The diagnosis of CBDS is more frequently achieved exclusively in patients with dilated CBD (diameter more than 8–10 mm). Furthermore, liver or pancreas pathologies are also detectable by this means.

Preoperative intravenous cholangiography (PIC) does not play a major role in the diagnosis of CBDS anymore. PIC has been reevaluated in patients without jaundice, using a new contrast reagent (meglumine iotroxate) with a reported risk of less than 1% of adverse reactions. Infusion yields a satisfactory bile duct opacification in 90–95% of patients. The negative predictive value (NPV) of a normal PIC is 0.98–1. The positive predictive value (PPV) of PIC for CBDS diagnosis was 0.94 for stones demonstrated at PIC but only 0.31 for stones suspected at PIC [16, 57]. Previous studies showed that PIC missed CBDS in an average of 40% of cases (range, 22–90% sensitivity). Therefore, it is not recommended as a routine procedure. It may be an option based on the local circumstances of a center.

Endoscopic retrograde cholangiopancreatography (ERCP) is a valid diagnostic tool (high sensitivity, specificity, accuracy in experienced hands). It should only be applied with the intention to treat in patients with a high probability of CBDS who are eligible for ES. It has to be recognized that the procedure is invasive and inconvenient for the patient. It requires sedation and has defined morbidity (5–10%) and mortality (less than 1% for diagnostic purpose) rates. The success rate for ERCP is 95%. The sensitivity is 0.84–0.89. Specificity is 0.97–1. PPV is 1 and NPV is 0.88.

Endoscopic ultrasonography (EUS) is another exclusively diagnostic procedure with a high accuracy rate, but currently there is no indication for its routine use in diagnosing CBDS. The sensitivity of endoscopic ultrasound is 93%; specificity is 97%. PPV is 98% and NPV is 88%.

Intraoperative cholangiography (IOC) and *laparoscopic ultrasound* are reliable diagnostic tools (more than 90% accuracy). Modern equipment and the use of fluoroscopy is required and may increase the accuracy in general practice. However, routine performance for the detection of symptomatic CBDS is questionable, although some of our panelists did recommend it. No final consensus was achieved regarding this point. The decision to perform routine or selective IOC during cholecystectomy depends both on the physician's personal beliefs regarding asymptomatic CBDS and his or her individual strategy for treatment. Reasons other than detection of CBDS for performing IOC, such as clarification of biliary anatomy, were considered outside the scope of the consensus. Invasive preoperative diagnostic tests should be avoided in patients scheduled for elective cholecystectomy.

Magnetic resonance cholangiopancreaticography (MRCP) seems to be an excellent diagnostic tool with high accuracy rates, so it might supersede other invasive diagnostic procedures such as ERCP. Disadvantages include inconvenience for the patient, low availability, and high costs. Furthermore, it is not applicable in every case (morbid obesity, pacemaker, etc.). In a first study from Italy [89], MRCP showed 91.6% sensitivity, 100% specificity, and an overall diagnostic accuracy of 96.8%.

Computer tomography (CT) has been evaluated only in biased populations. It plays no role in routine management. All patients with symptomatic gallbladder stones need to be assessed for CBDS, and the treatment of all diagnosed CBDS is mandatory (eight of 12 panelists were in favor of it). There are three options:

- Routine IOC requires no preoperative screening for CBDS. The rate of useless examinations is in correspondence with the prevalence of CBDS in the population scheduled for cholecystectomy.
- Selective contraindication for IOC is based on the negative predictive value of indicators for CBDS. It allows a 30–50% reduction in the number of IOC and yields a 2–3% rate of missed CBDS [61, 70]. Selective indication for IOC is based on the positive predictive value of preoperative indicators for CBDS. It limits diagnosis and treatment to preoperatively symptomatic CBDS. Limitations are related to the information provided by the predictors and uncertainty regarding the natural history of asymptomatic CBDS.

Question 3. Timing of Diagnostics

When Should CBDS Be Diagnosed?

The timing of diagnostics should be dependent on the status of the patient and the preferred treatment modality of the center – pre- or intraoperatively. A routine policy of postoperative diagnoses of patients with preoperative suspicion for CBDS is not advisable, since it entails the risk of a second operative intervention.

Question 4. Timing of Treatment

Should CBDS Be Treated Before, During, or After Cholecystectomy?

Depending on the clinical status of the patient, treatment can be performed before or during surgery. The policy of the specific center, as well as the experience and expertise of the medical team, may affect the choice of treatment modalities yet yield similar results (Table 15.2). Postoperative treatment of CBDS is only necessary if intraoperative clearance of the common bile duct fails or if patients develop symptoms of retained stones.

Table 15.2. Results of six prospective randomized trials comparing preoperative endoscopic retrograde cholangiography(*ERC*)/endoscopic sphincterotomy (*ES*) with open surgery alone for CBDS

	Surgery	Preop ERC/ES
Total number of patients	302	283
Endoscopic failures		15 (5%)
Successful primary extraction	275 (91%)	233 (82%)
Complications (range)		
Major	8% (4–15%)	8% (4–10)
Minor	15% (8–15%)	10% (6–17)
Total	23% (18–31%)	19% (12–26)
Deaths	4 (1.3%)	8 (2.8%)
Residual stones (range)	4.9% (2–12)	3.4% (0–12)

See Neoptolemos et al. [107], Stain et al. [151], Stiegmann et al. [154], Hammarström et al. [56], Targarona et al. [160], and Association universitaire de recherche en chirurgie [6]

Table 15.3. Evaluation of the status of CBDS therapy in 1997: strength of evidence

Stages in technology assessment[a]	ERCP	Open surgery	Laparoscopic surgery	ESWL	Transhepatic approach
Feasibility	III	III	III	III	0–I
Benefit for patient	III	III	III	III	0
Benefit for	III	III	I–III	0–III	0
surgeon	II	III	II	0–I	0–I
Effectivenes	III	0–I	0–II	0–I	0
Costs	III	III	III	I–III	0
Ethics recommendations	Yes	Yes	Yes	No	No

Grading of scientific evidence was done using the scale explained in Table 15.4 (III is strong evidence, 0 is no evidence)
ESWL extracorporeal shockwave lithotripsy
a) See Mosteller [105] and Troidl [164]

Question 5. Standard Treatment

Which Is the Best Treatment for CBDS and What Is the Appropriate Surgical Procedure for CBDS with Gallbladder in Situ?

There is no standard treatment today. In principle, three treatment regimens are available: endoscopic stone extraction during ERCP, laparoscopic bile duct exploration, and open bile duct exploration (Table 15.3). There is no strong evidence from controlled trials that one procedure is superior to another in experienced hands (Table 15.4). The majority of panel members saw no advantages to laparoscopic surgery over ERCP in terms of intraopera-

Table 15.4. Ratings of the literature on CBDS: strength of evidence

Study design	Strength of evidence	References
Clinical randomized controlled trial with power and relevant end points	III	[5, 6, 14, 24, 28, 35, 37, 44, 49, 52, 56, 60, 61, 77, 79, 81, 83, 86, 91, 103, 106–110, 112, 113, 118, 127, 134, 135, 141, 143, 146, 149–152, 154, 157, 159, 160, 168]
Prospective studies with parallel or historical controls Case-control studies	II	[2–4, 7, 8, 10, 11, 13, 15–21, 23, 25–27, 29, 30–34, 36, 38–43, 45–48, 50, 51, 53–55, 57–59, 62–69, 71–76, 79, 80, 84, 85, 87–89, 92–102, 104, 114–117, 119–126, 128–134, 136, 137, 139, 140, 142–145, 147, 148, 153, 155, 156, 158, 161–163, 165–167, 169–175]
Cohort studies with literature controls Database analyses Reports of expert committees	1	Numerous, not evaluated
Uncontrolled trials Case reports, case series Belief	0	Numerous, not evaluated

tive safety, postoperative complications, mortality, pain, hospital stay, return to work, or cosmesis.

Laparoscopic bile duct exploration or a combination of endoscopic stone removal and laparoscopic cholecystectomy might be better than open surgery in terms of such aspects as less pain and faster recovery.

The laparoscopic transcystic approach and laparoscopic choledochotomy are feasible. For ASA I/II patients, they might be preferable to preoperative ERCP and endoscopic sphincterotomy (ES) followed by laparoscopic cholecystectomy, since they shorten the duration of hospital stay.

Question 6. Treatment in Special Situations

Should Asymptomatic CBDS Be Treated?

Because of the impredictibility of the occurrence of symptoms or complications, diagnosed stones should be treated in all cases. It is additionally an ethical problem to knowingly leave stones behind. However, an expectant management for CBDS is acceptable in high-risk patients (ASA III/IV) and patients unfit for surgery. These patients may benefit from endoscopic treatment alone.

What Is the Appropriate Treatment for Large and/or Impacted CBDS?

Large and/or impacted stones are a rare and ill-defined condition. Their treatment is usually difficult and depends on individual expertise. Options include:

- Endoscopic treatment (with the adjunct of lithotripsy)
- Primary surgery (laparoscopic or open approach with the adjunct of intraoperative lithotripsy and/or hepaticojejunostomy)
- Extracorporeal shockwave lithotripsy (ESWL) with or without ES

How Should CBDS in Cholecystectomized Patients Be Managed?

All such patients should be first treated by endoscopy, if feasible, including lithotripsy as required. There is as yet no evidence that endoscopic sphincterotomy or dilation of the sphincter performed in younger patients has a long-term negative outcome with higher rates of cholangitis, papillary stenosis, or other sequelae.

Question 7. Cholecystectomy

Is Cholecystectomy Always Compulsory in Patients with CBDS?

Available data suggest that cholecystectomy should be recommended in patients with CBDS. In patients with major risk factors for surgery or in elderly patients, an individual management policy – e.g., leaving the gallbladder in situ – can be justified. In Oriental cholangitis and in patients without gallbladder stones, cholecystectomy is usually not indicated after clearance of the common bile duct.

Question 8. Consequences of Therapy

What Are the Long-Term Results and Sequelae of Therapeutic Interventions?

For both endoscopic sphincterotomy and open surgical common bile duct exploration, the long-term complication rates are reported to be in the same range (below 10%), and the procedures have a high success rate in experienced hands. There are no data on the long-term complication rate of laparoscopic bile duct exploration.

Closing Remarks

The closing remarks were delivered by J. Périssat, of France:

▪ The emerging success of MR cholangiopancreaticography, which has provided an excellent roadmap for the surgeon, should help to stem the debate over the diagnostic purpose of ERCP.

▪ The general population of surgeons should be brought up to date about the technology of laparoscopic bile duct exploration; furthermore, additional research is urgently needed.

▪ There should be a follow-up on the results of this conference in the year 2000.

References

1. Abboud PAC, Malet PF, Berlin JA, Staroscik R, Cabana MD, Clarke JR, Shea JA, Schwartz JS, Williams SV (1996) Predictors of common bile duct stones prior to cholecystectomy: a meta-analysis. Gastrointest Endosc 44:450–459
2. Adamek HE, Maier M, Jakobs R, Wessbecher FR, Neuhauser T, Riemann JF (1996) Management of retained bile duct stones: a prospective open trial comparing extracorporeal and intracorporeal lithotripsy. Gastrointest Endosc 44:40–47
3. Adamek HE, Riemann JF (1996) Extrakorporale Stoßwellenlithotripsie von Gallensteinen. Rückblick und Perspektive. Zeitschr Gesamte Inn Med Grenzgebiete 47:285–290
4. Adloff M, Ollier JC, Arnaud JP (1980) Place de la suture primitive du choledoque dans la chirurgie de la lithiase biliaire. Ann Chir 34:341–344
5. Alinder G, Nilsson U, Lunderquist A, Herlin P, Holmin T (1986) Pre-operative infusion cholangiography compared to routine operative cholangiography at elective cholecystectomy. Br J Surg 73:383–387
6. Association universitaire de recherche en chirurgie: Lenriot JP, Le Néel JC, Hay JM, Jaeck D, Millat B, Fagniez PL (1993) Cholangiopancréatographie rétrograde et sphinctérotomie endoscopique pour lithiase biliaire. Evaluation prospective en milieu chirurgical. Gastroenterol Clin Biol 17:244–250
7. Barkun AN, Barkun JS, Fried GM, Ghitulescu G, Steinmetz O, Pham C, Meakins JL, Goresky CA (1994) Useful predictors of bile duct stones in patients undergoing laparoscopic cholecystectomy. McGill Gallstone Treatment Group. Ann Surg 220:32–39
8. Barteau JA, Castro D, Arregui ME, Tetik C (1995) A comparison of intraoperative ultrasound versus cholangiography in the evaluation of the common bile duct during laparoscopic cholecystectomy. Surg Endosc 9:490–496
9. Berci G, Cuschieri A (1997) Bile ducts and bile duct stones. Saunders, Philadelphia
10. Berci G, Morgenstern L (1994) Laparoscopic management of common bile duct stones. A multi-institutional SAGES study. Society of American Gastrointestinal Endoscopic Surgeons. Surg Endosc 8:1174–1175
11. Berci G, Sakier JM, Paz-Partlow M (1991) Routine or selected intraoperative cholangiography during laparoscopic cholecystectomy? Am J Surg 161:355–360
12. Berci G, Shore JM, Hamlin JA, Morgenstern L (1978) Operative flouroscopy and cholangiography – the use of modern radiologic technics during surgery. Am J Surg 135:32–35
13. Berggren P, Farago I, Gabrielsson N, Thor K (1997) Intravenous cholangiography before 1000 consecutive laparoscopic cholecystectomies. Br J Surg 84:472–476
14. Bergman JJGHM, Rauws EAJ, Fockens P, van Berkel AM, Bossuyt PMM, Tijssen JGP, Tytgat GNJ, Huibregtse K (1997) Randomised trial of endoscopic balloon dilatation versus endoscopic sphincterotomy for removal of bile duct stones. Lancet 349:1124–1129
15. Bland KI, Scott-Jones R, Maher JW, Cotton PB, Pennell TC, Amerson JR, Munson JL, Berci G, Fuchs GJ, Way LW, Graham JB, Lindenau BU, Moody FG (1989) Extracorporeal

shock-wave lithotripsy of bile duct calculi – an interim report of the Dornier US bile duct lithotripsy prospective study. Ann Surg 209:743–755

16. Bloom IT, Gibbs SL, Keeling Roberts CS, Brough WA (1996) Intravenous infusion cholangiography for investigation of the bile duct: a direct comparison with endoscopic retrograde cholangiopancreatography. Br J Surg 83:755–757

17. Boender J, Nix GA, de Ridder MA, van Blankenstein M, Schutte HE, Dees J, Wilson JH (1994) Endoscopic papillotomy for common bile duct stones: factors influencing the complication rate. Endoscopy 26:209–216

18. Boey JH, Way LW (1980) Acute cholangitis. Ann Surg 191:264–270

19. Borge J (1977) Operative cholangiography – new cholangiogram catheter clamp and improved technique. Arch Surg 112: 340–342

20. Brocks H (1959/60) Choledochoscopy versus cholangiography – experience of a 12-month trial. Acta Chir Scand 118:434–438

21. Broome A, Jensen R, Thoerne J (1976) A new cholangiography catheter. Acta Chir Scand 142:421–422

22. Burhenne JH (1978) Nonoperative instrument extraction of retained bile duct stones. World J Surg 3:439–445

23. Burhenne JH (1980) Percutaneous extraction of retained biliary tract stones – 661 patients. Am J Radiol 134:888–898

24. Canto M, Chak A, Sivak MV, Blades E, Stellato T (1995) Endoscopic ultrasonography (EUS) versus cholangiography for diagnosing extrahepatic biliary stones – a prospective, blinded study in pre- and post-cholecystectomy patients [Abstract]. Gastrointest Endosc 41:391

25. Changchien C-S, Chuah S-K, Chiu K-W (1995) Is ERCP necessary for symptomatic gallbladder stone patients before laparoscopic cholecystectomy? Am J Gastroenterol 90:2124–2127

26. Chen YK, Foliente RL, Santoro MJ, Walter MH, Collen MJ (1994) Endoscopic sphincterotomy – induced pancreatitis: increased risk associated with nondilated bile ducts and sphincter of Oddi dysfunction. Am J Gastroenterol 89:327–333

27. Chijiiwa K, Kozaki N, Naito T, Kameoka N, Tanaka M (1995) Treatment of choice for choledocholithiasis in patients with acute obstructive suppurative cholangitis and liver cirrhosis. Am J Surg 170:356–360

28. Chopra KP, Peters RA, O'Toole PA, Williams SGJ, Gimson AES, Lombard MG, Westaby D (1996) Randomised study of endoscopic biliary endoprosthesis versus duct clearance for bileduct stones in high-risk patients. Lancet 348:791–793

29. Clair DG, Carr Locke DL, Becker JM, Brooks DC (1993) Routine cholangiography is not warranted during laparoscopic cholecystectomy. Arch Surg 128:554–555

30. Corlette MB, Schatzki S, Ackroyd F (1978) Operative cholangiography and overlooked stones. Arch Surg 113:729–734

31. Cotton PB, Vallon AG (1982) Duodenoscopic sphincterotomy for removal of bile duct stones in patients with gallbladders. Surgery 91:628–630

32. Cox MR, Wilson TG, Toouli J (1995) Peroperative endoscopic sphincterotomy during laparoscopic cholecystectomy for choledocholithiasis. Br J Surg 82:257–259

33. Cronan JJ (1986) US diagnosis of choledocholithiasis: a reappraisal. Radiology 161:133–134

34. Csendes A, Diaz JC, Burdiles P, Maluenda F, Morales E (1992) Risk factors and classification of acute suppurative cholangitis. Br J Surg 79:655–658

35. Cuschieri A, Croce E, Faggioni A, Jakimowicz J, Lacy A, Lezoche E, Morino M, Ribeiro VM, Toouli J, Visa J, Wayand W (1996) EAES ductal stone study – preliminary findings of a multi-center prospective randomized trial comparing two-stage vs single-stage management. Surg Endosc 10:1130–1135

36. Cuschieri A, Shimi S, Banting S, Nathanson LK, Pietrabissa A (1994) Intraoperative cholangiography during laparoscopic cholecystectomy – routine vs selective policy. Surg Endosc 8:302–305

37. Daly J, Fitzgerald T, Simpson CJ (1987) Pre-operative intravenous cholangiography as an alternative to routine operative cholangiography in elective cholecystectomy. Clin Radiol 38:161–163

38. Davidson BR, Neoptolemus JP, Carr-Locke DL (1988) Endoscopic sphincterotomy for common bile duct calculi in patients with gall bladder in situ considered unfit for surgery. Gut 29:114–120

39. De Palma GD, Angrisani L, Lorenzo M, Di Matteo E, Catanzano C, Persico G, Tesauro B (1996) Laparoscopic cholecystectomy (LC), intraoperative endoscopic sphincterotomy (ES), and common bile duct stones (CBDS) extraction for management of patients with cholecystocholedocholithiasis. Surg Endosc 10:649–652

40. de Watteville JC, Gailleton R, Gayral F, Testas P (1992) Role of routine preoperative intravenous cholangiography before laparoscopic cholecystectomy [Abstract]. Br J Surg 79:S10

41. DenBesten L, Berci G (1986) The current status of biliary tract surgery: an international study of 1072 consecutive patients. World J Surg 10:116–122

42. Dowsett JF, Polydorou AA, Vaira D, D'Anna LM, Ashraf M, Croker J, Salmon PR, Russell RCG, Hatfield ARW (1990) Needle knife papillotomy: how safe and how effective? Gut 31:905–908

43. Doyle PJ, Ward-McQuaid JN, McEwen-Smith A (1982) The value of routine peroperative cholangiography – a report of 4000 cholecystectomies. Br J Surg 69:617–619

44. Duron JJ, Roux JM, Imbaud P, Dumont JL, Dutet D, Validire J (1987) Biliary lithiasis in the over seventy-five age group – a new therapeutic strategy. Br J Surg 74:848–849

45. Ellul JPM, Wilkinson ML, McColl I, Dowling RH (1992) A predictive ERCP study of patients with gallbladder stones (GBS) and probable choledocholithiasis – predictive factors [Abstract]. Gastrointest Endosc 38:266

46. Erickson RA, Carlson B (1995) The role of endoscopic retrograde cholangiopancreatography in patients with laparoscopic cholecystectomies. Gastroenterology 109:252–263

47. Escarce JJ, Shea JA, Chen W, Qian Z, Schwartz JS (1995) Outcomes of open cholecystectomy in the elderly: a longitudinal analysis of 21,000 cases in the prelaparoscopic era. Surgery 117:156–164

48. Escourrou J, Cordova JA, Lazorthes F, Frexinos J, Ribet A (1994) Early and late complications after endoscopic sphincterotomy for biliary lithiasis with and without the gallbladder 'in situ.' Gut 25:598–602

49. Fan ST, Lai EC, Mok FP, Lo CM, Zheng SS, Wong J (1993) Early treatment of acute biliary pancreatitis by endoscopic papillotomy. N Engl J Med 328:228–232

50. Farha GJ, Pearson RN (1976) Transcystic duct operative cholangiography – personal experience with 500 consecutive cases. Am J Surg 131:228–231

51. Finnis D, Rowntree T (1977) Choledochoscopy in exploration of the common bile duct. Br J Surg 64:661–664

52. Fölsch UR, Nitsche R, Lüdtke R, Hilgers RA, Creutzfeldt W (1997) The German study group for acute biliary pancreatitis: early ERCP and papillotomy compared with conservative treatment for acute biliary pancreatitis. N Engl J Med 336:237–242

53. Gail K, Seifert E (1982) Cholecystectomy after endoscopic removal of common bile duct stones – a necessary procedure? [Abstract]. Scand J Gastroenterol 78:S142

54. Grace PA, Qureshi A, Burke P, Leahy A, Brindley N, Osborne H, Lane B, Broe P, Bouchier Hayes D (1993) Selective cholangiography in laparoscopic cholecystectomy. Br J Surg 80:244–246

55. Gunn A (1980) The use of tantalum clips during operative cholangiography. Br J Surg 67:146

56. Hammarström LE, Holmin T, Stridbeck H, Ihse I (1995) Long-term follow-up of a prospective randomized study of endoscopic versus surgical treatment of bile duct calculi in patients with gallbladder in situ. Br J Surg 82:1516–1521

57. Hammarström LE, Holmin T, Stridbeck H, Ihse I (1996) Routine preoperative infusion cholangiography at elective cholecystectomy: a prospective study in 694 patients. Br J Surg 83:750–754

58. Hammarström LE, Holmin T, Stridbeck H, Ihse I (1996) Routine preoperative infusion cholangiography versus intraoperative cholangiography at elective cholecystectomy: a prospective study in 995 patients. J Am Coll Surg 182:408–416

59. Hauer-Jensen M, Karesen R, Nygaard K, Solheim K, Amlie E, Havig Ø, Viddal O (1985) Predictive ability of choledocholithiasis indicators – a prospective evaluation. Ann Surg 202:64–68
60. Hauer-Jensen M, Karesen R, Nygaard K, Solheim K, Amlie E, Havig Ø, Viddal KO (1986) Consequences of routine peroperative cholangiography during cholecystectomy for gallstone disease – a prospective, randomized study. World J Surg 10:996–1002
61. Hauer-Jensen M, Karesen R, Nygaard K, Solheim K, Amlie EJB, Havig Ø, Rosseland AR (1993) Prospective randomized study of routine intraoperative cholangiography during open cholecystectomy – long-term follow-up and multivariate analysis of predictors of choledocholithiasis. Surgery 113:318–323
62. Heinerman M, Boeckl O, Pimpl W (1989) Selective ERCP and preoperative stone removal in bile duct surgery. Ann Surg 209:267–272
63. Heinerman M, Pimpl W, Waclawiczek W, Boeckl O (1987) Combined endoscopic and surgical approach to primary gallstone disease. Surg Endosc 1:195–198
64. Holbrook RF, Jacobson FL, Pezzuti RT, Howell DA (1991) Biliary patence imaging after endoscopic retrograde sphincterotomy with gallbladder in situ. Arch Surg 126:738–742
65. Hollis R (1993) Predictors of common bile duct (CBD) abnormalities in patients undergoing ERCP prior to laparoscopic cholecystectomy (LC) [Abstract]. Am J Gastroenterol 88:1531
66. Hopton D (1978) Common bile duct perfusion combined with operative cholangiography. Br J Surg 65:852–854
67. Houdart R, Brisset D, Perniceni T, Palau R (1990) La cholangiographie intraveineuse est inutile avant cholecystectomie pour lithiase non compliquee – etude prospective de 100 cas. Gastroenterol Clin Biol 14:652–654
68. Huang SM, Wu CW, Chau GY, Jwo SC, Lui WY, P'eng FK (1996) An alternative approach of choledocholithotomy via laparoscopic choledochotomy. Arch Surg 131:407–411
69. Huddy SPJ, Southam JA (1989) Is intravenous cholangiography an alternative to the routine per-operative cholangiogram? Postgrad Med J 65:896–899
70. Huguier M, Bornet P, Charpak Y, Houry S, Chastang C (1991) Selective contraindications based on multivariate analysis for operative cholangiography in biliary lithiasis. Surg Gynecol Obstet 172:470–474
71. Jakimowicz JJ, Carol EJ, Mak B, Roukema A (1986) An operative choledochoscopy using the flexible choledochoscope. Surg Gynecol Obstet 162:215–221
72. Johnson GK, Geenen JE, Venu RP, Schmalz MJ, Hogan WJ (1993) Treatment of non-extractable common bile duct stones with combination ursodeoxycholic acid plus endoprostheses. Gastrointest Endosc 39:528–531
73. Jones DB, Dunnegan DL, Soper NJ (1995) Results of a change to routine fluorocholangiography during laparoscopic cholecystectomy. Surgery 118:701–702
74. Joyce WP, Keane R, Burke GJ, Daly M, Drumm J, Egan TJ, Delaney PV (1991) Identification of bile duct stones in patients undergoing laparoscopic cholecystectomy. Br J Surg 78:1174–1176
75. Keighley MRB, Graham NG (1971) Infective complications of choledochotomy with T-tube drainage. Brit J Surg 58:764–768
76. Kitahama A, Kerstein MD, Overby JL, Kappelman MD, Webb WR (1986) Routine intraoperative cholangiogram. Surg Gynecol Obstet 162:317–322
77. Lacaine F, Corlette MB, Bismuth H (1980) Preoperative evaluation of the risk of common bile duct stones. Arch Surg 115:1114–1116
78. Lai CW, Tam P-C, Paterson IA, Ng MMT, Fan S-T, Choi T-K, Wong J (1990) Emergency surgery for severe acute cholangitis – the high risk patients. Ann Surg 211:55–59
79. Lai ECS, Mok FPT, Tan ESY, Lo C-ML, Fan S-T, You K-T, Wong J (1992) Endoscopic biliary drainage for severe acute cholangitis. N Engl J Med 326:1582–1586
80. Leese T, Neoptolemus JP, Carr-Locke DL (1985) Successes, failures, early complications and their management following endoscopic sphincterotomy: results in 394 consecutive patients from a single centre. Br J Surg 72:215–219

81. Lewis RT, Allan CM, Goodall RG, Marien B, Park M, Lloyd-Smith W, Wiegand FM (1984) A single preoperative dose of cefazolin prevents postoperative sepsis in high-risk biliary surgery. Can J Surg 27:44–47

82. Lezoche E, Paganini AM, Carlei F, Feliciotti F, Lomanto D, Guerrieri M (1996) Laparoscopic treatment of gallbladder and common bile duct stones: a prospective study. World J Surg 20:542

83. Liberman MA, Phillips EH, Carroll BJ, Fallas MJ, Rosenthal R, Hiatt J (1996) Cost-effective management of complicated choledocholithiasis: laparoscopic transcystic duct exploration or endoscopic sphincterotomy. J Am Coll Surg 182:488–494

84. Lillemoe KD, Yeo CJ, Talamini MA, Wang BH, Pitt HA, Gadacz TR (1992) Selective cholangiography. Current role in laparoscopic cholecystectomy. Ann Surg 215:674–676

85. Linder S, von Rosen A, Wiechel KL (1993) Bile duct pressure, hormonal influence and recurrent bile duct stones. Hepatogastroenterology 40:370–374

86. Lindsell DRM (1990) Ultrasound imaging of pancreas and biliary tract. Lancet 335:390–393

87. Little JM (1987) A prospective evaluation of computerized estimates of risk in the management of obstructive jaundice. Surgery 102:473–476

88. Liu CL, Lai ECS, Lo CM, Chu KM, Fan ST, Wong J (1996) Combined laparoscopic and endoscopic approach in patients with cholelithiasis and choledocholithiasis. Surgery 119:534–537

89. Lomanto D, Pavone P, Laghi A, Panebianco V, Mazzocchi P, Fiocca F, Lezoche E, Passariello R, Speranza V (1997) Magnetic resonance cholangiopancreatography in the diagnosis of biliopancreatic diseases. Am J Surg 174:33–38

90. Lorimer JW, Lauzon J, Fairfull-Smith RJ, Yelle J-D (1997) Management of choledocholithiasis in the time of laparoscopic cholecystectomy. Am J Surg 174:68–71

91. Lygidakis NJ (1982) A prospective randomized study of recurrent choledocholithiasis. Surg Gynecol Obstet 155:679–684

92. MacMathuna P, White P, Clarke E, Lennon J, Crowe J (1994) Endoscopic sphincteroplasty: a novel and safe alternative to papillotomy in the management of bile duct stones. Gut 35:127–129

93. Madden JL (1978) Primary common bile duct stones. World J Surg 2:465–471

94. Madhavan KK, MacIntyre IMC, Wilson RG, Saunders JH, Nixon SJ, Hamer-Hodges DW (1995) Role of intraoperative cholangiography in laparoscopic cholecystectomy. Br J Surg 82:249–252

95. Masci E, Toti G, Cosentino F, Mariani A, Guerini S, Meroni E, Missale G, Lomazzi A, Prada A, Comin U, Crosta C, Tittobello A (1997) Prospective studies on post ERCP/ES acute pancreatitis [Abstract]. Gastrointest Endosc 45:AB139

96. Mazariello RM (1978) A fourteen-year experience with nonoperative instrument extraction of retained bile duct stones. World J Surg 2:447–455

97. McEvedy BV (1970) Routine operative cholangiography. Br J Surg 57:277–279

98. Metcalf AM, Ephgrave KS, Dean TR, Maher JW (1992) Preoperative screening with ultrasonography for laparoscopic cholecystectomy: an alternative to routine intraoperative cholangiography. Surgery 112:813–817

99. Meyers WC (1991) A prospective analysis of 1518 laparoscopic cholecystectomies – the Southern Surgeons Club. N Engl J Med 324:1073–1078

100. Michotey G, Signouret B, Argeme M, Ages M (1981) Les complications du drain de Kehr – a propos de quatre observations. Ann Chir 35:351–355

101. Millat B, Atger J, Deleuze A, Briandet H, Fingerhut A, Guillon F, Marrel E, de Seguin C, Soulier P (1997) Laparoscopic treatment for choledocholithiasis: a prospective evaluation in 247 consecutive unselected patients. Hepatogastroenterology 44:28–34

102. Millat B, Fingerhut A, Deleuze A, Briandet H, Marrel E, de Seguin C, Soulier P (1995) Prospective evaluation in 121 consecutive unselected patients undergoing laparoscopic treatment of choledocholithiasis. Br J Surg 82:1266–1269

103. Minami A, Nakatsu T, Uchida N, Hirabayashi S, Fukuma H, Morshed SA, Nishioka M (1995) Papillary dilation vs sphincterotomy in endoscopic removal of bile duct stones. A randomized trial with manometric function. Dig Dis Sci 40:2550–2554
104. Mofti AB, Ahmed I, Tandon RC, Al-Tameen MM, Al-Khudairy NN (1986) Routine or selective peroperative cholangiography. Br J Surg 73:548–550
105. Mosteller F (1985) Assessing medical technologies. National Academic Press, Washington, DC
106. Murison MS, Gartell PC, McGinn FP (1993) Does selective peroperative cholangiography result in missed common bile duct stones? J R Coll Surg Edinb 38:220–224
107. Neoptolemus JP, Carr-Locke DL, Fossard DP (1987) Prospective randomised study of preoperative endoscopic sphincterotomy versus surgery alone for common bile duct stones. Br Med J 294:470–474
108. Neoptolemus JP, Carr-Locke DL, London NJ, Bailey IA, James D, Fossard DP (1988) Controlled trial of urgent endoscopic retrograde cholangiopancreatography and endoscopic sphincterotomy versus conservative treatment for acute pancreatitis due to gallstones. Lancet 2:979–983
109. Neoptolemus JP, Davidson BR, Shaw DE, Lloyd D, Carr-Locke DL, Fossard DP (1987) Study of common bile duct exploration and endoscopic sphincterotomy in a consecutive series of 438 patients. Br J Surg 74:916–921
110. Neoptolemus JP, Shaw DE, Carr-Locke DL (1989) A multivariate analysis of preoperative risk factors in patients with common bile duct stones. Ann Surg 209: 157–161
111. Neugebauer E, Troidl H, Kum CK, Eypasch E, Miserez M, Paul A (1995) The E.A.E.S. Consensus Development Conferences on laparoscopic cholecystectomy, appendectomy, and hernia repair. Consensus statements – September 1994. The Educational Committee of the European Association for Endoscopic Surgery. Surg Endosc 9:550–563
112. Neuhaus H, Feussner H, Ungeheuer A, Hoffmann W, Siewert JR, Classen M (1992) Prospective evaluation of the use of endoscopic retrograde cholangiography prior to laparoscopic cholecystectomy. Endoscopy 24:745–749
113. Neuhaus H, Ungeheuer A, Feussner H, Classen M, Siewert JR (1992) Laparoskopische Cholezystektomie: ERCP als präoperative Standarddiagnostik? Dtsch Med Wochenschr 117:1863–1867
114. Nilson U (1987) Adverse reactions to iotroxate at intravenous cholangiography. Acta Radiol 28:571–575
115. Nora PJ, Berci G, Dorazio RA, Kirshenbaum G, Shore JM, Tompkins RK, Wilson SD (1977) Operative choledochoscopy – results of a prospective study in several institutions. Am J Surg 133:105–110
116. Nowak A, Nowakowska-Dulawa E, Marek TA, Rybicka J (1996) Résultat d'une étude prospective contrôlée et randomisée comparant le traitment endoscopique par rapport au traitement conventionnel en cas de pancréatite aigue biliaire [Abstract]. Gastroenterol Clin Biol 20:A2
117. Osnes M, Larsen S, Lowe P, Grønseth K, Løtveit T, Nordshus T (1978) Comparison of endoscopic retrograde and intravenous cholangiography in diagnosis of biliary calculi. Lancet 2:230
118. Panis Y, Fagniez P-L, Brisset D, Lacaine F, Levard H, Hay J-M (1993) Long-term results of choledochoduodenostomy versus choledochojejunostomy for choledocholithiasis. Surg Gynecol Obstet 177:33–37
119. Pencev D, Brady PG, Pinkas H, Boulay J (1994) The role of ERCP in patients after laparoscopic cholecystectomy. Am J Gastroenterol 89:1523–1527
120. Périssat J (1996) Laparoscopic treatment of bile duct stones. In: Brune IB (ed) Laparoendoscopic surgery, 2d ed. Blackwell, London, pp 57–63
121. Périssat J, Huibregtse K, Keane FB, Russell RC, Neoptolemos JP (1994) Management of bile duct stones in the era of laparoscopic cholecystectomy. Br J Surg 81:799–810
122. Petelin JB (1993) Laparoscopic approach to common duct pathology. Am J Surg 165:487–491

123. Phillips EH, Carroll BJ, Pearlstein AR, Daykhovsky L, Fallas MJ (1993) Laparoscopic choledochoscopy and extraction of common bile duct stones. World J Surg 17:22–28

124. Phillips EH, Liberman M, Carroll BJ, Fallas MJ, Rosenthal RJ, Hiatt JR (1995) Bile duct stones in the laparoscopic era. Is preoperative sphincterotomy necessary? Arch Surg 130:885–886

125. Planells Roig M, Garćýa Espinosa R, Moya Sanz A, Pastor P, Rodero D (1992) Laparoscopic cholecystectomy and selective intraoperative cholangiography: a prospective series of 70 patients [Abstract]. Br J Surg 79:S11

126. Podolsky I, Kortan P, Haber GB (1989) Endoscopic sphincterotomy in outpatients. Gastrointest Endosc 35:372–376

127. Ponchon T, Bory R, Chavaillon A, Fouillet P (1989) Biliary lithiasis – combined endoscopic and surgical treatment. Endoscopy 21:15–18

128. Ponchon T, Genin G, Mitchell R, Henry L, Bory RM, Bodnar D, Valette P-J (1996) Methods, indications, and results of percutaneous choledochoscopy – a series of 161 procedures. Ann Surg 223:26–36

129. Prasad JK, Daniel O (1971) A comparison of the value of measurement of flow and pressure as aids to bile-duct surgery [Abstract]. Br J Surg 58:868

130. Prat F, Malak NA, Pelletier G, Buffet C, Fritsch J, Choury AD, Altman C, Liguory C, Etienne JP (1996) Biliary symptoms and complications more than 8 years after endoscopic sphincterotomy for choledocholithiasis. Gastroenterology 110:894–899

131. Regan F, Fradin J, Khazan R, Bohlman M, Magnoson T (1996) Choledocholithiasis: evaluation with MR cholangiography. Am J Roentgenol 167:1441–1445

132. Rhodes M, Nathanson L, O'Rourke N, Fielding G (1995) Laparoscopic exploration of the common bile duct: lessons learned from 129 consecutive cases. Br J Surg 82:666–668

133. Rijna H, Borgstein PJ, Meuwissen SG, de Brauw LM, Wildenborg NP, Cuesta MA (1995) Selective preoperative endoscopic retrograde cholangiopancreatography in laparoscopic biliary surgery. Br J Surg 82:1130–1133

134. Röthlin MA, Schlumpf R, Largiader F (1994) Laparoscopic sonography. An alternative to routine intraoperative cholangiography? Arch Surg 129:694–700

135. Röthlin MA, Schob O, Schlumpf R, Largiader F (1996) Laparoscopic ultrasonography during cholecystectomy. Br J Surg 83:1512–1516

136. Salomon J, Roseman DL (1978) Intraoperative measurement of common bile duct resistance. Arch Surg 113:650–653

137. Santucci L, Natalini G, Sarpi L, Fiorucci S, Solinas A, Morelli A (1996) Selective endoscopic retrograde cholangiography and preoperative bile duct stone removal in patients scheduled for laparoscopic cholecystectomy: a prospective study. Am J Gastroenterol 91:1326–1330

138. Sauerbruch T, Feussner H, Frimberger E, Hasegawa H, Ihse I, Riemann JF, Yasuda H (1994) Treatment of common bile duct stones. A consensus report. Hepatogastroenterology 41:513–515

139. Sauerbruch T, Holl J, Sackmann M, Paumgartner G (1992) Fragmentation of bile duct stones by extracorporeal shock-wave lithotripsy: a five-year experience. Hepatology 15:208–214

140. Schwab G, Pointner R, Wetscher G, Glaser K, Foltin E, Bodner E (1992) Treatment of calculi of the common bile duct. Surg Gynecol Obstet 175:115–120

141. Seifert E, Gail K, Weismüller J (1982) Langzeitresultate nach endoskopischer Sphinkerotomie. Dtsch Med Wochenschr 107:610–614

142. Shaffer EA, Braasch JW, Small DM (1972) Bile composition at and after surgery in normal persons and patients with gallstones. N Engl J Med 287:1317–1322

143. Sheen Chen SM, Chou FF (1995) Intraoperative choledochoscopic electrohydraulic lithotripsy for difficulty retrieved impacted common bile duct stones. Arch Surg 130:430–432

144. Sheridan WG, Williams HOL, Lewis MH (1987) Morbidity and mortality of common bile duct exploration. Br J Surg 74:1095–1099

145. Siegel JH, Safrany L, Ben-Zvi JS, Pullano WE, Cooperman A, Stenzel M, Ramsey WH (1988) Duodenoscopic sphincterotomy in patients with gallbladders in situ: report of a series of 1272 patients. Am J Gastroenterol 83:1255–1258

146. Sigel B, Machi J, Beitler JC, Donahue PE, Bombeck T, Baker RJ, Duarte B (1983) Comparative accuracy of operative ultrasonography and cholangiography in detecting common duct calculi. Surgery 94:715–720

147. Simmons F, Ross APJ, Bouchier IAD (1972) Alterations in hepatic bile composition after cholecystectomy. Gastroenterology 63:466–471

148. Skar V, Skar AG, Osnes M (1989) The duodenal bacterial flora in the region of papilla of Vater in patients with and without duodenal diverticula. Scand J Gastroenterol 24:649–656

149. Soper NJ, Dunnegan DL (1992) Routine versus selective intraoperative cholangiography during laparoscopic cholecystectomy. World J Surg 16:1133–1140

150. Soto JA, Barish MA, Yucel EK, Siegenberg D, Ferrucci JT, Chuttani R (1996) Magnetic resonance cholangiography – comparison with endoscopic retrograde cholangiopancreatography. Gastroenterology 11:589–597

151. Stain SC, Cohen H, Tsuishoysha M, Donovan AJ (1991) Choledocholithiasis – endoscopic sphincterotomy or common bile duct exploration. Arch Surg 213:627–634

152. Stark ME, Loughry CW (1980) Routine operative cholangiography with cholecystectomy. Surg Gynecol Obstet 151:657–658

153. Steele RJC, Park K, Gilbert F (1991) Prediction of common bile duct stones: the importance of ultrasonic duct visualisation [Abstract]. Gut 32:A1253–A1254

154. Stiegmann GV, Goff JS, Mansour A, Pearlman N, Reveille RM, Norton L (1992) Precholecystectomy endoscopic cholangiography and stone removal is not superior to cholecystectomy, cholangiography, and common duct exploration. Am J Surg 163:227–230

155. Stiegmann GV, Pearlman N, Goff JS, Sun JH, Norton L (1989) Endoscopic cholangiography and stone removal prior to cholecystectomy – a more cost-effective approach than operative duct exploration. Arch Surg 124:787–790

156. Stiegmann GV, Soper NJ, Filipi CJ, McIntyre RC, Callary MP, Cordova JF (1995) Laparoscopic ultrasonography as compared with static or dynamic cholangiography at laparoscopic cholecystectomy. Surg Endosc 9:1269–1273

157. Stoker ME (1995) Common bile duct exploration in the era of laparoscopic surgery. Arch Surg 130:268–269

158. Swanstrom LL, Marcus DR, Kenyon T (1996) Laparoscopic treatment of known choledocholithiasis. Surg Endosc 10:526–528

159. Tanaka M, Sada M, Eguchi T, Konomi H, Naritomi G, Takeda T, Ogawa Y, Chijiwa K, Deenitchin GP (1996) Comparison of routine and selective endoscopic retrograde cholangiography before laparoscopic cholecystectomy. World J Surg 20:267–271

160. Targarona EM, Perez-Ayuso RM, Bordas JM, Ros E, Pros I, Martinez J, Teres J, Trias M (1996) Randomized trial of endoscopic sphincterotomy with gallbladder left in situ versus open surgery for common bile duct calculi in high-risk patients. Lancet 347:926–929

161. Taylor TV, Armstrong CP, Rimmer S, Lucas SB, Jeacock J, Gunn AA (1988) Prediction of choledocholithiasis using a pocket microcomputer. Br J Surg 75:138–140

162. Tham TCK, Collins JSA, Watson RGP, Ellis PK, McIllrath EM (1996) Diagnosis of common bile duct stones by intravenous cholangiography: prediction by ultrasound and liver function tests compared with endoscopic retrograde cholangiography. Gastrointest Endosc 44:158–163

163. Thurston OG, McDougall RM (1976) The effect of hepatic bile on retained common duct stones. Surg Gynecol Obstet 143:625–627

164. Troidl H (1994) Endoscopic surgery – a fascinating idea requires responsibility in evaluation and handling. In: Szabo Z, Kerstein MD, Lewis JE (eds) Surgical technology. Universal Medical Press, San Francisco, pp 111–117

165. Van Dam J, Sivak MV (1993) Mechanical lithotripsy of large common bile duct stones. Cleve Clin J Med 60:38–42
166. Welbourn CR, Haworth JM, Leaper DJ, Thompson MH (1995) Prospective evaluation of ultrasonography and liver function tests for preoperative assessment of the bile duct. Br J Surg 82:1371–1373
167. Wenckert A, Robertson B (1966) The natural course of gallstone disease – eleven-year review of 781 nonoperated cases. Gastroenterology 50:376–381
168. Wermke W, Schulz H-J (1987) Sonographische Diagnostik von Gallenwegskonkrementen. Ultraschall 8:116–120
169. White TT, Waisman H, Hopton D, Kavlie H (1972) Radiomanometry, flow rates, and cholangiography in the evaluation of common bile duct disease. Am J Surg 123:73–79
170. Widdison AL, Longstaff AJ, Armstrong CP (1994) Combined laparoscopic and endoscopic treatment of gallstones and bile duct stones: a prospective study. Br J Surg 81:595–597
171. Wilson TG, Hall JC, Watts JM (1986) Is operative cholangiography always necessary? Br J Surg 73:637–640
172. Wilson TG, Jeans PL, Anthony A, Cox MR, Toouli J (1993) Laparoscopic cholecystectomy and management of choledocholithiasis. Aust N Z J Surg 63:443–450
173. Wolloch Y, Feigenberg Z, Zer M, Dintsman M (1977) The influence of biliary infection on the postoperative course after biliary tract surgery. Am J Gastroenterol 67:456–462
174. Worthley CS, Watts JM, Toouli J (1989) Common duct exploration or endoscopic sphincterotomy for choledocholithiasis? Aust N Z J Surg 59:209–215
175. Zaninotto G, Costantini M, Rossi M, Anselmino M, Pianalto S, Oselladore D, Pizzato D, Norberto L, Ancona E (1996) Sequential intraluminal endoscopic and laparoscopic treatment for bile duct stones associated with gallstones. Surg Endosc 10:644–648

Common Bile Duct Stones – Update 2006

Jürgen Treckmann, Stefan Sauerland, Andreja Frilling, Andreas Paul

Definition, Epidemiology and Clinical Course

There are no obvious changes in epidemiology of common bile duct stones (CBDS). As less invasive treatment options for CBDS are now well established, even older patients with significant comorbidities and pediatric patients who present with symptomatic cholecystolithiasis and CBDS are reported to be treated with increasing success [3, 25, 34]. In contrast, some prospective data suggest that in selected patients older than 80 years of age an expectant attitude can be justified, because symptoms are rare (below 15%) and in over one third of patients spontaneous passages of calculi were observed [4, 25].

Diagnosis of Common Bile Duct Stones

The ongoing unsolved crucial issue in diagnosis and treatment of CBDS is whether one should favour a high rate of negative examinations or a higher rate of retained stones. The benefit or harm of either strategy short and long term remains to be settled. Further studies [1, 32] underlined that cholangitis, dilated common bile duct with evidence of stones by ultrasound, elevated conjugated bilirubin, and less likely elevated asparate transaminase were predictive as individual factors and jointly excellent indicators (positive predictive value 99%) for CBDS. No new predictive factors for CBDS have been described in the literature and the 1997 statement is still valid for the identification of high-, medium- and low-risk groups for CBDS.

No new diagnostic tools have been established, but some of the existing diagnostic tools have been improved. Conventional percutaneous ultrasound continues to be useful, but still serves just as a screening tool. Intravenous cholangiography is of very limited value and the routine use of intravenous cholangiography cannot be advocated [14, 21]. Besides the technical advances, for example in evaluation of living related liver transplantation ("all-in-one" CT), CT continues to play a major role in routine diagnosis and management of CBDS [16]. Intraoperative ultrasound has a high accuracy (above 95%), but requires sufficient expertise and normally has its place only in centres performing one-stage procedures either by an open approach or by laparoscopy [2, 28].

Endoscopic ultrasound is an excellent diagnostic tool for CBDS with a sensitivity of more than 95% and a specificity of more than 90%, but is an invasive procedure and no controlled trials were published in the last 5 years, indicating that there is no widespread acceptance of endoscopic ultrasound in diagnosis of CBDS in general practice [24, 30]. The technology of magnetic resonance cholangiopancreatography (MRCP) is evolving rapidly and is increasingly gaining acceptance. Sensitivities and specificities for diagnosis of CBDS are reported to be 97 and 95%, respectively. Furthermore, there are data available showing that differentiated use of short and long-sequence MRI and half-Fourier acquired single-shot turbo spin echo (HASTE) vs rapid acquisition with relaxation enhancement (RARE) can increase diagnostic accuracy and decrease costs [6, 7, 13, 19, 20, 27, 36]. Currently, MRC(P), whenever available, should be the standard diagnostic test for patients with medium or high risk for CBDS. Endoscopic retrograde cholangiopancreatography (ERCP) provides an accuracy of at least more than 90% but owing to its invasiveness and complication rate ERCP is only indicated for confirming diagnosis of CBDS and whenever there is an intention to treat CBDS by endoscopic papillotomy (EPT) and stone extraction in the same session, or when magnetic resonance cholangiography (MRC) or endoscopic ultrasound are not available. Alternatively, CBDS are diagnosed by intraoperative cholangiography, whenever preoperative diagnosis is uncertain, or when there is an intention to treat CBDS intraoperatively [2, 21, 28].

Operative vs Conservative (Interventional) Treatment

According to published (external) evidence there is no option which can be identified as a "gold standard". Endoscopic stone extraction via endoscopic retrograde cholangiography/papillotomy, laparoscopic transcystic or laparoscopic common bile duct revision, and open duct exploration are applied. All three treatment options can be very effective and safe in experienced hands; however, all three treatment principles have their specific disadvantages [5]. Results of three randomized controlled trials comparing therapeutic splitting with one-stage procedures including laparoscopic common bile duct exploration (LCBDE) are available. Depending on the study design, some arguments in favour of laparoscopic bile duct revision [5, 26, 29] can be derived from these studies. Furthermore, in some published series, single-stage procedures including LCBDE are safe and effective, and can result in shorter hospital stay and less frequent procedures, although a clear advantage could not be shown [8, 23]. However, preoperative ERCP and clearance of the common bile duct followed by laparoscopic cholecystectomy is the most frequently applied technique, at least in surveys in Scotland (96.2%) and Germany (94.2%) [12, 17].

CBDS following cholecystectomy should be primarily treated by endoscopy. In the absence of cholangitis, indication for "routine" cholecystectomy after endoscopic duct clearance can be individualized in high-risk patients. In order to potentially reduce long-term complications of endoscopic sphincterotomy, endoscopic dilatation for stone clearance showed similar clearance rates, less bleeding, and preservation of sphincter function in controlled trials [15, 22, 33].

Choice of Surgical Approach and Procedure

If single-stage procedures are performed or operative bile duct exploration is otherwise indicated, there is no clear recommendation whether to perform open or laparoscopic common bile duct revision. LCBDE has possible advantages concerning hospital stay and postoperative pain, while being equally safe in experienced hands. Concerning technical aspects of LCBDE, descriptions of various techniques exist. Especially, concerning closure of the common bile duct over T-tubes, an endoprothesis, or no drainage at all, no recommendations can be given [9, 10, 35].

General Comments

In general, it remains uncertain what are the exclusively best diagnostic and therapeutic strategies for CBDS. Personal expertise and experience of the surgical, medical, and radiology team and costs or socioeconomics still seem to be dominating factors in general practice. Nevertheless the currently existing diagnostic tools have a high accuracy and the existing treatment options are effective concerning clearance of CBDS, while usually being safe.

In patients who have a medium risk for the presence of CBDS they are best diagnosed by MRC. Although there has been a continuous trend in the last decade from large incisions towards "closed-cavity" treatment options, up to now, only a minority of surgeons prefer the LCBDE. Most frequently, the also minimally invasive treatment option of combining laparoscopy and conventional interventional endoscopy is applied. Possible reasons are that laparoscopic bile duct surgery requires demanding technical skills, has a longer learning curve, and new methods of adequate training in advanced endoscopic surgery still have to be developed, evaluated, and introduced in general practice [11, 31]. Additionally specialization is already high and increasing, and for example, ERCP and EPT are rather performed by physicians and percutaneous transhepatic cholangiography with drainage by interventional radiologists and not by surgeons. Therefore, an interdisciplinary team approach is usually necessary and overall success may depend on the strength of the team. Training and continuous education should be intensified, especially in academic institutions. Surgeons should be preferably trained in academic institutions which are independent.

References

1. Alponat A, Kum CK, Rajnakova A, Koh BC, Goh PM (1997) Predictive factors for synchronous common bile duct stones in patients with cholelithiasis. Surg Endosc 11(9):928–932
2. Birth M, Ehlers KU, Delinikolas K, Weiser HF (1998) Prospective randomized comparison of laparoscopic ultrasonography using a flexible-tip ultrasound probe and intraoperative dynamic cholangiography during laparoscopic cholecystectomy. Surg Endosc 12(1):30–36
3. Bonnard A, Seguier-Lipszyc E, Liguory C, Benkerrou M, Garel C, Malbezin S, Aigrain Y, de Lagausie P (2005) Laparoscopic approach as primary treatment of common bile duct stones in children. J Pediatr Surg 40(9):1459–1463
4. Collins C, Maguire D, Ireland A, Fitzgerald E, O'Sullivan GC (2004) A prospective study of common bile duct calculi in patients undergoing laparoscopic cholecystectomy: natural history of choledocholithiasis revisited. Ann Surg 239(1):28–33
5. Cuschieri A, Lezoche E, Morino M, Croce E, Lacy A, Toouli J, Faggioni A, Ribeiro VM, Jakimowicz J, Visa J, Hanna GB (1999) EAES multicenter prospective randomized trial comparing two-stage vs single-stage management of patients with gallstone disease and ductal calculi. Surg Endosc 13(10):952–957
6. de Ledinghen V, Lecesne R, Raymond JM, Gense V, Amouretti M, Drouillard J, Couzigou P, Silvain C (1999) Diagnosis of choledocholithiasis: EUS or magnetic resonance cholangiography? A prospective controlled study. Gastrointest Endosc 49(1):26–31
7. Demartines N, Eisner L, Schnabel K, Fried R, Zuber M, Harder F (2000) Evaluation of magnetic resonance cholangiography in the management of bile duct stones. Arch Surg 135(2):148–152
8. Ebner S, Rechner J, Beller S, Erhart K, Riegler FM, Szinicz G (2004) Laparoscopic management of common bile duct stones. Surg Endosc 18(5):762–765
9. Fanelli RD, Gersin KS (2001) Laparoscopic endobiliary stenting: a simplified approach to the management of occult common bile duct stones. J Gastrointest Surg 5(1):74–80
10. Griniatsos J, Karvounis E, Arbuckle J, Isla AM (2005) Cost-effective method for laparoscopic choledochotomy. ANZ J Surg 75(1–2):35–38
11. Hamdorf JM, Hall JC (2000) Acquiring surgical skills. Br J Surg 87(1):28–37
12. Hamouda A, Khan M, Mahmud S, Sharp CM, Nassar AHM (2004) Management trends for suspected ductal stones in Scotland (abstract). 9th world congress of endoscopic surgery, Cancun
13. Hintze RE, Adler A, Veltzke W, Abou-Rebyeh H, Hammerstingl R, Vogl T, Felix R (1997) Clinical significance of magnetic resonance cholangiopancreatography (MRCP) compared to endoscopic retrograde cholangiopancreatography (ERCP). Endoscopy 29(3):182–187
14. Holzinger F, Baer HU, Wildi S, Vock P, Buchler MW (1999) The role of intravenous cholangiography in the era of laparoscopic cholecystectomy: is there a renaissance? Dtsch Med Wochenschr 124(46):1373–1378
15. Ido K, Tamada K, Kimura K, Ohashi A, Ueno N, Kawamoto C (1997) The role of endoscopic balloon sphincteroplasty in patients with gallbladder and bile duct stones. J Laparoendosc Adv Surg Tech A 7(3):151–156
16. Kondo S, Isayama H, Akahane M, Toda N, Sasahira N, Nakai Y, Yamamoto N, Hirano K, Komatsu Y, Tada M, Yoshida H, Kawabe T, Ohtomo K, Omata M (2005) Detection of common bile duct stones: comparison between endoscopic ultrasonography, magnetic resonance cholangiography, and helical-computed-tomographic cholangiography. Eur J Radiol 54(2):271–275
17. Ludwig K, Lorenz D, Koeckerling F (2002) Surgical strategies in the laparoscopic therapy of cholecystolithiasis and common duct stones. ANZ J Surg 72(8):547–552
18. Millat B, Atger J, Deleuze A, Briandet H, Fingerhut A, Guillon F, Marrel E, De Seguin C, Soulier P (1997) Laparoscopic treatment for choledocholithiasis: a prospective evaluation in 247 consecutive unselected patients. Hepatogastroenterology 44(13):28–34

19. Montariol T, Msika S, Charlier A, Rey C, Bataille N, Hay JM, Lacaine F, Fingerhut A (1998) Diagnosis of asymptomatic common bile duct stones: preoperative endoscopic ultrasonography versus intraoperative cholangiography – a multicenter, prospective controlled study. French Associations for Surgical Research. Surgery 124(1):6–13
20. Morrin MM, Farrell RJ, McEntee G, MacMathuna P, Stack JP, Murray JG (2000) MR cholangiopancreatography of pancreaticobiliary diseases: comparison of single-shot RARE and multislice HASTE sequences. Clin Radiol 55(11):866–873
21. Nies C, Bauknecht F, Groth C, Clerici T, Bartsch D, Lange J, Rothmund M (1997) Intraoperative cholangiography as a routine method? A prospective, controlled, randomized study. Chirurg 68(9):892–897
22. Ochi Y, Mukawa K, Kiyosawa K, Akamatsu T (1999) Comparing the treatment outcomes of endoscopic papillary dilation and endoscopic sphincterotomy for removal of bile duct stones. J Gastroenterol Hepatol 14(1):90–96
23. Paganini AM, Feliciotti F, Guerrieri M, Tamburini A, Beltrami E, Carlei F, Lomanto D, Campagnacci R, Nardovino M, Sottili M, Rossi C, Lezoche E (2000) Single-stage laparoscopic surgery of cholelithiasis and choledocholithiasis in 268 unselected consecutive patients. Ann Ital Chir 71(6):685–692
24. Prat F, Edery J, Meduri B, Chiche R, Ayoun C, Bodart M, Grange D, Loison F, Nedelec P, Sbai-Idrissi MS, Valverde A, Vergeau B (2001) Early EUS of the bile duct before endoscopic sphincterotomy for acute biliary pancreatitis. Gastrointest Endosc 54(6):724–729
25. Pring CM, Skelding-Millar L, Goodall RJ (2005) Expectant treatment or cholecystectomy after endoscopic retrograde cholangiopancreatography for choledocholithiasis in patients over 80 years old? Surg Endosc 19(3):357–360
26. Rhodes M, Sussman L, Cohen L, Lewis MP (1998) Randomised trial of laparoscopic exploration of common bile duct versus postoperative endoscopic retrograde cholangiography for common bile duct stones. Lancet 17; 351(9097):159–161
27. Shamiyeh A, Lindner E, Danis J, Schwarzenlander K, Wayand W (2005) Short-versus long-sequence MRI cholangiography for the preoperative imaging of the common bile duct in patients with cholecystolithiasis. Surg Endosc 19(8):1130–1134. Epub 2005 May 26
28. Siperstein A, Pearl J, Macho J, Hansen P, Gitomirsky A, Rogers S (1999) Comparison of laparoscopic ultrasonography and fluorocholangiography in 300 patients undergoing laparoscopic cholecystectomy. Surg Endosc 13(2):113–117
29. Suc B, Escat J, Cherqui D, Fourtanier G, Hay JM, Fingerhut A, Millat B (1998) Surgery vs endoscopy as primary treatment in symptomatic patients with suspected common bile duct stones: a multicenter randomized trial. French Associations for Surgical Research. Arch Surg 133(7):702–708
30. Sugiyama M, Atomi Y (1997) Endoscopic ultrasonography for diagnosing choledocholithiasis: a prospective comparative study with ultrasonography and computed tomography. Gastrointest Endosc 45(2):143–146
31. Troidl H (1999) "How do I get a good surgeon?" "How do I become a good surgeon?". Zentralbl Chir 124(10):868–875
32. Trondsen E, Edwin B, Reiertsen O, Faerden AE, Fagertun H, Rosseland AR (1998) Prediction of common bile duct stones prior to cholecystectomy: a prospective validation of a discriminant analysis function. Arch Surg 133(2):162–166
33. Tsujino T, Isayama H, Komatsu Y, Ito Y, Tada M, Minagawa N, Nakata R, Kawabe T, Omata M (2005) Risk factors for pancreatitis in patients with common bile duct stones managed by endoscopic papillary balloon dilation. Am J Gastroenterol 100(1):38–42
34. Vrochides DV, Sorrells DL Jr, Kurkchubasche AG, Wesselhoeft CW Jr, Tracy TF Jr, Luks FI (2005) Is there a role for routine preoperative endoscopic retrograde cholangiopancreatography for suspected choledocholithiasis in children? Arch Surg 140(4):359–361
35. Wani MA, Chowdri NA, Naqash SH, Wani NA (2005) Primary closure of the common duct over endonasobiliary drainage tubes. World J Surg 29(7):865–868
36. Zidi SH, Prat F, Le Guen O, Rondeau Y, Rocher L, Fritsch J, Choury AD, Pelletier G (1999) Use of magnetic resonance cholangiography in the diagnosis of choledocholithiasis: prospective comparison with a reference imaging method. Gut 44(1):118–122

The EAES Clinical Practice Guidelines on Laparoscopy for Abdominal Emergencies (2006)

Stefan Sauerland, Ferdinando Agresta, Roberto Bergamaschi,
Guiseppe Borzellino, Andrzej Budzynski, Gerard Champault, Abe Fingerhut,
Alberto Isla, Mikael Johansson, Per Lundorff, Benoit Navez, Stefano Saad,
Edmund A. M. Neugebauer

Introduction

Acute complaints referable to the abdomen are common presentations in surgical emergency departments. Abdominal pain is the leading symptom in this context. In the context of these guidelines, we define acute abdominal pain as any medium or severe abdominal pain with a duration of less than 7 days. Some of the conditions that cause abdominal pain prove to be self-limiting and benign, whereas others are potentially life-threatening. Since it is often difficult to identify patients who have critical problems early in the course of their disease, laparoscopy offers a superior overview of the abdominal cavity with minimal trauma to the patient. On the other hand, the risks of applying laparoscopy to emergency patients include delay to definitive open surgical treatment, missed diagnoses, and procedure-related complications.

Principally, two different clinical scenarios have to be considered. Either a specific condition can be assumed after diagnostic workup or the reason for the abdominal pain has remained uncertain. Therefore, laparoscopy has a diagnostic but also a therapeutic role. The history of diagnostic laparoscopy covers several decades. In an early study from 1975, Sugarbaker et al. [256] showed that in more than 90% of patients a diagnosis can be established by laparoscopy, thereby avoiding non-therapeutic laparotomy in the majority of cases. Table 17.1 summarizes several cohort studies of diagnostic laparoscopy, which show that over the years increasingly more patients could be successfully managed exclusively by means of laparoscopic surgery. In parallel, specific laparoscopic procedures were evaluated with regard to their effectiveness in the elective and emergency setting. Today, it is possible to hypothesize that all patients with acute abdominal pain would benefit from laparoscopic surgery. It is the aim of these guidelines to define which subgroups of patients should undergo laparoscopic instead of open surgery for abdominal pain.

Table 17.1. Observational studies on the routine use of laparoscopy in unselected patient cohorts

Study year[a]	No. of patients	Percentages of appendicitis/ gynecological disorders	Definitive diagnosis possible (%)	Percentage of laparoscopic/ open surgical/ conservative therapy	Avoidance of open surgery (%)
Reiertsen et al. [225] 1985	81	23/0/23	86	0/35/38	38
Paterson-Brown et al. [211] 1986	125	NA	91	0/30/70	9
Nagy and James [193] 1989	31	29/3/23	90	6/45/48	55
Graham et al. [99] 1991	79	32/NA/35	99	NA/34/NA	66
Schrenk et al. [236] 1994	15	67/7/7	93	80/20/0	80
Geis and Kim [94] 1995	155	66/5/1	99	96/4/0	80
Navez et al. [198] 1995	255	18/48/5	93	73/27/0	73
Waclawiczek et al. [282] 1997	172	17/28/NA	NA	65/28/7	72
Chung et al. [57] 1998	55	22/15/11	100	62/38/0	62
Salky and Edye [231] 1998	121	50/0/13	98	43/19/38	91
Sözüer et al. [252] 2000	56	38/4/32	95	64/13/23	87
Ou and Rowbotham [207] 2000	77	7/1/52	NA	87/12/1	88
Ahmad et al. [4] 2001	100	37/23/29	NA	81/19/0	81
Lee and Wong [157] 2002	137	25/9/39	91	41/16/43	84
Kirshtein et al. [130] 2003	277	23/1/9	99	75/25/0	75
Sanna et al. [232] 2003	94	20/6/26	98	88/12/0	88
Agresta et al. [2] 2004	602	NA/27/61	96	94/16/0	94
Golash and Willson [98] 2005	1320	69/1/19	90	83/7/10	93
Majewski [176] 2005	108	41/11/15	100	87/13/0	87

NA not assessed.
[a] Studies are ordered according to year of publication

Methods

Consensus Development

In their meeting on September 11, 2004, the Scientific and Educational Committee of the European Association for Endoscopic Surgery (EAES) decided to focus new clinical guidelines for the role of laparoscopy in abdominal emergencies. These guidelines were primarily intended to supplement the existing guidelines on specific diseases (e.g., appendicitis and diverticulitis) and secondly to define the role of laparoscopy for other, more rare conditions. Based on a review of the current literature, European experts were invited to participate in the development of the guidelines. All members of the expert panel were asked to define the role of laparoscopy in the various diseases that may underlie abdominal emergencies. For each disease, two experts summarized independently the current state of the art. From these papers and the results of the literature review, a preliminary document with recommendations was compiled.

In April 2005, the expert panel met for 1 day to discuss the text of the guideline recommendations. All key statements were reformulated until a 100% consensus within the group was achieved [190]. Next, these statements were presented to the audience of the annual congress of EAES in June 2005. Comments from the audience were collected and partly included in the manuscript. The final version of the guidelines was approved by all experts in the panel. Each "chapter" consists of a key statement with a grade of recommendation (GoR) followed by a commentary to explain the rationale and evidence behind the statement.

Literature Searches and Appraisal

We used the Oxford hierarchy for grading clinical studies according to levels of evidence. Literature searches were aimed at finding randomized (i.e., level 1b evidence) or nonrandomized controlled clinical trials (i.e., level 2b evidence). Alternatively, low-level evidence (mainly case series and case reports; i.e., level 4 evidence) was reviewed. Studies containing severe methodological flaws were downgraded. For each intervention, we considered the validity and homogeneity of study results, effect sizes, safety, and economic consequences.

Systematic literature searches were conducted on Medline and the Cochrane Library until June 2005. There were no restrictions regarding the language of publication. Database searches combined the key word laparoscopy (or laparosc* as title word) with a condition-specific keyword (e.g., diverticulitis). We also paid attention to studies that were referenced in systematic reviews or previous guidelines [35, 134, 214, 275].

Results

General Remark

The wide variability in experience with laparoscopy makes it necessary to state that the following recommendations are valid only for surgeons or surgical teams with sufficient expertise in laparoscopic surgery.

Gastroduodenal Ulcer

If symptoms and diagnostic findings are suggestive of perforated peptic ulcer, diagnostic laparoscopy and laparoscopic repair are recommended (GoR A).

Perforation is the most dangerous complication of gastroduodenal ulcer disease and accounts for approximately 5% of all abdominal emergencies [208, 298]. In perforated peptic ulcer, surgery is generally superior to conservative treatment evidence level (EL) 1b [27, 61]), also because surgical procedures have improved considerably (EL 1a [184]).

Laparoscopic repair of perforated ulcer was first reported in 1990 by Mouret et al. [188].

In two randomized trials, laparoscopic surgery was found to be superior to open surgery for perforated ulcers (EL 1b [153, 246]), and other nonrandomized comparison studies are in accordance with these two trials (Table 17.2). Complication rates in these studies are strongly influenced by the selection of patients for surgery. Contradictory results were found on postoperative pain levels because there appears to be no difference in pain immediately after surgery (when pain is mainly caused by peritoneal inflammation), but laparoscopic patients seemingly experienced less pain later on (when pain is mainly caused by the incision) (EL 2b [21, 135, 185, 191]). Decreased pain may also account for shorter hospital stay and earlier return to normal activities. Long-term results of both procedures showed no major differences in complication or recurrence rates. Mortality was marginally higher after open surgery, although revisional surgery was more frequently required after laparoscopic surgery (EL 2a [152]).

Many patients in these studies received omental patch repair rather than simple suture, but there is nearly no comparative evidence available to decide which repair technique is superior (EL 2b [155]; EL 4 [44, 137, 178, 194, 247]). One trial by Lau et al. [153] compared patch repair with fibrin sealing without finding any differences (El 1b). Conversion to an upper midline incision may be necessary in approximately 10–20% of operations, usually for multiple, large, or rear side perforations and for advanced peritonitis (EL 4 [60, 62, 66, 110, 244]), Nevertheless, conversion does not seem to worsen the clinical outcome compared to open surgery (EL 2b [57]). The treatment of bleeding gastroduodenal ulcers was considered to fall outside the field of the current guidelines.

Table 17.2. Randomized and nonrandomized controlled trials comparing laparoscopic and open repair for perforated gastroduodenal ulcers

Study year	LoE	No. of patients	Leak agerates (%)	Total complication rates (%)	Difference in hospital stay (days)
Lau et al. [153] 1996	1b	48/45	2/2	23/22	±0 NS [a]
Siu et al. [246] 2002	1b	63/58	2/2	25/50	−1 sign [b]
Johansson et al. [119] 1996	2b	10/17	10/7	30/20	−1 NS [a]
Sø et al. [250] 1996	2b	15/38	0/0	7/24	−2 NS [a]
Miserez et al. [74, 185] 1996	2b	18/16	NA	50/9	−1 NS [a]
Chung et al. [57] 1998	2b	3/3	NA	NA	−4 sign [b]
Kok et al. [135] 1999	2b	13/20	NA	8/15	−1 NS [a]
Næsgaard et al. [191] 1999	2b	25/49	4/0	28/14	±0 NS [a]
Bergamaschi et al. [21] 1999	2b	17/62	0/0	29/34	−2 NS [a]
Mehendale et al. [180] 2002	2b	34/33	0/0	3/6	−5 sign [b]
Lee et al. [155] 2001	3b [c]	155/219	13/2	NA	−1 NS [a]
Nicolau et al. [202] 2002	3b [c]	51/105	0/0	6/7	−2 sign [b]
Seelig et al. [240] 2003	3b [c]	24/31	4/3	13/26	−2 NS [a]
Tsamura et al. [272] 2004	3b [c]	58/13	NA	5/23	−12 sign [b]
Lam et al. [148] 2005	3b [c]	523/1737	NA	3/13	−3 sign [b]

Data are shown for laparoscopic/open group. Studies are ordered according to level of evidence (*LoE*) and year of publication
NS not significant, *sign* significant
[a] Data are difference of medians
[b] Data are difference of means
[c] Study was downgraded because type of surgery was selected according to the patient's status or because converted cases were not analyzed within the laparoscopic group

Acute Cholecystitis

Patients with acute cholecystitis should undergo laparoscojoic cholecystec-tomy (GoR A). Surgery should be carried out as early as possible after admis-sion (GoR A). In patients unsuitable for early surgery, conservative treatment or percutaneous cholecystostomy should be considered (GoR B).

Laparoscopy is of minor importance in terms of diagnosis of acute chole-cystitis. Studies have shown that the following diagnostic criteria define cho-lecystistis with nearly 100% specificity: (1) acute right upper quadrant ten-derness for more than 6 h and ultrasound evidence of acute cholecystitis (the presence of gallstones with a thickened and edematous gallbladder wall, positive Murphy's sign on ultrasound examination, and pericholecystic fluid collections) or (2) acute right upper quadrant tenderness for more than 6 h, an ultrasound image showing the presence of gallstones, and one or more of the following: temperature above 38°C, leukocytosis greater than 10×10/L, and/or C-reactive protein level greater than 10 mg/L (EL 1 a [270]).

Traditional treatment consisted of open cholecystectomy, which was per-formed several weeks after an attack or in the acute setting. With the intro-duction of laparoscopy for the surgical approach to gallstone disease acute, cholecystitis was initially considered a contraindication. However, with in-creasing experience, a number of reports became available demonstrating the feasibility of the laparoscopic approach with an acceptable morbidity [143, 144, 286]. Today, there is sufficient evidence to state that laparoscopy is a safe approach, but the question to ask is if it is clearly superior to an open approach. There are several published studies comparing laparoscopic and open cholecystectomy for acute cholecystitis (Table 17.3). Only two of them are randomized trials (EL 1 b [122, 131]). Nearly all comparative studies dem-onstrated faster recovery and shorter hospital stay in favor of laparoscopy (EL 1 a [152]). Similarly, a minilaparotomic cholecystectomy was studied by Assalia et al. (EL 1 b [14]), who were able to reduce hospital stay from 4.7 days with open surgery to 3.1 days with minilaparotomy. However, in the most recently published study, the outcome was very similar in the laparo-scopic and conventional groups (EL 1 b [122]).

The question remains whether the favorable outcome for laparoscopy is a result of altered pathophysiological response to the operation or whether this is due to concomitant changes in postoperative care due to the expected faster recovery from laparoscopic surgery. There is a clear possibility that trials com-paring open and laparoscopic procedures contain traditional care regimens that have not been revised in the open treatment groups but have been modi-fied in the laparoscopic groups, thereby favoring, the expected improved out-come after minimally invasive surgery. Several studies in which hospital stay and convalescence were utilized as endpoints may merely reflect traditions of

Table 17.3. Randomized and nonrandomized controlled trials comparing laparoscopic and open cholecystectomy for acute cholecystitis

Study year	LoE	No. of patients	Preoperative duration of symptoms	Total complication rates (%)	Difference in hospital stay (days)
Kiviluoto et al. [131] 1998	1 b	32/31	4 days (mean)	3/42	−2 sign[a]
Johansson et al. [122] 2005	1 b	35/35	72 h (mean)	2/3	−0 sign[a]
Kum et al. [144] 1994	2 b	66/43	24–96 h	10/9	−0 sign[a]
Rau et al. [224] 1994	2 b	102/114	NA	9/11	−2 sign[b]
Carbajo Caballero et al. [41] 1998	2 b	30/30	NA	NA	−7 sign[b]
Lujan et al. [170] 1998	2 b	114/110	<72 h	14/23	−5 sign[b]
Araujo-Teixeira et al. [12] 1999	2 b	100/100	Variable	10/32	−7 sign[b]
Pessaux et al. [218] 2001	2 b	50/89	NA	18/21	−5 sign[b]
Chau et al. [48] 2002	2 b	31/42	Surgery performed 2 days (mean) after admission	13/40	−3 sign[b]
Eldar et al. [71] 1997	3 b[c]	97/146	72 h (median)	17/26	−4 sign[a]
Glavic et al. [97] 2001	3 b[c]	94/115	72 h (mean)	10/17	−4 sign[b]
Bove et al. [33] 2004	3 b[c]	87/153	NA	14/NA	NA
Lam et al. [148] 2005	3 b[c]	1223/1408	NA	1/5	−4 sign[b]

Data are shown for laparoscopic/open group. Studies are ordered according to LoE and year of publication

[a] Data are difference of medians

[b] Data are difference of means

[c] Study was downgraded because type of surgery was selected according to the patient's status or because converted cases were not analyzed within the laparoscopic group

postoperative care and patient expectations associated with open procedures rather than differences between open and laparoscopic surgical techniques. However, even after the advent of fast-track surgery, the existing evidence supports the use of laparoscopy in terms of earlier postoperative recovery. The basic recommendation should therefore be to offer all patients a laparoscopic approach. If there is no laparoscopically trained surgeon available, the patient should be treated with an open operation in the acute phase of the disease.

The optimal timing of the operation, regardless of whether performed laparoscopically or conventionally, is of major importance. In fact, timing of surgery seems more important than choice of surgical approach. A large number of studies have compared early versus late cholecystectomy for acute cholecystitis (EL 1a [23, 210]; EL 1b [45, 120, 121, 136, 146, 169], EL 2b [24, 25, 49, 69, 93, 102, 133, 139, 173, 199, 215, 220, 242, 258, 273, 285, 295]). However, the time intervals for early, delayed, or interval surgery were inconsistently defined in these studies. It can be concluded from these studies that conversion rates, complication rates, convalescence times, and hospital costs rise in parallel with an increasing delay between admission and operation (EL 5 [96]). Unfortunately, it is impossible to define the exact time limit until which surgery should be performed, but the majority of studies considered a delay of more than 48 or 72 h to be suboptimal. Delaying surgery is considered potentially harmful, especially in patients with a clinical presentation of gangrenous or hemorrhagic cholecystitis (EL 2b [105, 181]), but laparoscopic surgery in these advanced stages of cholecystitis is technically very demanding.

When performing laparoscopic cholecystectomy, the threshold for conversion should be quite low (EL 4 [168]). In many patient series, conversion rates were between 5 and 40% (EL 4 [15, 33, 36, 48, 70, 80, 95, 105, 140, 168, 199, 215, 230, 242, 258, 268, 295]) – much higher than in elective cholecystectomy for uncomplicated cholecystolithiasis. A set of prognostic variables have been identified that predict the need for conversion, such as degree of inflammation, number of previous gallbladder colics, gallstone size, higher age, male gender, obesity, and surgical, expertise (EL 4 [12, 102, 156, 168, 241]). However, these variables do not allow a completely reliable identification of patients in whom laparoscopic cholecystectomy is impossible. Therefore, every surgical procedure for acute cholecystitis should be started laparoscopically, except for patients with general contraindications.

Despite its general superiority, early laparoscopic cholecystectomy may not be possible in all patients. In elderly patients, comorbidities often render early surgery too risky or they simply preclude anesthesia (EL 5 [39]). These cases can only undergo delayed or interval cholecystectomy, although a small study (EL 1b [280]) suggested that a fully conservative treatment can be tried. In the acute phase, precutaneous cholecystostomy has been proposed as a means of alleviating symptoms until definitive treatment can take place (EL 1b [115]; EL 4 [20, 28, 31, 40, 47, 100, 126, 145, 213, 217, 288]). However, one randomized trial from Greece (EL 1b [109]) found that cholecystostomy and conservative treatment performed similarly well, thus justifying the use of both approaches in an individually tailored manner. On the other hand, the benefits of early surgery should not be generally denied to elderly or comorbid patients. With careful anesthesiologic and surgical management, satisfactory results can be achieved in these difficult subgroups (EL 2b [48]; EL 4 [219]).

Acute Pancreatitis

Patients with acute biliary pancreatitis should undergo definitive management of gallstones during the same admission (GoR B). After assessment of severity, mild cases should be done within 2 weeks, whereas severe cases should be done when the general condition has significantly improved (GoR C). The bile duct should be imaged to ensure it is clear of stones (intraoperative cholangiography, magnetic resonance cholangiopancreatography, (MRCP), or endoscopic ultrasound) (GoR B).

Acute pancreatitis is a disease entity with manifold etiologies and large differences in clinical appearance but with high morbidity and mortality in more severe cases. Therefore, classification of acute pancreatitis according to severity is crucial for clinical management. Severe disease requires intensive care and CT imaging (EL 5 [195]). Laparoscopy for diagnostic reasons is unnecessary since diagnosis and classification can be based on other criteria and imaging results (EL 5 [34, 65]).

Early pancreatic necrosectomy compared to late or no surgery has been found to be detrimental in various studies (EL 1 b [125, 182]; EL 2 b [6, 19, 75, 108, 274]). Whenever possible, necrotic tissue should be allowed to demarcate over a few weeks before necrosectomy takes place. Although some situations (e.g. hemorrhage or compartment syndrome) render surgical exploration inevitable, the majority of cases with severe pancreatitis can and should be spared early surgery (EL 1 b [167, 237]). If surgery is necessary, minimally invasive techniques can be chosen for exploration, irrigation, necrosectomy, and drainage (EL 2 b [91]; EL 4 [107, 209, 297]), but the open approach is still considered the gold standard (EL 4 [195]).

In biliary pancreatitis, two different approaches may be chosen depending on disease severity. In mild biliary pancreatitis, early laparoscopic cholecystectomy with intraoperative cholangiography is the preferred approach (EL 1 b [46, 227, 255]; EL 4 [114, 263]; EL 5 [30, 214]). Bile duct clearance is essential to prevent recurrent disease.

Therefore, all patients with biliary pancreatitis should undergo definitive treatment at the next best opportunity, preferably during the same hospital admission. There are no studies available to compare a wait-and-see policy versus early removal of bile duct stones, but the risk of a potentially life-threatening recurrent pancreatitis when delaying bile duct clearance is generally considered to be unwarrantable.

There are three different options available to clear the bile duct: endoscopic stone extraction during endoscopic retrograde cholangiopancreatography (ERCP), laparoscopic exploration, and open exploration. Neither the 1998 EAES guidelines on common bile duct stones nor the 2005 UK guidelines on acute pancreatitis, favored one approach over the others (EL 5 [214,

275]). Because the scientific basis for these recommendations is unchanged, all three strategies are still equally recommendable. In general, surgery should only be started after the bile duct has been cleared, unless there is expertise available for intraoperative duct clearance (EL 2b [276]). If MRCP is available for imaging, it allows detection of choledocholithiasis with sensitivity and specificity both over 90% (EL 2a [124]), although the performance of MRCP may be inferior in acute pancreatitis. In most patients, a negative MRCP is sufficient to exclude bile duct stones, thus obviating the necessity of intraoperative clearance (EL 1b [106]). In conclusion, the optimal strategy in most hospitals will depend on the availability of imaging modalities, on the one hand, and surgical expertise with laparoscopic bile duct exploration, on the other hand.

Severe cases of biliary pancreatitis have a high risk of organ failure and death, which usually contraindicates early surgery. Again, bile duct clearance is necessary, but the timing and methods of definitive therapy are different than in mild disease forms. In severe cases, ERCP with or without endoscopic sphincterotomy followed by interval laparoscopic cholecystectomy is common (EL 1a [16]; EL 1b [76, 87, 200, 269], EL 4 [228]; EL 5 [1, 59]). After the publication of several diagnostic accuracy studies with good results (EL 1b [5, 42, 166, 221, 234]), the role of endoscopic ultrasonography (EUS) increased, but the advantage of EUS depends on the prior probability of bile duct stones (EL 2b [13, 229]). As already mentioned, disease classification is the cornerstone of successful therapy (EL 2b [201]). Several different systems have been proposed for defining a presumably severe case of pancreatitis and for describing the clinical course (Ranson score, APACHE II score, inflammatory markers, etc.), but the difficult choice of an optimal system is beyond the scope of these recommendations. The UK guidelines recommend delaying surgery "until signs of lung injury and systemic disturbance have resolved," which aptly describes the subjective nature of this decision on timing.

Acute Appendicitis

Patients with symptoms and diagnostic findings suggestive of acute appendicitis should undergo diagnostic laparoscopy (GoR A) and, if the diagnosis is confirmed, laparoscopic appendectomy (GoR A). If diagnostic laparoscopy shows that symptoms cannot be ascribed to appendicitis, the appendix may be left in situ (GoR B).

Appendicitis is a very common disease, but its symptoms are often equivocal and many other causative pathologies can be responsible. Despite improved imaging with sonography or CT, the rates of false-negative appendectomy are still high, especially in women (El 4 [29, 86]). Among the 56 randomized trials that have compared laparoscopic and conventional approaches for suspected appendicitis (EL 1a [233]; EL 1b [186]), only a few studies have explicitly used the findings of diagnostic laparoscopy to guide further surgical therapy. Most of these studies included only female patients of fertile age and documented a large reduction in the rate of negative appendectomy (EL 1b [37, 117, 147, 151, 205, 277]). However, the diagnostic advantages in men and children seem to be smaller and less consistent since appendicitis is much easier to diagnose in these subgroups.

The relative advantage of laparoscopic over conventional appendectomy has been under under debate for more than a decade. According to the most recent Cochrane Review (EL 1a [233]), laparoscopic appendectomy offers certain advantages, although the difference compared to open appendectomy is not major. The EAES guidelines on appendectomy clearly favor the laparoscopic approach (EL 5 [72]), mainly because of the significantly reduced risk of wound infection and the faster postoperative recovery. This recommendation also pertains to perforated cases.

If the appendix looks normal on laparoscopy but another pathology is found to be the cause of the patient's symptom, then the appendix should be left in situ (EL 4 [278]). The 10-year follow-up by van Dalen et al. [277] (EL 1b) demonstrated the safety of this approach in women. The situation is more complicated when the appendix shows no signs of inflammation and no other pathology can be found. Different groups have provided contradictory data on the reliability of macroscopic diagnosis of appendicitis (EL 4 [51, 103, 141, 266]). Weighing the disadvantage of a negative appendectomy against the risk of overlooking a case of appendicitis is difficult. If symptoms and signs are severe and typical for appendicitis, most surgeons will consider appendectomy to be indicated because in early appendicitis inflammation may be limited to intramural layers.

Acute Diverticulitis

Patients with presumed acute uncomplicated diverticulitis should not undergo emergency laparoscopic surgery (GoR C). Although colonic resection remains standard treatment for perforated diverticulitis, laparoscopic lavage and drainage may be considered in some selected patients (GoR C).

After physical examination and a blood count, CT is especially useful to diagnose diverticulitis. If complicated disease is likely, CT is able to visualize inflammation of the pericolic fat, thickening of the bowel wall, or peridiverticular abscess. Diagnostic laparoscopy is therefore unnecessary. Resection of the diseased segment should be performed in an elective rather than an emergency setting since the risk of conversion and the rate of primary reanastomosis strongly depend on the presence and severity of acute inflammation. The value of elective laparoscopic sigmoid resection has been addressed in guidelines issued by the EAES in 1999 [134].

Complicated cases of diverticular disease are classified according to the modified Hinchey classification. Stage I indicates the presence of a pericolic abscess, stage IIa indicates distant abscess amenable to percutaneous drainage, and stage IIb Indicates complex abscess associated with or without fistula. Diffuse peritonitis is classified as stage III (purulent) or IV (fecal). Peritonitis or pneumoperitoneum usually require emergency surgical exploration (EL 1b [142, 294]; EL 5 (10, 212)). In Hinchey stages III and IV, laparoscopic abdominal exploration and peritoneal lavage have been successfully used, but there are only limited data available (EL 2b [77]; EL 4 [88, 206, 223, 235]). A laparoscopic approach may be especially advantageous in high-risk patients, who would probably not survive Hartmann's procedure. In such patients, perforation may be closed by an omental patch (EL 4 [88]). In stage IIb, abscesses can be drained and fistula can be closed laparoscopically (EL 4 [88, 223, 238]), but it must be taken into account that only very few surgeons are experienced enough to perform these operations. It is therefore too early to generally recommend laparoscopic emergency surgery for complicated diverticular disease, despite promising results.

Small Bowel Obstruction due to Adhesions

In the case of clinical and radiological evidence of small bowel obstruction nonresponding to conservative management, laparoscopy may be performed using an open access technique (GoR C). If adhesions are found at laparoscopy, cautious laparoscopic adhesiolysis can be attempted for release of small bowel obstruction (GoR C).

The clinical value and the potential complications of adhesiolysis are highly debated. A blinded trial by Swank et al. [262] found similar levels of pain after diagnostic laparoscopy with or without adhesiolysis (El 1b). Although this trial was performed in patients with chronic recurrent abdominal pain, it also has implications for the acute pain situation. On the other hand, laparoscopic adhesiolysis is sometimes performed at diagnostic laparoscopy for acute abdominal pain, to enable complete visualization of the abdominal content. Therefore, the term adhesiolysis covers a wide spectrum of invasiveness. Furthermore, the natural variability of adhesions and their sequelae determines possible success and failure rates of adhesiolysis. Therefore, the decision for adhesiolysis in the acute setting is a balance of these factors (EL 2b [284]). As a rule, adhesiolysis in an abdomen without intestinal obstruction should be kept to a minimum.

Radiographically confirmed small bowel obstruction requires emergency surgery (EL 2b [82–84] when nonoperative therapy is unsucessful. Laparoscopic treatment of acute small bowel obstruction was first described by Bastug et al. [18] (EL 4) and has since been reported by others (EL 4 [3, 8, 17, 32, 55, 56, 89, 90, 111, 129, 160, 163, 197, 243, 254, 259, 261]). Studies comparing the results of laparoscopic and conventional treatment of this condition are nearly lacking, except for the matched-pair analysis by Wullstein and Gross [289] (EL 2b). The benefits of the laparoscopic approach that have been reported consist of a more rapid postoperative recovery with faster return of bowel movements, lower morbidity, and shorter hospital stay. However, there is concern that laparoscopic treatment of small bowel obstruction may lead to a higher rate of bowel injury than conventional surgery. In the single comparative study (EL 2b [289]), the risk of perforation was clearly higher in the laparoscopic group (27%). The high conversion rate is also an issue. Complete laparoscopic treatment seems to be possible in only 50–60% of patients (EL 4 [3, 8, 17, 32, 55, 56, 89, 111, 129, 160, 163, 197, 243, 254, 259, 261]). The remaining patients have to be converted to open surgery for malignant disease, iatrogenic bowel perforation, or other reasons. Some studies have examined predictive factors for successful laparoscopy (EL 2b [163, 259]). A history of two or more surgical abdominal operations, late operation (after 24 h), and bowel diameter exceeding 4 cm have been reported to be predictors of conversion. An isolated scar from a previous appendicectomy seems to be favorable in terms of avoiding a conversion. To avoid the possibility of intraabdominal injuries during laparoscopic access, open rather than laparoscopic surgery should be performed if scars or other findings indicate the presence of severe or extended adhesions (EL 4 [85, 192]).

Incarcerated Hernia

Although the open approach remains standard treatment for incarcerated hernia, laparoscopic surgery may be considered in carefully selected patients (GoR C).

The available evidence for the use of laparoscopic surgery in inguinal, incisional, and other hernias is very good, but all these studies have excluded symptomatic and emergency surgery cases. It seems unjustified to adopt the principle of transferable evidence to delineate the treatment of incarcerated hernia from the results obtained in the elective setting. With regard to the laparoscopic treatment of incarcerated hernias, so far only case reports (EL 4 [38, 58, 78, 123, 150, 164, 271, 283, 290]) and small case series (EL 4 [81, 113, 149, 154, 165, 239]) have been published. The largest series is from Leibl et al. [158] (EL 4) and reports on 220 patients. The authors – highly experienced laparoscopic surgeons – found their results in incarcerated groin hernias to be similar to those elective for hernia repair. Because there are no comparative studies available to compare open and laparoscopic surgery, one should be very reluctant to choose a laparoscopic approach to hernia sac, abdominal wall, or peritoneum. Although early clinical results are promising, these techniques should be restricted to surgeons with maximum expertise in laparoscopic hernia surgery.

Mesenteric Ischemia

If mesenteric ischemia is clinically suspected, conventional imaging is preferable over diagnostic laparoscopy in defining therapeutic management (GoR C).

Acute mesenteric ischemia is caused by arterial occlusion (approxiamately 50% of cases), nonocclusive arterial ischemia (20–30%), or venous occlusion (5–15%) [253]. A clinical diagnosis of mesenteric ischemia is usually confirmed by the use of conventional angiography, CT scanning, or duplex sonography [132, 204, 216]. Traditional surgical therapy consists of resection of infarcted bowel segments or embolectomy, depending on duration and extent of ischemia. The benefit of surgery needs to be considered on a case-by-case basis since there is no good evidence available to compare surgical and medical treatment for those patients with a salvageable condition (EL 2 b [26, 68, 296]).

The potential value of emergency laparoscopy in these patients relates to its diagnostic rather than its therapeutic opportunities. However, the rate of mesenteric ischemia among patients with acute abdomen is only approximately 1% [112]. Furthermore, laparoscopic viewing does not guarantee correct recognition of ischemia. Since radiographic imaging accurately identifies most cases of mesenteric ischemia, it is very unlikely that diagnostic laparoscopy will prevent a negative laparotomy in these patients. In the literature, only a few cases have been published (EL 4 [52, 54, 73, 292]; EL 5 [159]), although there are more reports concerning second-look laparoscopies.

Gynecologic Disorders

If gynecologic disorders are the suspected cause of abdominal pain, diagnostic laparoscopy should follow conventional diagnostic investigations (GoR A), and, if needed, a laparoscopic therapy for the disease should be performed (GoR A). A close cooperation with the gynecologist is strongly recommended.

Many acute gynecologic disorders can be approached safely and effectively by laparoscopy with the intent not only to correctly diagnose the patient but also to render treatment (EL 4 [138, 174, 196, 207]). The most common diagnoses encountered in women with acute pelvic pain are ectopic pregnancy (approximately 20% of cases), salpingo-oophoritis (20%), pelvic adhesions (20%), endometriosis (15%), and ovarian cysts (15%). In gynecological emergencies, CT scans are very seldom helpful. After a pregnancy test, transvaginal and conventional ultrasound can aid in formulating a differential diagnosis. However, diagnostic laparoscopy is superior to other diagnostic tools (EL 2 b [183]) and may lead to the correction of an erroneous preoperative diagnosis in up to 40% of patients (EL 4 [7, 67, 138, 264]).

Ectopic pregnancy (EP) is a life-threatening condition. In early pregnant women presenting with acute pelvic pain and/or vaginal bleeding, a diagnostic laparoscopy should always be considered to exclude EP. In the vast majority of cases, a pregnancy test can exclude the diagnosis in cases with only minor symptoms. When serum human chorionic gonadotropin (hCG) levels reach 1,000 IU/L, transvaginal ultrasonography can differentiate between an EP or an intrauterine pregnancy (IUP) because all IUPs can clearly be seen in cases with hCG > 1,000 IU/L. A normal IUP will have a hCG doubling rate of 2 days. Thus, vaginal ultrasound and hCG go hand in hand in the diagnosis of EP in cases of minor or no abdominal symptoms (EL 5 [222]). In cases with EP, laparoscopic surgery should be undertaken also because of its total cost is cheaper (EL 1 b [101]). It is fast, and fertility outcome is comparable to laparotomy. Furthermore, sick leave and hospitalization are shorter and adhesion development is minor compared to laparotomy (EL 1 b [171, 172, 279]; EL 2 b [79, 189]). Laparoscopic salpingectomy should be performed in cases of ruptured tubal pregnancy. In cases of unruptured tubal pregnancy, a tube-preserving operation should be considered. Hemodynamic instability is a contraindication for laparoscopy.

Torsion of ovarian cysts is an organs-threatening disease. Patients often present with acute abdominal pain. After excluded pregnancy, a transvaginal ultrasound is mandatory to exclude ovarian cyst formation. In the majority of patients, free fluid can be seen in the abdomen, and if symptoms decline, an expectative attitude can be undertaken. In cases with persistent pain and/ or if a larger cyst is seen on ultrasound, a diagnostic laparoscopy must be performed to exclude adnexal torsion. Ovarian cysts that are found during diagnostic laparoscopic should be treated laparoscopically (EL 1 b [175, 291]). Pregnant women with acute pelvic pain and clinical signs of torsion of ovarian cyst should be offered laparoscopic repair. Laparoscopic surgery was also reported to be superior compared to open surgery for resecting other types of ovarian cysts (EL 1 b [203]).

Endometriosis often causes infertility and pain. Pain is usually chronic and recurrent, but some patients present with acute symptoms. Surgical treatment may be indicated in some patients and may be performed as an open procedure or laparoscopically. Only one trial has compared the two approaches (EL 1b [175]) and documented a significantly faster and less painful recovery after laparoscopy. More evidence is available on the comparative effectiveness of laparoscopic excision versus conservative treatment of endometriosis. Although these studies included elective rather than emergency patients, their results indicate that laparoscopic excision results in clear and patient-relevant advantages as opposed to conservative treatment (EL 1 a [116]; EL 1 b [1, 260]).

Salpingo-oophoritis commonly causes acute pelvic pain and often mimics other diseases. Conservative treatment consists of antibiotics. Laparoscopy is useful to exclude other pathologies, which may be present in approximately 20% of patients (EL 4 [22]). Furthermore, microbiological specimens can be taken to guide antibiotic therapy. Depending on the severity of symptoms, laparoscopy is therefore considered to be advantageous for acute salpingitis (EL 4 [22, 251]) and pyosalpinx (EL 4 [267]).

Nonspecific Abdominal Pain

Patients with severe nonspecific abdominal pain (NSAP) after full conventional investigations should undergo diagnostic laparoscopy if symptoms persist (GoR A). Patients with NSAP of medium severity may undergo diagnostic laparoscopy after a period of observation (GoR C).

According to symptoms and diagnostic findings, most patients with acute abdominal pain can easily be categorized into different groups of presumed diagnoses, but some patients will not fit into these diagnostic categories due to unclear or equivocal findings. In these cases, of NSAP, the severity of symptoms determines the necessity of emergency surgery. Some patients definitely require surgical exploration, a second group can safely be monitored under conservative therapy, and in a third group the decision between operative or conservative management is unclear. If symptoms are severe enough to require surgical exploration, this should be done laparoscopically. The reason lies more in the therapeutic than the diagnostic value of laparoscopic surgery. As described previously, laparoscopic surgery is advantageous for many intraabdominal diseases, which may also turn out to be the underlying cause of an unclear abdomen. Also, because converted cases have a similar outcome compared to primarily open cases (EL 2 b [57]), the benefits of a laparoscopic approach outweigh its potential negative effects.

Four randomized controlled trials have compared early laparoscopy versus observation for nononspecific acute abdominal pain (Table 17.4). Three trials focused exclusively on right iliac fossa pain in women after excluding clear cases of appendicitis (EL 1 b [43, 92, 187]). The fourth trial included 120 men and women with acute abdominal pain regardless of pain localization (EL 1 b [64]). Three out of four trials found that early laparoscopy clearly facilitated the establishment of a diagnosis with subsequent therapy, whereas more patients in the control group left the hospital without a clear diagnosis. More important, hospital stay was shorter in two of the trials (EL 1 b [43, 92]). At 1-year follow-up, recurrent pain episodes were less frequent (EL 1 b [187]) and health-related quality of life was better (EL 1 b [64])

Table 17.4. Randomized controlled trials comparing laparoscopic surgery and conservative management for acute nonspecific abdominal pain

Study year	LoE	No. of patients	Patients in conservative group receiving surgical exploration (%)	Patients remaining without a final diagnosis (%)	Difference in hospital stay (days)
Champault et al. [43] 1993	1 b	33/32	50	3/72	−2 sign[a)]
Decadt et al. [64] 1999	1 b	59/61	28	19/64	±0 NS[b)]
Gaitán et al. [92] 2002	1 b	55/55	40	5/2	−1 sign[a)]
Morino et al. [187] 2003	1 b[c)]	24/29	31	12/55	NA

Data are shown for laparoscopic/conservative group. Studies are ordered according to year of publication
[a)] Data are difference of means
[b)] Data are difference of medians
[c)] Only published abstract available

in the laparoscopic group. Based on these data, it seems justified to lower the threshold for surgical exploration when using a laparoscopic rather than an open approach. However, it seems advisable to observe patients over some hours because abdominal symptoms may become more specific over time or simply disappear in some cases (EL 4 [128]).

Abdominal Trauma

For suspected penetrating trauma, diagnostic laparoscopy is a useful tool to assess the integrity of the peritoneum and avoid a nontherapeutic laparotomy in stable patients (GoR B). Stable patients with blunt abdominal trauma may undergo diagnostic laparoscopy to exclude relevant injury (GoR C).

Laparotomy for abdominal trauma used to be negative or nontherapeutic in approximately one-third of patients (EL 4 [162, 226]), but modern imaging techniques have reduced this figure to less than 10% (EL 4 [104]). The literature contains approximately 40 prospective or retrospective cohort studies on the diagnostic role of laparoscopy in trauma (EL 4 [281]). The major advantage of laparoscopy as identified in these studies was the obviation of unnecessary laparotomy in approximately 60% of cases. However, relevant injuries went undetected in 1% of all laparoscopies, particularly after blunt trauma affecting solid organs or hollow viscus (EL 4 [281]). Because the majority of the available evidence derives from patients with stab or gunshot wounds, diagnostic laparoscopy seems to be recommendable as a screening tool for patients with a moderate to high index of suspicion for intraabdominal injuries. However, in hemodynamically unstable patients, emergency surgical exploration of the abdomen may be life-saving. In this situation, delaying definitive therapy by laparoscopy is contraindicated.

Two randomized studies have been published on laparoscopy in trauma. A small study compared laparoscopy with peritoneal lavage and found higher diagnostic specificity in the laparoscopic group (EL 1b [63]). The second trial was, in fact, a double trial (EL 1b [161]). First, it compared exploratory laparotomy and diagnostic laparoscopy for stab wounds that had penetrated the peritoneum. Second, patients with equivocal peritoneal violation were randomized to diagnostic laparoscopy or expectant nonoperative management. Not unexpectedly, laparoscopy reduced hospital stay compared to laparotomy but prolonged hospital stay compared to conservative management (EL 1b [161]). Although laparoscopy saved more than half of patients from laparotomy, the postoperative clinical course and costs failed to differ between laparoscopic and laparotomic group. Because the study was relatively small and did not report on the potential long-term advantages of laparoscopy, further research is needed. Accordingly, the panel believes that the available evidence does not justify a high-grade recommendation.

Although the trials mentioned previously did not use laparoscopy for therapeutic reasons, it is clearly possible to treat certain injuries laparoscopically. Bleeding from minor injuries to the liver or the spleen can be controlled through the laparoscope (EL 4 [50, 53, 293]). Diaphragmatic lacerations (EL 4 [179, 248, 249]) and perforating stab wounds of the gastrointestinal tract can be sewn or stapled (EL 4 [53, 177, 293]). Nevertheless, the scarceness of clinical data prohibits a clear recommendation in favor of therapeutic laparoscopy for trauma.

Discussion

Available evidence clearly demonstrates the superiority of a laparoscopic approach in various emergency situations, but laparoscopy offers less or unclear benefit in other acute conditions. Therefore, a policy of laparoscopy for all patients with acute abdominal pain still seems unjustified, although laparoscopy will be to the advantage of the majority of patients. The initial usage of diagnostic procedures and imaging should aim to identify those patients who would probably not benefit from laparoscopy. On the other hand, it usually carries only minor disadvantages for a patient if a diagnostic laparoscopy has to be converted to an open procedure. Because the current guidelines deal with complex laparoscopic procedures, a low threshold toward early conversion is generally useful in order to avoid delays in the operating room.

Although the current recommendations address the most common diagnoses, some less prevalent causes of acute abdominal pain were not specifically discussed. Some of the more rare diagnoses were encountered in the cohort studies summarized in Table 17.1. These diseases include abdominal abscess, peritoneal tuberculosis, and intestinal volvulus. Due to their low occurrence, these diseases will probably never be studied in a randomized trial, but their relative importance in the treatment of an average patient is low. Laparoscopic therapy has been described to be useful for many of these conditions (EL 2b [265]; EL 4 [9, 127, 245]).

The panel also decided not to prepare separate recommendations on the usage of laparoscopy in children with acute abdominal pain. The disease spectrum of pediatric acute abdominal pain is completely different compared to that of adults, but older children and adolescents are good candidates for laparoscopy (EL 4 [118, 287]). The value of specific procedures in pediatric surgery, such as laparoscopic appendectomy, is still under intensive debate. In consequence, these guidelines are valid only for adult patients. Also, there was no pediatric surgeon on the panel to define the possible role of laparoscopic surgery for pyloric stenosis, congenital malformations, and other disorders of the newborn or small child.

Future research should concentrate on those fields or which only low-level evidence is available. The current guidelines have identified some topics that have been described only in feasibility studies. It is highly desirable to supplement these studies with additional comparative data on effectiveness and cost-effectiveness. Because the EAES updates its guidelines regularly, such data are also important before stronger recommendations can be issued. On the other hand, in those fields for which there is good evidence, laparoscopic surgery has been shown to be highly beneficial. Therefore, optimism with regard to laparoscopy may prove to be justified. Laparoscopy has already had a major impact on the management of abdominal emergencies and has become an indispensable technique.

References

1. Abbott J, Hawe J, Hunter D, Holmes M, Finn P, Garry R (2004) Laparoscopic excision of endometriosis; a randomized, placebo-controlled trial. Fertil Steril 82:878–884
2. Agresta F, De Simone P, Bedin N (2004) The laparoscopic approach in abdominal emergencies: a single-center 10-year experience. J Soc Laparoendosc Surg 8:25–30
3. Agresta F, Piazza A, Michelet I, Bedin N, Sartori CA (2000) Small bowel obstruction. Laparoscopic approach. Surg Endosc 14:154–156
4. Ahmad TA, Shelbaya E, Razek SA, Mohamed RA, Tajima Y, Ali SM, Sabet MM, Kanematsu T (2001) Experience of laparoscopic management in 100 patients with acute abdomen. Hepatogastroenterology 48:733–736
5. Ainsworth AP, Rafaelsen SR, Wamberg PA, Durup J, Pless TK, Mortensen MB (2003) Is there a difference in diagnostic accuracy and clinical impact between endoscopic ultrasonography and magnetic resonance cholangiopancreatography? Endoscopy 35:1029–1032

6. Alimoglu O, Ozkan OV, Sahin M, Akcakaya A, Eryilmaz R, Bas G (2003) Timing of cholecystectomy for acute biliary pancreatitis: outcomes of cholecystectomy on first admission and after current biliary pancreatitis. World J Surg 27:256–259

7. Allen LA, Schoon MG (1983) Laparoscopic diagnosis of acute pelvic inflammatory disease. Br J Obstet Gynaecol 90:966–968

8. Al-Mulhim AA (2000) Laparoscopic management of acute small bowel obstruction. Experience from a Saudi teaching hospital. Surg Endosc 14:157–160

9. Al-Mulhim AA (2004) Laparoscopic diagnosis of peritoneal tuberculosis. Surg Endosc 18:1757–1761

10. American Society of Colon and Rectal Surgeons (2000) Practice parameters for the treatment of sigmoid diverticulitis. Dis Colon Rectum 43:289–297

11. Anonymous (2002) NIH state-of-the-science statement on endoscopic retrograde cholangiopancreatography (ERCP) for diagnosis and therapy. NIH Consens State Sci Statements 19:1–26

12. Araujo-Teixeira JP, Rocha-Reis J, Costa-Cabral A, Barros H, Saraiva AC, Araujo-Teixeira AM (1999) Laparoscopie ou laparotomie dans la cholecystite aigue (200 cas). Comparaison des resultats et facteurs predisposant a la conversion. Chirurgie 124:529–535

13. Arguedas MR, Dupont AW, Wilcox CM (2001) Where do ERCP, endoscopic ultrasound, magnetic resonance cholangiopancreatography, and intraoperative cholangiography fit in the management of acute biliary pancreatitis? A decision analysis model. Am J Gastroenterol 96:2892–2899

14. Assalia A, Kopelman D, Hashmonai M (1997) Emergency minilaparotomy cholecystectomy for acute cholecystitis: prospective randomized trials – implications for the laparoscopic era. World J Surg 21:534–539

15. Avrutis O, Friedman SJ, Meshoulm J, Haskel L, Adler S (2000) Safety and success of early laparoscopic cholecystectomy for acute cholecystitis. Surg Laparosc Endosc Percutan Tech 10:200–207

16. Ayub K, Imada R, Slavin J (2004) Endoscopic retrograde cholangiopancreatography in gallstone-associated acute pancreatitis. Cochrane Database Syst Rev CD003630

17. Bailey IS, Rhodes M, O'Rourke N, Nathanson L, Fielding G (1998) Laparoscopic management of acute small bowel obstruction. Br J Surg 85:84–87

18. Bastug DF, Trammell SW, Boland JP, Mantz EP, Tiley EH 3rd (1991) Laparoscopic adhesiolysis for small bowel obstruction. Surg Laparosc Endosc 1:259–262

19. Bedirli A, Sözüer EM, Sakrak O, Babayigit H, Yilmaz Z (2003) Comparison of the results of early, delayed and elective surgery in biliary pancreatitis. Turk J Gastroenterol 14:97–101

20. Berber E, Engle KL, String A, Garland AM, Chang G, Macho J, Pearl JM, Siperstein AE (2000) Selective use of tube cholecystostomy with interval laparoscopic cholecystectomy in acute cholecystitis. Arch Surg 135:341–346

21. Bergamaschi R, Marvik R, Johnsen G, Thoresen JE, Ystgaard B, Myrvold HE (1999) Open vs laparoscopic repair of perforated peptic ulcer. Surg Endosc 13:679–682

22. Bevan CD, Johal BJ, Mumtaz G, Ridgway GL, Siddle NC (1995) Clinical, laparoscopic and microbiological findings in acute salpingitis; report on a United Kingdom cohort. Br J Obstet Gynaecol 102:407–414

23. Bhattacharya D, Ammori BJ (2005) Contemporary minimally invasive approaches to the management of acute cholecystitis: a review and appraisal. Surg Laparosc Endosc Percutan Tech 15:1–8

24. Bhattacharya D, Senapati PS, Hurle R, Ammori BJ (2002) Urgent versus interval laparoscopic cholecystectomy for acute cholecystitis: a comparative study. J Hepatobiliary Pancreat Surg 9:538–542

25. Bittner R, Leibl B, Kraft K, Butters M, Nick G, Ulrich M (1997) Laparoskopische Cholecystektomie in der Therapie der akuten Cholecystitis; Sofort-versus Intervalloperation. Chirurg 68:237–243

26. Bjorck M, Acosta S, Lindberg F, Troeng T, Bergqvist D (2002) Revascularization of the superior mesenteric artery after acute thromboembolic occlusion, Br J Surg 89:923–927

27. Boey J, Lee NW, Koo J, Lam PH, Wong J, Ong GB (1982) Immediate definitive surgery for perfof rated duodenal ulcers: a prospective controlled trial. Ann Surg 196:338–344
28. Boggi U, Di Candio G, Campatelli A, Oleggini M, Pietrabissa A, Filipponi F, Bellini R, Mazzotta D, Mosca F (1999) Percutaneous cholecystostomy for acute cholecystitis in critically ill patients, Hepatogastroenterology 46:121–125
29. Borgstein PJ, Gordijn RV, Eijsbouts QAJ, Cuesta MA (1997) Acute appendicitis – clearcut case in men, a guessing game in young women. A prospective study on the role of taparoscopy. Surg Endosc 11:923–927
30. Borie F, Fingerhut A, Millat B (2003) Acute biliary pancreatitis, endoscopy, and laparoscopy. Surg Endosc 17:1175–1180
31. Borzellino G, de Manzoni G, Ricci F, Castaldini G, Guglielmi A, Cordiano C (1999) Emergency cholecystostomy and subsequent cholecystectomy for acute gallstone cholecystitis in the elderly. Br J Surg 86:1521–1525
32. Borzellino G, Tasselli S, Zerman G, Pedrazzani C, Manzoni G (2004) Laparoscopic approach to postoperative adhesive obstruction. Surg Endosc 18:686–690
33. Bove A, Bongarzoni G, Serafini FM, Bonomo L, Dragani G, Palone F, Scotti U, Corbellini L (2004) L'approccio laparoscopico alla colecistite acuta. Risultati e fattori predittivi di conversione. G Chir 25:75–79
34. Bradley EL 3rd (1993) A clinically based classification system for acute pancreatitis. Summary of the International Symposium on Acute Pancreatitis, Atlanta, Ga, September 11 through 13, 1992, Arch Surg 128:586–590
35. British Society of Gastroenterology (1998) United Kingdom guidelines for the management of acute pancreatitis. Gut 42:S1–S13
36. Brodsky A, Matter I, Sabo E, Cohen A, Abrahamson J, Eldar S (2000) Laparoscopic cholecystectomy for acute cholecystitis: can the need for conversion and the probability of complications be predicted. A prospective study. Surg Endosc 14:755–760
37. Bruwer F, Coetzer M, Warren BL (2003) Laparoscopic versus open surgical exploration in menopausal women with suspected acute appendicitis. S Afr J Surg 41:82–85
38. Bryant TL, Umstot RK Jr (1996) Laparoscopic repair of an incarcerated obturator hernia. Surg Endosc 10:437–438
39. Budzynski A, Bobizynski A, Rembiasz K, Biesiada Z (2003) Laparoscopic emergency surgery. Przegl Lek 607:20–24
40. Byrne MF, Suhock Pp, Mitchell RM, Pappas TN, Stiffler HL, Jowell PS, Branch MS, Baillie J (2003) Percutaneous cholecystostomy in patients with acute cholecystitis: experience of 45 patients at a US referral center. J Am Coll Surg 197:206–211
41. Carbajo Caballero MA, Martín del Olmo JC, Blanco Álvarez JI, Cuesta de la Llave C, Atienza Sánchez R, Inglada Galiana L, Vaquero Puerta C (1998) Surgical treatment of the acute cholecystitis in the laparoscopic age. A comparative study: laparoscopy against laparatomy. Rev Esp Enferm Dig 90:788–793
42. Chak A, Hawes RH, Cooper GS, Hoffman B, Catalano MF, Wong RC, Herbener TE, Sivak MV Jr (1999) Prospective assessment of the utility of EUS in the evaluation of gallstone pancreatitis. Gastrointest Endosc 49:590–604
43. Champault G, Rizk N, Lauroy J, Olivares P, Belhassen A, Boutelier P (1993) Douleurs iliaques droites de la femme. Approche diagnostique conventionelle versus laparoscopie-première. Étude contrôlée (65 cas). Ann Chir 47:316–319
44. Champault GG (1994) Laparoscopic treatment of perforated peptic ulcer, Endosc Surg Allied Technol 2:117–118
45. Chandler CF, Lane JS, Ferguson P, Thompson JE, Ashley SW (2000) Prospective evaluation of early versus delayed laparoscopic cholecystectomy for treatment of acute cholecystitis. Am Surg 66:896–900
46. Chang L, Lo S, Stabile BE, Lewis RJ, Toosie K, de Virgilio C (2000) Preoperative versus postoperative endoscopic retrograde cholangiopancreatography in mild to moderate gallstone pancreatitis; a prospective randomized trial. Ann Surg 231:82–87
47. Chang L, Moonka R, Stelzner M (2000) Percutaneous cholecystostomy for acute cholecystitis in veteran patients. Am J Surg 180:198–202

48. Chau CH, Tang CM, Siu WT, Ha JP, Li MK (2002) Laparoscopic cholecystectomy versus open cholecystectomy in elderly patients with acute cholecystitis: retrospective study. Hong Kong Med J8:394–399

49. Cheema S, Brannigan AE, Johnson S, Delaney PV, Grace PA (2003) Timing of laparoscopic cholecystectomy in acute cholecystitis. Ir J Med Sci 172:128–131

50. Chen RJ, Fang JF, Lin BC, Hsu YB, Kao JL, Kao YC, Chen MF (1998) Selective application of laparoscopy and fibrin glue in the failure of nonoperative management of blunt hepatic trauma. J Trauma 44:691–695

51. Chiarugi M, Buccianti P, Decanini L, Balestri R, Lorenzetti L, Ranceschi M, Cavina E (2001) "What you see is not what you get". A plea to remove a "normal" appendix during diagnostic laparoscopy. Acta Chir Belg 101:243–245

52. Cho YP, Jung SM, Han MS, Jang HJ, Kim JS, Kim YH, Lee SG (2003) Role of diagnostic laparoscopy in managing acute mesenteric venous thrombosis. Surg Laparosc Endosc Percutan Tech 13:215–217

53. Chol YB, Lim KS (2003) Therapeutic laparoscopy for abdominal trauma. Surg Endosc 17:421–427

54. Chong AK, So JB, Ti TK (2001) Use of laparoscopy in the management of mesenteric venous thrombosis. Surg Endosc 15:1042

55. Chopra R, McVay C, Phillips E, Khalili TM (2003) Laparoscopic lysis of adhesions. Am Surg 69:966–968

56. Chosidow D, Johanet H, Montariol T, Kielt R, Manceau C, Marmuse JP, Benhamou G (2000) Laparoscopy for acute small-bowel obstruction secondary to adhesions. J Laparoendosc Adv Surg Tech A 10:155–159

57. Chung RS, Diaz JJ, Chari V (1998) Efficacy of routine laparoscopy for the acute abdomen. Surg Endosc 12:219–222

58. Cloyd DW (1994) Laparoscopic repair of incarcerated paraesophageal hernias. Surg Endosc 8:893–897

59. Consensus Panel, Society for Surgery of the Alimentary Tract, American Gastroenterological Association, American Society for Gastrointestinal Endocospy (2001) Management of the biliary tract in acute necrotizing pancreatitis. J Gastrointest Surg 5:221–222

60. Cougar P, Barras C, Gayral F et al (2000) Societé Francaise de Chirurgie Laparoscopique Le traitement laparoscopique de l'ulcère duodénal perforé. Résultats d'une étude rétrospective multicentrique. Ann Chir 125:726–731

61. Crofts TJ, Park KG, Steele RJ, Chung SS, Li AK (1989) A randomized trial of nonoperative treatment for perforated peptic ulcer. N Engl J Med 320:970–973

62. Cueto J, Díaz O, Garteiz D, Rodriguez M, Weber A (1997) The efficacy of laparoscopic surgery in the diagnosis and treatment of peritonitis. Experience with 107 cases in Mexico City. Surg Endosc 11:366–370

63. Cuschieri A, Hennessy TP, Stephens RB, Berci G (1988) Diagnosis of significant abdominal trauma after road traffic accidents: preliminary results of a multicentre clinical trial comparing minilaparoscopy with peritoneal lavage. Ann R Coll Surg Engl 70:153–155

64. Decadt B, Sussman L, Lewis MPN, Seeker A, Cohen L, Rogers C, Patel A, Rhodes M (1999) Randomized clinical trial of early laparoscopy in the management of acute nonspecific abdominal pain. Br J Surg 86:1383–1386

65. Dervenis C, Johnson CD, Bassi C, Bradley E, Imrie CW, McMadlin MJ, Modlin I (1999) Diagnosis, objective assessment of severity, and management of acute pancreatitis. Santorini consensus conference. Int J Pancreatol 25:195–210

66. Druart ML, Van Hee R, Etienne J et al (1997) Laparoscopic repair of perforated duodenal ulcer. A prospective multicenter clinical trial. Surg Endosc 11:1017–1020

67. Easter DW, Cuschieri A, Nathanson LK, Lavelle-Jones M (1992) The utility of diagnostic laparoscopy for abdominal disorders. Audit of 120 patients. Arch Surg 127:379–383

68. Edwards MS, Cherr GS, Craven TE, Olsen AW, Plonk GW, Geary RL, Ligush JL, Hansen KJ (2003) Acute occlusive mesenteric ischemia: surgical management and outcomes. Ann Vasc Surg 17:72–79

69. Eldar S, Eltan A, Bickel A, Sabo E, Cohen A, Abrahamson J, Matter I (1999) The impact of patient delay and physician delay on the outcome of laparoscopic cholecystectomy for acute cholecystitis. Am J Surg 178:303–307
70. Eldar S, Sabo E, Nash E, Abrahamson J, Matter I (1997) Laparoscopic cholecystectomy for acute cholecystitis: prospective trial. World J Surg 21:540–545
71. Eldar S, Sabo E, Nash E, Abrahamson J, Matter I (1997) Laparoscopic versus open cholecystectomy in acute cholecystitis. Surg Laparosc Endosc 7:407–414
72. Eypasch E, Kum CK, Neugebauer E et al Laparoscopic appendectomy: EAES consensus development conference (1997) and updating comments (2000). In: Neugebauer H, Sauerland S, Troidi H (eds) Recommendations for evidence-based surgery. Springer, Berlin Heidelberg New York pp 15–23
73. Eypasch E, Menninger R, Paul A, Troidl H (1993) Die Bedeutung der Laparoskopie bei der Diagnostik und Therapie des akuten Abdomens. Zentralbl Chir 118:726–732
74. Eypasch E, Spangenberger W, Ure B, Mennigen R, Troidl H (1994) Laparoskopische und konventionelle Übernähung perforierter peptischer Ulcera: eine Gegenüberstellung, Chirurg 65:445–450
75. Fagniez PL, Rotman N, Association de Recherche en Chirurgie (1998) Influence de la date de l'intervention chirurgicale sur le pronostic des pancreatites aigues biliaires graves. Chirurgie 123:368–372
76. Fan ST, Lai ECS, Mok FPT, Lo CML, Zheng SS, Wong J (1993) Early treatment of acute biliary pancreatitis by endoscopic papillotomy. N Engl J Med 328:228–232
77. Faranda C, Barrat C, Catheline JM, Champault GG (2000) Two-stage laparoscopic management of generalized peritonitis due to perforated sigmoid diverticula; eighteen cases. Surg Laparosc Endosc Percutan Tech 10:135–141
78. Feigel M, Thalmann C, Blessing H (1996) Laparoskopisch endoskopisch-präperitoneale kombinierte Hernien-Operation bei incarcerierter indirekter Inguinalhernie. Chirurg 67:188–189
79. Fernandez H, Marchal L, Vincent Y (1998) Fertility after radical surgery for tubal pregnancy. Fertil Steril 70:680–686
80. Ferrozzi L, Lippolis G, Petitti T, Carnevale D, Masi M (2004) La colecistectomia videolaparoscopica nella colecistite acuta: nostra esperienza. G Chir 25:80–82
81. Ferzli G, Shapiro K, Chaudry G, Patel S (2004) Laparoscopic extraperitoneal approach to acutely incarcerated inguinal hernia. Surg Endosc 18:228–231
82. Fevang BT, Fevang J, Lie SA, Soreide O, Svanes K, Viste A (2004) Long-term prognosis after operation for adhesive small bowel obstruction. Ann Surg 240:193–201
83. Fevang BT, Fevang JM, Soreide O, Svanes K, Viste A (2003) Delay in operative treatment among patients with small bowel obstruction. Scand J Surg 92:131–137
84. Fevang BT, Jensen D, Svanes K, Viste A (2002) Early operation or conservative management of patients with small bowel obstruction? Eur J Surg 168:475–481
85. Fischer CP, Doherty D (2002) Laparoscopic approach to small bowel obstruction. Semin Laparosc Surg 9:40–45
86. Flum DR, Morris A, Koepsell T, Dellinger EP (2001) Has misdiagnosis of appendicitis decreased over time? A population-based analysis. J Am Med Assoc 286:1748–1753
87. Fölsch UR, Nitsche R, Ludtke R, Hilgers RA, Creutzfeldt W, the German Study Group on Acute Biliary Pancreatitis (1997) Early ERCP and papillotomy compared with conservative treatment for acute biliary pancreatitis. N Engl J Med 336:237–242
88. Franklin ME Jr, Dorman JP, Jacobs M, Plasencia G (1997) Is laparoscopic surgery applicable to complicated colonic diverticular disease? Surg Endosc 11:1021–1025
89. Franklin ME Jr, Dorman JP, Pharand D (1994) Laparoscopic surgery in acute small bowel obstruction. Surg Laparosc Endosc 4:289–296
90. Franklin ME Jr, Gonzalez JJ Jr, Miter DB, Glass JL, Paulson D (2004) Laparoscopic diagnosis and treatment of intestinal obstruction. Surg Endosc 18:26–30
91. Gagner M (1996) Laparoscopic treatment of acute necrotizing pancreatitis. Semin Laparosc Surg 3:21–28

92. Gaitán H, Angel E, Sánchez J, Gómez I, Sánchez L, Agudelo C (2002) Laparoscopic diagnosis of acute lower abdominal pain in women of reproductive age. Int J Gynaecol Obstet 76:149–158

93. Garber SM, Korman J, Cosgrove JM, Cohen JR (1997) Early laparoscopic cholecystectomy for acute cholecystitis. Surg Endosc 11:347–350

94. Geis WP, Kim HC (1995) Use of laparoscopy in the diagnosis and treatment of patients with surgical abdominal sepsis. Surg Endosc 9:178–182

95. Gharaibeh KI, Qasaimeh GR, Al-Heiss H, Ammari F, Bani-Hani K, Al-Jaberi TM, Al-Natour S (2002) Effect of timing of surgery, type of inflammation, and sex on outcome of laparoscopic cholecystectomy for acute cholecystitis. J Laparoendosc Adv Surg Tech A 12:192–198

96. Giger U, Michel JM, Vonlanthen R, Becker K, Kocher T, Krähenbühl L (2005) Laparoscopic cholecystectomy in acute cholecystitis: indication, technique, risk and outcome. Langenbecks Arch Surg 390:373–380

97. Glavic Z, Begic L, Simlesa D, Rukavina A (2001) Treatment of acute cholecystitis. A comparison of open vs laparoscopic cholecystectomy. Surg Endosc 15:398–401

98. Golash V, Willson PD (2005) Early laparoscopy as a routine procedure in the management of acute abdominal pain: a review of 1320 patients. Surg Endosc 19:882–885

99. Graham A, Henley C, Mobley J (1991) Laparoscopic evaluation of acute abdominal pain. J Laparoendosc Surg 1:165–168

100. Granlund A, Karlson BM, Elvin A, Rasmussen I (2001) Ultrasound-guided percutaneous cholecystostomy in high-risk surgical patients. Langenbecks Arch Surg 386:212–217

101. Gray DT, Thorburn J, Lundorff P, Strandell A, Lindblom B (1995) A cost-effectiveness study of a randomised trial of laparoscopy versus laparotomy for ectopic pregnancy. Lancet 345:1139–1143

102. Greenwald JA, McMullen HF, Coppa GF, Newman RM (2000) Standardization of surgeon-controlled variables: impact on outcome in patients with acute cholecystitis. Ann Surg 231:339–344

103. Grunewald B, Keating J (1993) Should the "normal" appendix be removed at operation for appendicitis? J R Coll Surg Edinb 38:158–160

104. Haan J, Kole K, Brunetti A, Kramer M, Scalea TM (2003) Nontherapeutic laparotomies revisted. Am Surg 69:562–565

105. Habib FA, Kolachaiam RB, Khilnani R, Preventza O, Mittal VK (2001) Role of laparoscopic cholel cystectomy in the management of gangrenous cholecystitis. Am J Surg 181:71–75

106. Hallal AH, Amortegui JD, Jeroukhimov IM, Casillas J, Schulman CI, Manning RJ, Habib FA, Lopez PP, Cohn SM, Sleeman D (2005) Magnetic resonance cholangiopancreatography accurately detects common bile duct stones in resolving gallstone pancreatitis. J Am Coll Surg 200:869–875

107. Hamad GG, Broderick TJ (2000) Laparoscopic pancreatic necrosectomy. J Laparoendosc Adv Surg Tech A 10:115–118

108. Hartwig W, Maksan SM, Foitzik T, Schmidt J, Herfarth C, Klar E (2002) Reduction in mortality with delayed surgical therapy of severe pancreatitis. J Gastrointest Surg 6:481–487

109. Hatzidakis AA, Prassopoulos P, Petinarakis I, Sanidas E, Chrysos E, Chalkiaoakis G, Tsiftsis D, Gourtsoyiannis NC (2002) Acute cholecystitis in high-risk patients: percutaneous cholecystostomy vs conservative treatment. Eur Radiol 12:1778–1784

110. Heiss MM, Hüttl TP, Spelsberg FW, Lang RA, Jauch KW (2003) Möglichkeiten und Grenzen der laparoskopischen Magenchirurgie. Viszeralchirurgie 38:107–117

111. Ibrahim IM, Wolodiger F, Sussman B, Kahn M, Silvestri F, Sabar A (1996) Laparoscopic management of acute small-bowel obstruction. Surg Endosc 10:1012–1015

112. Irvin TT (1989) Abdominal pain; a surgical audit of 1190 emergency admissions. Br J Surg 76:1121–1125

113. Ishihara T, Kubota K, Eda N, Ishibashi S, Haraguchi Y (1996) Laparoscopic approach to incarcerated inguinal hernia. Surg Endosc 10:1111–1113
114. Isla A, Griniatsos J, Rodway A (2003) Single-stage definitive laparoscopic management in mild acute biliary pancreatitis. J Laparoendosc Adv Surg Tech A 13:77–81
115. Ito K, Fujita N, Noda Y, Kobayashi G, Kimura K, Sugawara T, Horaguchi J (2004) Percutaneous cholecystostomy versus gallbladder aspiration for acute cholecystitis: a prospective randomized controlled trial. Am J Roentgenol 183:193–196
116. Jacobson TZ, Barlow DH, Garry R, Koninckx P (2001) Laparoscopic surgery for pelvic pain associated with endometriosis. Cochrane Database Syst Rev CD001300
117. Jadallah FA, Abdul-Ghani AA, Tibblin S (1994) Diagnostic laparoscopy reduces unnecessary appendicectomy in fertile women. Eur J Surg 160:41–45
118. Jawad AJ, Al-Meshari A (1998) Laparoscopy for ovarian pathology in infancy and childhood. Pediatr Surg Int 14:62–65
119. Johansson B, Hallerbäck B, Glise H, Johnsson E (1996) Laparoscopic suture closure of perforated peptic ulcer. A nonrandomized comparison with open surgery. Surg Endosc 10:656–658
120. Johansson M, Thune A, Blomqvist A, Nelvin L, Lundell L (2003) Management of acute cholecystitis in the laparoscopic era: results of a prospective, randomized clinical trial. J Gastrointest Surg 7:642–645
121. Johansson M, Thune A, Blomqvist A, Nelvin L, Lundell L (2004) Impact of choice of therapeutic strategy for acute cholecystitis on patinet's health-related quality of life: results of a randomized, controlled clinical trial. Dig Surg 21:359–362
122. Johansson M, Thune A, Nelvin L, Stiernstam M, Westman B, Lundell L (2005) Randomized clinical trial of open versus laparoscopic cholecystectomy in the treatment of acute cholecystitis. Br J Surg 92:44–49
123. Kaiwa Y, Namiki K, Matsumoto H (2003) Laparoscopic relief of reduction en masse of incarcerated inguinal hernia. Surg Endosc 17:352
124. Kaltenthaler E, Vergel YB, Chilcott J, Thomas S, Blakeborough T, Walters SJ, Bouchier H (2004) A systematic review and economic evaluation of magnetic resonance cholangiopancreatography compared with diagnostic endoscopic retrograde cholangiopancreatography. Health Technol Assess 8:iii, 1–89
125. Kelly TR, Wagner DS (1988) Gallstone pancreatitis; a prospective randomized trial of the timing of surgery. Surgery 104:600–605
126. Kim HJ, Lee SK, Kim MH, Yoo KS, Lim BC, Seo DW, Min YI (2000) Safety and usefulness of percutaneous transhepatic cholecystoscopy examination in high-risk surgical patients with acute cholecystitis. Gastrointest Endosc 52:645–649
127. Kim SY, Moore JT (2003) Volvulus of the gallbladder: laparoscopic detorsion and removal. Surg Endosc 17:1849
128. Kirby CP, Sparnon AL (2001) Active observation of children with possible appendicitis does not increase morbidity. ANZ J Surg 71:412–413
129. Kirshtein B, Roy-Shapira A, Lantsberg L, Avinoach E, Mizrahi S (2005) Laparoscopic management of acute small bowel obstruction. Surg Endosc, 19:464–467
130. Kirshtein B, Roy-Shapira A, Lantsberg L, Mandel S, Avinoach E, Mizrahi S (2003) The use of laparocopy in abdominal emergencies. Surg Endosc 17:1118–1124
131. Kiviluoto T, Sirén J, Luukkonen P, Kivilaakso E (1998) Randomised trial of laparoscopic versus open cholecystectomy for acute and gangrenous cholecystitis. Lancet 351:321–325
132. Klein HM, Lensing R, Klosterhalfen B, Tons C, Gunther RW (1995) Diagnostic imaging of mesenteric infarction. Radiology 197:79–82
133. Knight JS, Mercer SJ, Somers SS, Walters AM, Sadek SA, Toh SK (2004) Timing of urgent laparoscopic cholecystectomy does not influence conversion rate. Br J Surg 91:601–604
134. Köhler L, Sauerland S, Neugebauer E, for the Scientific Committee of the European Association for Endoscopic Surgery (1999) Diagnosis and treatment of diverticular disease; results of a consensus development conference. Surg Endosc 13:430–436

135. Kok KYY, Mathew VV, Yapp SKS (1999) Laparoscopic omental patch repair for perforated duodenal ulcer. Am Surg 65:27–30
136. Kolla SB, Aggarwal S, Kumar A, Kumar R, Chumber S, Parshad R, Seenu V (2004) Early versus delayed laparoscopic cholecystectomy for acute cholecystitis: a prospective randomized trial. Surg Endosc 18:1323–1327
137. Köninger J, Böttinger P, Redecke J, Butters M (2004) Laparoscooic repair of perforated gastroduodenal ulcer by running suture. Langenbecks Arch Surg 389:11–16
138. Kontoravdis A, Chryssikopoulos A, Hassiakos D, Liapis A, Zourlas PA (1996) The diagnostic value of laparoscopy in 2365 patients with acute and chronic pelvic pain. Int J Gynaecol Obstet 52:243–248
139. Koo KP, Thirlby RC (1996) Laparoscopic cholecystectomy in acute cholecystitis. What is the optimal timing for operation? Arch Surg 131:540–545
140. Koperna T, Kisser M, Schulz F (1999) Laparoscopic versus open treatment of patients with acute cholecystitis. Hepatogastroenterology 46:753–757
141. Kraemer M, Ohmann C, Leppert R, Yang Q (2000) Macroscopic assessment of the appendix at diagnostic laparoscopy is reliable. Surg Endosc 14:625–633
142. Kronborg O (1993) Treatment of perforated sigmoid diverticulitis: a prospective randomized trial. Br J Surg 80:505–507
143. Kum CK, Eypasch E, Lefering R, Paul A, Neugebauer E, Troidl H (1996) Laparoscopic cholecystectomy for acute cholecystitis: is it really safe? World J Surg 20:43–49
144. Kum CK, Goh PMY, Isaac JR, Tekant Y, Ngoi SS (1994) Laparoscopic cholecystectomy for acute cholecystitis. Br J Surg 81:1651–1654
145. Kuster GG, Domagk D (1996) Laparoscopic cholecystostomy with delayed cholecystectomy as an alternative to conversion to open procedure. Surg Endosc 10:426–428
146. Lai PBS, Kwong KH, Leung KL, Kwok SPY, Chan ACW, Chung SCS, Lau WY (1998) Randomized trial of early versus delayed laparoscopic cholecystectomy for acute cholecystitis. Br J Surg 85:764–767
147. Laine S, Rantala A, Gullichsen R, Ovaska J (1997) Laparoscopic appendectomy is it worthwhile? A prospective, randomized study in young women. Surg Endosc 11:95–97
148. Lam CM, Yuen AW, Chik B, Wai AC, Fan ST (2005) Laparoscopic surgery for common surgical emergencies: a population-based study. Surg Endosc 19:774–779
149. Landau O, Kyzer S (2004) Emergent laparoscopic repair of incarcerated incisional and venral hernia. Surg Endosc 18:1374–1376
150. Lanzafame RJ (1993) Techniques for the simultaneous management of incarcerated ventral herniae and cholelithiasis via laparoscopy. J Laparoendosc Surg 3:193–201
151. Larsson PG, Henriksson G, Olsson M, Boris J, Stroberg P, Tronstad SE, Skuilman S (2001) Laparoscopy reduces unnecessary appendicectomies and improves diagnosis in fertile women. A randomized study. Surg Endosc 15:200–202
152. Lau H (2004) Laparoscopic repair of perforated peptic ulcer: a meta-analysis. Surg Endosc 18:1013–1021
153. Lau WY, Leung KL, Kwong KH, Davey IC, Robertson C, Dawson JJ, Chung SC, Li AK (1996) A randomized study comparing laparoscopic versus open repair of perforated peptic ulcer using suture or sutureless technique. Ann Surg 224:131–138
154. Lavonius MI, Ovaska J (2000) Laparoscopy in the evaluation of the incarcerated mass in groin hernia. Surg Endosc 14:488–489
155. Lee FYJ, Leung KL, Lai PBS, Lau JWY (2001) Selection of patients for laparoscopic repair of perforated peptic ulcer. Br J Surg 88:133–136
156. Lee HK, Han HS, Min SK, Lee JH (2005) Sex-based analysis of the outcome of laparoscopic cholecystectomy for acute cholecystitis. Br J Surg 92:463–466
157. Lee KB, Wong SK (2002) Emergency laparoscopic surgery – the Changi General Hospital experience. Ann Acad Med Singapore 31:155–157
158. Leibl BJ, Schmedt CG, Kraft K, Kraft B, Bittner R (2001) Laparoscopic transperitoneal hernia repair of incarcerated hernias: is it feasible? Results of a prospective study. Surg Endosc 15:1179–1183

159. Leister I, Markus PM, Becker H (2003) Mesenteriale Ischämie: Hat die diagnostische Laparokopie einen Stellenwert? Chirurg 74:407–412
160. Leon EL, Metzger A, Tsiotos GG, Schlinkert RT, Sarr MG (1998) Laparoscopic management of small bowel obstruction; indications and outcome, J Gastrointest Surg 2:132–140
161. Leppäniemi A, Haapiainen R (2003) Diagnostic laparoscopy in abdominal stab wounds: a prospective, randomized study. J Trauma 55:636–645
162. Leppaniemi A, Salo J, Haapiainen R (1995) Complications of negative laparotomy for truncal stab wounds. J Trauma 38:54–58
163. Levard H, Boudet MJ, Msika S, Molkhou JM, Hay JM, Laborde Y, Gillet M, Fingerhut A (2001) Laparoscopic treatment of acute small bowel obstruction: a multicentre retrospective study. ANZ J Surg 71:641–646
164. Liao K, Ramirez J, Carryl S, Shaftan GW (1997) A new approach in the management of incarcety ated hernia. Emergency laparoscopic hernia repair. Surg Endosc 11:944–945
165. Lin E, Wear K, Tiszenkel HI (2002) Planned reduction of incarcerated groin hernias with hernia sac laparoscopy. Surg Endosc 16:936–938
166. Liu CL, Lo CM, Chan JK, Poon RT, Lam CM, Fan ST, Wong J (2001) Detection of choledocholithiasis by EUS in acute pancreatitis: a prospective evaluation in 100 consecutive patients. Gastrointest Endosc 54:325–330
167. Liu S, Chen F, Chen H (1995) An evaluation of nonsurgical treatment for severe acute pancreatitis. Zhonghua Wai Ke Za Zhi 33:545–547
168. Lo CM, Fan ST, Liu CL, Lai EC, Wong J (1997) Early decision for conversion of laparoscopic to open cholecystectomy for treatment of acute cholecystitis. Am J Surg 173:513–517
169. Lo CM, Liu CL, Fan ST, Lai EC, Wong J (1998) Prospective randomized study of early versus delayed laparoscopic cholecystectomy for acute cholecystitis. Ann Surg 227:461–467
170. Lujan JA, Parrilla P, Robles R, Marin P, Torralba JA, Garcia-Ayllon J (1998) Laparoscopic chole? cystectomy vs open cholecystectomy in the treatment of acute cholecystitis: a prospective study. Arch Surg 133:173–175
171. Lundorff P, Thorburn J, Hahlin M, Kallfelt B, Lindblom B (1991) Laparoscopic surgery in ectopic pregnancy. A randomized trial versus laparotomy. Acta Obstet Gynecol Scand 70:343–348
172. Lundorff P, Thorburn J, Lindblom B (1992) Fertility outcome after conservative surgical treatment of ectopic pregnancy evaluated in a randomized trial. Fertil Steril 57:998–1002
173. Madan AK, Aliabadi-Wahle S, Tesi D, Flint LM, Steinberg SM (2002) How early is early laparoscopic treatment of acute cholecystitis? Am J Surg 183:232–236
174. Magos AL, Baumannn R, Burnbull AC (1989) Managing gynaecological emergencies with laparoscopy. Br Med J 299:371–374
175. Mais V, Ajossa S, Piras B, Marongiu D, Guerriero S, Melis GB (1995) Treatment of nonendometriotic benign adnexal cysts; a randomized comparison of laparoscopy and laparotomy. Obstet Gynecol 86: 770–774
176. Majewski WD (2005) Long-term outcome, adhesions, and quality of life after laparoscopic open surgical therapies for acute abdomen: follow-up of a prospective trial. Surg Endosc 19:81–90
177. Mathonnet M, Peyrou P, Gainant A, Bouvier S, Cubertafond P (2003) Role of laparoscopy in blunt perforations of the small bowel. Surg Endosc 17:641–645
178. Matsuda M, Nishiyama M, Hanai T, Saeki S, Watanabe T (1995) Laparoscopic omental patch repair for perforated peptic ulcer. Ann Surg 221:236–240
179. Matthews BD, Bui H, Harold KL, Kercher KW, Adrales G, Park A, Sing RF, Heniford BT (2003) Laparoscopic repair of traumatic diaphragmatic injuries. Surg Endosc 17:254–258

180. Mehendale VG, Shenoy SN, Joshi AM, Chaudhari NC (2002) Laparoscopic versus open surgical closure of perforated duodenal ulcers: a comparative study. Indian J Gastroenterol 21:222–224
181. Merriam LT, Kanaan SA, Dawes LG, Angelos P, Prystowsky JB, Rege RV, Joehl RJ (1999) Gangrenous cholecystitis: analysis of risk factors and experience with laparoscopic cholecystectomy. Surgery 126:680–686
182. Mier J, Luque-de León E, Castillo A, Robledo F, Blanco R (1997) Early versus late necrosectomy in severe necrotizing pancreatitis. Am J Surg 173:71–75
183. Mikkelsen AL, Felding C (1990) Laparoscopy and ultrasound examination in women with acute pelvic pain. Gynecol Obstet Invest 30:162–164
184. Millat B, Fingerhut A, Borie F (2000) Surgical treatment of complicated duodenal ulcers: co trolled trials. World J Surg 24:299–306
185. Miserez M, Eypasch E, Spangenberger W, Lefering R, Troidl H (1996) Laparoscopic and conventional closure of perforated peptic ulcer. A comparison. Surg Endosc 10:831–836
186. Moberg AC, Berndsen F, Palmquist I, Petersson U, Resch T, Montgomery A (2005) Randomized clinical trial of laparoscopic versus open appendicectomy for confirmed appendicitis. Br J Surg 92:298–304
187. Morino M, Castagna E, Rosso E, Mao P (2004) Non-specific acute abdominal pain: a randomized controlled trial comparing early laparoscopy vs observation [abstract]. Surg Endosc 18:S2
188. Mouret P, Francois Y, Vignal J, Barth X, Lombard-Platet R (1990) Laparoscopic treatment of perforated peptic ulcer. Br J Surg 77:1006
189. Murphy AA, Nager CW, Wujek JJ, Kettel LM, Torp VA, Chin HG (1992) Operative laparoscopy versus laparotomy for the management of ectopic pregnancy: a prospective trial. Fertil Steril 57:1180–1185
190. Murphy MK, Black NA, Lamping DL, McKee CM, Sanderson CFB, Askham J, Marteau T (1998) Consensus development methods, and their use in clinical guideline development Health Technol Assessment 2:i–iv, 1–88
191. Naesgaard JM, Edwin B, Reiertsen O, Trondsen E, Frden AE, Rosseland AR (1999) Laparoscopic and open operation in patients with perforated peptic ulcer. Eur J Surg 165:209–214
192. Nagle A, Ujiki M, Denham W, Murayama K (2004) Laparoscopic adhesiolysis for small bowel obstruction. Am J Surg 187:464–470
193. Nagy AG, James D (1989) Diagnostic laparoscopy. Am J Surg 157:490–493
194. Nathanson LK, Easter DW, Cuschieri A (1990) Laparoscopic repair peritoneal toilet of perforated duodenal ulcer. Surg Endosc 4:232–233
195. Nathens AB, Gurtis JR, Beale RJ, Cook DJ, Moreno RP, Romand JA, Skerrett SJ, Stapleton RD, Ware LB, Waldmann CS (2004) Management of the critically ill patient with severe acute pancreatitis. Crit Care Med 32:2524–2536
196. Navarrete Aulestia S, Cantele H, Leyba JL, Navarrete M, Navarrete Llopla S (2003) Laparoscopic diagnosis and treatment in gynecologic emergencies. J Soc Laparoendosc Surg 7:239–242
197. Navez B, Arimont JM, Guiot P (1998) Laparoscopic approach in acute small bowel obstruction. A review of 68 patients. Hepatogastroenterology 45:2146–2150
198. Navez B, d'Udekem Y, Cambier E, Richir C, de Pierpont B, Guiot P (1995) Laparoscopy for management of nontraumatic acute abdomen. World J Surg 19:382–386
199. Navez B, Mutter D, Russier Y, Vix M, Jamali F, Lipski D, Cambier E, Guiot P, Leroy J, Marescaux J (2001) Safety of laparoscopic approach for acute cholecystitis: retrospective study of 609 cases. World J Surg 25:1352–1356
200. Neoptolemos JP, Carr-Locke DL, London NJ, Bailey IA, James D, Fossard DP (1988) Controlled trial of urgent endoscopic retrograde cholangiopancreatography and endoscopic sphincterotomy versus conservative treatment for acute pancreatitis due to gallstones. Lancet 2:979–983

201. Neoptolemos JP, Shaw DE, Carr-Locke DL (1989) A multivariate analysis of preoperative risk factors in patients with common bile duct stones. Implications for treatment Ann Surg 209:157–161
202. Nicolau AE, Ionescu G, Iordache F, Mehic R, Spataru A (2002) Sutura laparoscopica sau sutura deschisa in ulcerul duodenal recent perforat la tineri. Chirurgia (Bucur) 97:305–311
203. Nitke S, Goldman GA, Fisch B, Kaplan B, Ovadia J (1996) The management of dermoid cysts – a comparative study of laparoscopy and laparotomy. Isr J Med Sci 32:1177–1179
204. Nordback I, Sisto T (1991) Ultrasonography and computed tomography in the diagnosis of por; tomesenteric vein thrombosis. Int Surg 76:179–182
205. Olsen JB, Myrén CJ, Haahr PE (1993) Randomized study of the value of laparoscopy before appendicectomy. Br J Surg 80:922–923
206. O'Sullivan GC, Murphy D, O'Brien MG, Ireland A (1996) Laparoscopic management of generalized peritonitis due to perforated colonic diverticula. Am J Surg 171:432–434
207. Ou CS, Rowbotham R (2000) Laparoscopic diagnosis and treatment of nontraumatic acute abdominal pain in women. J Laparoendosc Adv Surg Tech A 10:41–45
208. Paimela H, Oksala NK, Kivilaakso E (2004) Surgery for peptic ulcer today. A study on the incidence, methods and mortality in surgery for peptic ulcer in Finland between 1987 and 1999. Dig Surg 21:186–191
209. Pamoukian VN, Gagner M (2001) Laparoscopic necrosectomy for acute necrotizing pancreatitis, J Hepatobiliary Pancreat Surg 8:221–223
210. Papi C, Catarci M, D'Ambrosjo L, Gili L, Koch M, Grassi GB, Capurso L (2004) Timing of cholecystectomy for acute calculous cholecystitis: a meta-analysis. Am J Gastroenterol 99:147–155
211. Paterson-Brown S, Eckersley JRT, Sim AJW, Dudley HAF (1986) Laparoscopy as an adjunct to decision making in the "acute abdomen". Br J Surg 73:1022–1024
212. Patient Care Committee of the Society for Surgery of the Alimentary Tract (1999) Surgical treatment of diverticulitis. J Gastrointest Surg 3:212–213
213. Patterson EJ, McLoughlin RF, Mathieson JR, Cooperberg PL, MacFarlane JK (1996) An alternative approach to acute cholecystitis. Percutaneous cholecystostomy and interval laparoscopic cholecystectomy. Surg Endosc 10:1185–1188
214. Paul A, Millat B, Holthausen U, Sauerland S, Neugebauer E, for the Scientific Committee of the European Association for Endoscopic Surgery (1998) Diagnosis and treatment of common bile duct stones (CBDS). Results of a consensus development conference. Surg Endosc 12:856–864
215. Peng WK, Sheikh Z, Nixon SJ, Paterson-Brown S (2005) Role of laparoscopic cholecystectomy in the early management of acute gallbladder disease. Br J Surg 92:586–591
216. Perko MJ (2001) Duplex ultrasound for assessment of superior mesenteric artery blood flow. Eur J Vasc Endovasc Surg 21:106–117
217. Pessaux P, Lebigot J, Tuech JJ, Regenet N, Aubé C, Ridereau C, Arnaud JP (2000) Cholécystostomie percutanee dans les cholécystites aiguës chez les patients à haut risque. Ann Chir 125:738–743
218. Pessaux P, Regenet N, Tuech JJ, Rouge C, Bergamaschi R, Arnaud JP (2001) Laparoscopic versus open cholecystectomy: a prospective comparative study in the elderly with acute cholecystitis. Surg Laparosc Endosc Percutan Tech 11:252–255
219. Pessaux P, Tuech JJ, Derouet N, Rouge C, Regenet N, Arnaud JP (2000) Laparoscopic cholecystectomy in the elderly: a prospective study. Surg Endosc 14:1067–1069
220. Pessaux P, Tuech JJ, Rouge C, Duplessis R, Cervi C, Arnaud JP (2000) Laparoscopic cholecystectomy in acute cholecystitis. A prospective comparative study in patients with acute vs chronic cholecystitis. Surg Endosc 14:358–361
221. Prat F, Edery J, Meduri B et al (2001) Early EUS of the bile duct before endoscopic sphincterometry for acute biliary pancreatitis. Gastrointest Endosc 54:724–729
222. Promecene PA (2002) Laparoscopy in gynecologic emergencies. Semin Laparosc Surg 9:64–75

223. Pugliese R, Di Lernia S, Sansonna F, Scandroglio I, Maggioni D, Ferrari C, Costanzi A, Chiara O (2004) Laparoscopic treatment of sigmoid diverticulitis: a retrospective review of 103 cases. Surg Endosc 18:1344–1348

224. Rau HG, Meyer G, Maiwald G, Schardey M, Merkle R, Lange V, Schildberg FW (1994) Konventionelle oder laparoskopische Cholecystektomie zur Behandlung der akuten Cholecystitis? Chirurg 65:1121–1125

225. Reiertsen O, Rosseland AR, Hoivik B, Solheim K (1985) Laparoscopy in patients admitted for acute abdominal pain. Acta Chir Scand 151:52–524

226. Renz BM, Feliciano DV (1995) Unnecessary laparotomies for trauma; a prospective study of morbidity. J Trauma 38:350–356

227. Rhodes M, Sussman L, Cohen L, Lewis MP (1998) Randomised trial of laparoscopic exploration of common bile duct versus postoperative endoscopic retrograde cholangiography for common bile duct stones. Lancet 351:159–161

228. Ricci F, Castaldini G, de Manzoni G, Botzellino G, Rodella L, Kind R (1997) Minimally invasive treatment acute biliary pancreatitis. Surg Endosc 1179–1182

229. Romagnuolo J, Currie G (2005) Noninvasive vs selective invasive biliary imaging for acute biliary pancreatitis: an economic evaluation by using decision tree analysis. Gastrointest Endosc 61:86–87

230. Rutledge D, Jones D, Reqe R (2000) Consequences of delay in surgical treatment of biliary disease. Am J Surg 180:466–469

231. Salky BA, Edye MB (1998) The role of laparoscopy in the diagnosis and treatment of abdominal pain syndromes. Surg Endosc 12:911–914

232. Sanna A, Adani GL, Anania G, Donini A (2003) The role of laparoscopy in patients with suspected peritonitis: experience of a single institution. J Laparoendosc Adv Surg Tech A 13:17–19

233. Sauerland S, Lefering R, Neugebauer E (2004) Laparoscopic versus open surgery for suspected appendicitis [Cochrane Review]. In: The Cochrane Collaboration (ed). The cochrane database of systematic reviews, Vol. IV/2004 [CD-ROM]. Oxford Update Software

234. Scheiman JM, Carlos RC, Barnett JL, Elta GH, Nostrant TT, Chey WD, Francis IR, Nandi PS (2001) Can endoscopic ultrasound or magnetic resonance cholangiopancreatography replace ERCP in patients with suspected biliary disease? A prospective trial and cost analysis. Am J Gastroenterol 96:2900–2904

235. Schlachta CM, Mamazza J, Poulin EC (1999) Laparoscopic sigmoid resection for acute and chronic diverticulitis. An outcomes comparison with laparoscopic resection for nondiverticular disease. Surg Endosc 13:649–653

236. Schrenk P, Woisetschlager R, Wayand WU, Rieger R, Sulzbacher H (1994) Diagnostic laparoscopy: a survey of 92 patients. Am J Surg 168:348–351

237. Schroder T, Sainio V, Kivisaari L, Puolakkainen P, Kivilaakso E, Lempinen M (1991) Pancreatic resection versus peritoneal iavage in acute necrotizing pancreatitis. A prospective randomized trial. Ann Surg 214:663–666

238. Schwandner O, Farke S, Fischer F, Eckmann C, Schiedeck TH, Bruch HP (2004) Laparoscopic colectomy for recurrent and complicated diverticulitis: a prospective study of 396 patients, Langenbecks Arch Surg 389:97–103

239. Scierskl A (2004) Laparoscopic operations of incarcerated inguinal and femoral hernias. Wiad Lek 57:245–248

240. Seelig MH, Seelig SK, Behr C, Schonleben K (2003) Comparison between open and lapardscopic technique in the management of perforated gastroduodenal ulcers. J Clin Gastroenterol 37:226–229

241. Senapati PS, Bhattarcharya D, Harinath G, Ammori BJ (2003) A survey of the timing and approach to the surgical management of cholelithiasis in patients with acute biliary pancreatitis and acute cholecystitis in the UK. Ann R Coll Surg Engl 85:306–312

242. Serralta AS, Bueno JL, Planells MR, Rodero DR (2003) Prospective evaluation of emergency versus delayed laparoscopic cholecystectomy for early cholecystitis. Surg Laparosc Endosc Percutan Tech 13:71–75

243. Shalaby R, Desoky A (2001) Laparoscopic approach to small intestinal obstruction in children: a preliminary experience. Surg Laparosc Endosc Percutan Tech 11:301–305
244. Siu WT, Chau CH, Law BK, Tang CN, Ha PY, Li MK (2004) Routine use of laparoscopic repair for perforated peptic ulcer. Br J Surg 91:481–484
245. Siu WT, Law BK, Tang CN, Chau CH, Li MK (2003) Laparoscopic management of omental torsion secondary to an occult inguinal hernia. J Laparoendosc Adv Surg Tech A 13:199–201
246. Siu WT, Leong HT, Law BKB, Chau CH, Li ACN, Fung KH, Tai YP, Li MKW (2002) Laparoscopic repair for perforated peptic ulcer: a randomized controlled trial. Ann Surg 235:313–319
247. Siu WT, Leong HT, Li MK (1997) Single stitch laparoscopic omental patch repair of perforated peptic ulcer. JR Coll Surg Edinb 42:92–94
248. Smith CH, Novick TL, Jacobs DG, Thomason MH (2000) Laparoscopic repair of a ruptured diaphragm secondary to blunt trauma. Surg Endosc 14:501–502
249. Smith RS, Fry WR, Morabito DJ, Koehler RH, Organ CH Jr (1995) Therapeutic laparoscopy in trauma. Am J Surg 170:632–637
250. Sø JBY, Kum CK, Fernanes ML, Goh P (1996) Comparison between laparoscopic and conventional omental patch repair for perforated duodenal ulcer. Surg Endosc 10:1060–1063
251. Soper DE (1991) Diagnosis and laparoscopic grading of acute salpingitis, Am J Obstet Gynecol 164:1370–1376
252. Sözüer EM, Bedirli A, Ulusal M, Kayhan E, Yilmaz Z (2000) Laparoscopy for diagnosis and treatment of acute abdominal pain. J Laparoendosc Adv Surg Tech A 10:203–207
253. Sreenarasimhaiah J (2003) Diagnosis and management of intestinal ischaemic disorders. Br Med J 326:1372–1376
254. Strickland P, Lourie DJ, Suddleson EA, Blitz JB, Stain SC (1999) Is laparoscopy safe and effective for treatment of acute small-bowel obstruction? Surg Endosc 13:695–698
255. Suc B, Escat J, Cherqui P, Fourtanier G, Hay JM, Fingerhut A, Millat B, French Associations for Surgical Research (1998) Surgery endoscopy as primary treatment in symptomatic patients with suspected common bile duct stones; a multicenter randomized trial. Arch Surg 133:702–708
256. Sugarbaker PH, Sanders JH, Bloom BS, Wilson RE (1975) Preoperative laparoscopy in diagnosis of acute abdominal pain. Lancet 1:442–445
257. Sugiyama M, Tokuhara M, Atomi Y (1998) Is percutaneous cholecystostorpy the optimal treatment for acute cholecystitis in the very elderly. World J Surg 22:459–463
258. Suter M, Meyer A (2001) A 10-year experience with the use of laparoscopic cholecystectomy for acute cholecystitis: is it safe? Surg Endosc 15:1187–1192
259. Suter M, Zermatten P, Halkic N, Martinet O, Bettschart V (2000) Laparoscopic management of mechanical small bowel obstruction: are there predictors of success or failure? Surg Endosc 14:478–483
260. Sutton CJG, Pooley AS, Ewen SP, Haines P (1997) Follow-up report on a randomized controlled trial of laser laparoscopy in the treatment of pelvic pain associated with minimal to moderate endometriosis. Fertil Steril 68:1070–1074
261. Suzuki K, Umehara Y, Kimura T (2003) Elective laparoscopy for small bowel obstruction. Surg Laparosc Endosc Percutan Tech 13:254–256
262. Swank DJ, Swank-Bordewijk SC, Hop WC, van Erp WF, Janssen IM, Bonjer HJ, Jeekel J (2003) Laparoscopic adhesiolysis in patients with chronic abdominal pain: a blinded randomised controlled multi-centre trial, Lancet 361:1247–1251
263. Targarona EM, Balague C, Espert JJ, Perez Ayuso RM, Ros E, Navarro S, Bordas J, Teres J, Trias M (1995) Laparoscopic treatment of acute biliary pancreatitis, Int Surg 80:365–368
264. Taylor EW, Kennedy CA, Dunham RH, Bloch JH (1995) Diagnostic laparoscopy in women with acute abdominal pain. Surg Laparosc Endosc 5:125–128
265. Teague WJ, Ackroyd R, Watson DI, Devitt PG (2000) Changing patterns in the management of gastric volvulus over 14 years. Br J Surg 87:353–361

266. Teh SH, O'Ceallaigh S, McKeon JG, O'Donohoe MK, Tanner WA, Keane FB (2000) Should an appendix that look "normal" be removed at diagnostic laparoscopy for acute right iliac fossa pain? Eur J Surg 166:388–389

267. Teisala K, Heinonen PK, Punnonen R (1990) Laparoscopic diagnosis and treatment of acute pyosalpinx. J Reprod Med 35:19–21

268. Teixeira JP, Saraiva AC, Cabral AC, Barros H, Reis JR, Teixeira A (2000) Conversion factors in laparoscopic cholecystectomy for acute cholecystitis. Hepatogastroenterology 47:626–630

269. Trias M, Targarona EM, Ros E, Bordas JM, Perez Ayuso RM, Balague C, Pros I, Teres J (1997) Prospective evaluation of a minimally invasive approach for treatment of bile-duct calculi in the high-risk patient. Surg Endosc 11:632–635

270. Trowbridge RL, Rutkowski NK, Shojania KG (2003) Does this patient have acute cholecystitis? J Am Med Assoc 289:80–86

271. Tschudi J, Wagner M, Klaiber C (1993) Laparoskopische Operation einer incarcerierten Obturatoriushernie mit assistierter Darmresektion. Chirurg 64:827–828

272. Tsumura H, Ichikawa T, Hiyama E, Murakami Y (2004) Laparoscopic and open approach in perforated peptic ulcer. Hepatogastroenterology 51:1536–1539

273. Uchiyama K, Onishi H, Tani M, Kinoshita H, Ueno M, Yamaue H (2004) Timing of laparoscopic cholecystectomy for acute cholecystitis with cholecystolithiasis. Hepatogastroenterology 51:346–348

274. Uhl W, Müller CA, Krähenbühl L, Schmid SW, Scholzel S, Büchler MW (1999) Acute gallstone pancreatitis: timing of laparoscopic cholecystectomy in mild and severe disease. Surg Endosc 13:1070–1076

275. UK Working Party on Acute Pancreatitis (2005) UK guidelines for the management of acute pancreatitis. Gut 54:iii1–iii9

276. Urbach DR, Khajanch YS, Jobe BA, Standage BA, Hansen PD, Swanstrom LL (2001) Cost-effective management of common bile duct stones: a decision analysis of the use of endoscopic retrograde cholangiopancreatography (ERCP), intraoperative cholangiography, and laparoscopic bile duct exploration. Surg Endosc 15:4–13

277. van Dalen R, Bagshaw PF, Dobbs BR, Robertson GM, Lynch AC, Frizelle FA (2003) The utility of laparoscopy in the diagnosis of acute appendicitis in women of reproductive age. Surg Endosc 17:1311–1313

278. van den Broek WT, Bijnen AB, de Ruiter P, Gouma DJ (2001) A normal appendix found during diagnostic laparoscopy should not be removed. Br J Surg 88:251–254

279. Vermesh M, Silva PD, Rosen GF, Stein AL, Fossum GT, Sauer MV (1989) Management of ruptured ectopic gestation by linear salpingostomy: a prospective, randomized clinical trial of laparoscopy versus laparotomy. Obstet Gynecol 73:400–404

280. Vetrhus M, Soreide O, Nesvik I, Sondenaa K (2003) Acute cholecystitis: delayed surgery or observation. A randomized clinical trial. Scand J Gastroenterol 38:985–990

281. Villavicencio RT, Aucar JA (1999) Analysis of laparoscopy in trauma. J Am Coll Surg 189:11–20

282. Waclawiczek HW, Schneeberger V, Bekk A, Dinnewitzer A, Sungler P, Boeckl O (1997) Der Stellenwert der diagnostischen Laparoskopie und minimal-invasiver Verfahren beim akuten Abdomen. Zentralbl Chir 122:1108–1112

283. Watson SD, Saye W, Hollier PA (1993) Combined laparoscopic incarcerated herniorrhaphy and small bowel resection. Surg Laparosc Endosc 3:106–108

284. Williams SB, Greenspon J, Young HA, Orkin BA (2005) Small bowel obstruction: conservative vs surgical management Dis Colon Rectum 48:1140–1146

285. Willsher PC, Sanabria JR, Gallinger S, Rossi L, Strasberg S, Litwin DE (1999) Early laparoscopic cholecystectomy for acute cholecystitis: a safe procedure. J Gastrointest Surg 3:50–53

286. Wilson RG, Macintyre IM, Nixon SJ, Saunders JH, Varma JS, King PM (1992) Laparoscopic cholecystectomy as a safe and effective treatment for severe acute cholecystitis. Br Med J 305:394–396

287. Wolfman WL, Kreutner K (1984) Laparoscopy in children and adolescents. J Adolesc Health Care 5:261–265
288. Wong SK, Yu SC, Lam YH, Chung SS (1999) Percutaneous cholecystostomy and endoscopic cholecystolithotripsy in the management of acute cholecystitis. Surg Endosc 13:48–52
289. Wullstein C, Gross E (2003) Laparoscopic compared with conventional treatment of acute adhesive small bowel obstruction, Br J Surg 90:1147–1151
290. Yau KK, Siu WT, Chau CH, Yang PC, Li MK (2005) Laparoscopic management of incarcerated obturator hernia, Can J Surg 48:76–77
291. Yuen PM, Yu KM, Yip SK, Lau WC, Rogers MS, Chang A (1997) A randomized prospective study of laparoscopy and laparotomy in the management of benign ovarian masses. Am J Obstet Gynecol 177:109–114
292. Zamir G, Reissman P (1998) Diagnostic laparoscopy in mesenteric ischemia. Surg Endosc 12:390–396
293. Zantut LF, Ivatury RR, Smith RS, Kawahara NT, Porter JM, Fry WR, Poggetti R, Birolini D, Organ CH Jr (1997) Diagnostic and therapeutic laparoscopy for penetrating abdominal trauma: a multicenter experience. J Trauma 42:825–831
294. Zeitoun G, Laurent A, Rouffet F, Hay J, Fingerhut A, Paquet J, Peillon C; Association de Recherche en Chirurgie (2000) Multicentre, randomized clinical trial of primary versus secondary moid resection in generalized peritonitis complicating sigmoid diverticulitis. Br J Surg 87:1366–1374
295. Z'Graggen K, Metzger A, Birrer S, Klaiber C (1995) Die laparoskopische Cholecystektomie als Standardtherapie bei der akuten Cholecystitis. Eine prospektive Studie. Chirurg 66:366–370
296. Zhang J, Duan ZQ, Song QB, Luo YW, Xin SJ, Zhang Q (2004) Acute mesenteric venous thrombosis: a better outcome achieved through improved imaging techniques and a changed policy of clinical management. Eur J Vasc Endovasc Surg 28:329–334
297. Zhu JF, Fan Zhang XH (2001) Laparoscopic treatment of severe acute pancreatitis. Surg Endosc 15:146–148
298. Zittel TT, Jehle EC, Becker HD (2000) Surgical management of peptic ulcer disease today – indication, technique and outcome. Langenbecks Arch Surg 385:84–96

Perforated Peptic Ulcer – Update 2006

Dejan Ignjatovic, Roberto Bergamaschi

Definition

Perforated peptic ulcer is a relatively uncommon condition characterized by local or general peritonitis due to perforation of a gastric, duodenal, jejunal or ileal ulcer.

Epidemiology and Clinical Course

Perforated peptic ulcer accounts for about 5% of all abdominal emergencies. After simple surgical closure and *Helicobacter pylori* eradication, ulcer relapse and reperforation rates are 6.1 and 4.1%, respectively [5]. All three reperforations were in gastric locations. Crude rates for duodenal ulcer recurrence were 2.6% at 2 years and for duodenal ulcer reperforation rates were nil at 2 years. These results imply that laparoscopic suture repair and *H. pylori* eradication is safe in duodenal ulcers, however with recurrence in gastric ulcers [5].

Operative Versus Conservative Treatment

No new data are available. Surgery is indicated.

Choice of Surgical Approach and Procedure

A recent Cochrane systematic review suggests that a decrease in septic abdominal complications may occur when laparoscopic surgery is performed to repair a perforated peptic ulcer [6]. However, it is necessary to develop more randomized-controlled trials that include a greater number of patients to confirm such an assumption. Such trials should exclude the surgical learning curve in order to be valid. With the evidence at hand, the results of laparoscopic surgery are not clinically different from those of open surgery [3]. Other studies provide data on significantly shorter hospital stay and shorter operating time in the case of laparoscopic access [1]. In summary, we still believe that laparoscopic surgery is advantageous in the hands of an experienced surgeon.

Technical Aspects of Surgery

Omental patch–repair, patch–repair with fibrin sealing and simple suture are reported without enough comparative evidence on which repair technique is superior. Conversion to an upper midline incision may be necessary in 10–20% of operations, usually for multiple, large, or rear-side perforations and for advanced peritonitis. Conversion does not seem to worsen the clinical outcome [1, 2]. It seems that the size of the perforation is a significant risk factor influencing the conversion and complication rates [2].

Peri- and Postoperative Care

Laparoscopic surgery seems to have the benefit of shorter duration of postoperative nasogastric aspiration and time to resume oral intake, fewer postoperative analgesic requirements, and lower overall complications rate [2]. There was no statistically significant difference in mortality rate between open and laparoscopic access. Patients who developed suture leakage had acute symptoms for more than 9 h preoperatively [4]. Conversions seemed to occur with surgeons whose previous experience involved 1.8±2.3 cases compared with 3.9±2.9 cases in successful laparoscopic repair [4].

References

1. Kirshtein B, Bayme M, Mayer T, Lantsberg L, Avinoach E, Mizrahi S (2005) Laparoscopic treatment of gastroduodenal perforations: comparison with conventional surgery. Surg Endosc 19:1487–1490
2. Lunevicius R, Morkevicius M (2005) Comparison of laparoscopic versus open repair for perforated duodenal ulcers. Surg Endosc 19:1565–1571
3. Lunevicius R, Morkevicius M (2005) Systematic review comparing laparoscopic and open repair for perforated peptic ulcer. Br J Surg 92:1195–1207
4. Lunevicius R, Morkevicius M (2005) Risk factors influencing the early outcome results after laparoscopic repair of perforated duodenal ulcer and their predictive value. Langenbecks Arch Surg 390:413–420
5. Rodriguez-Sanjuan JC, Fernandez-Santiago R, Garcia RA, Trugeda S, Seco I, la de Torre F, Naranjo A, Gomez-Fleitas M (2005) Perforated peptic ulcer treated by simple closure and Helicobacter pylori eradication. World J Surg 29:849–852
6. Sanabria AE, Morales CH, Villegas MI (2005) Laparoscopic repair for perforated peptic ulcer disease. Cochrane Database Syst Rev CD004778

Acute Cholecystitis – Update 2006

Giuseppe Borzellino, Ivan Tomasi, Claudio Cordiano

This update is based on a systematic literature search in Medline. The search strategy is available from the authors on request.

Definition

Acute cholecystitis is defined as an acute inflammation of the gallbladder wall. Gallstone cholecystitis is differentiated from alithiasic cholecystitis on the basis of its aetiology, when bile outflow is obstructed by gallstones or biliary sludge.

Epidemiology and Clinical Course

Epidemiology

Epidemiological data are reported in a recent review [13] and are therefore based on previous studies. Gallstone cholecystitis is the most common form since it is reported in 90% of cases of acute cholecystitis [7], women up to 50 years old are 3 times more likely to develop an acute gallstone cholecystitis than men [7] and 10–30% of patients with acute cholecystitis develop severe complications such as gangrene, empyema or perforation [3, 8, 18]. A more recent retrospective study [10] confirmed results of previous retrospective or prospective studies [3, 6, 12] for which severe acute cholecystitis was observed more frequently in male and old patients, with reported odds ratios of 1.76 ($P=0.029$) for the former and 2.24 ($P=0.004$) for the latter. A Canadian study [17] reported an 18% reduction in the rate of acute cholecystitis after the introduction of laparoscopic cholecystectomy in 1991. The average annual rate of acute cholecystitis per 100,000 population was reported to be 109 (95% confidence interval 107–110) in the period 1988–1991 and 88 (87–89) in the period 1992–2000. The interpretation of the authors is that this highly significant reduction may be explained by an increase of 35% of elective cholecystectomies after the introduction of laparoscopy. However, the postlaparoscopic period is about 3 times longer than the prelaparoscopic one and since a greater number of elective cholecystectomies were performed in the early laparoscopic period, a division of the latter into another two 4-year periods for final comparison would have given a more precise measure of the effects registered.

Clinical Course

The clinical course of acute cholecystitis may be explained by its pathogenesis. There have been no new data since those reported in the review by Indar and Beckingham [7]. Increase in the intraluminal pressure and distension of the gallbladder wall due to bile obstruction outflow stimulates synthesis of prostaglandins, the mediators of the inflammatory response. Intraluminal pressure may rise up to a value above the arterial perfusion pressure of the gallbladder wall, with ischemia, necrosis and possible perforation as a result. The percentage of patients which develop such complications and therefore need urgent surgical intervention is reported to be 20% [7]. Another possible evolution of the cholecystitis is secondary bacterial infection, with enteric bacteria observed in about 20% of cases, with possible empyema formation as a result [7].

Diagnostics

There are no new data available on the diagnosis of cholecystitis other than those in one retrospective study [2] published with the aim to predict bile infection. However, no clinical, biological nor radiological parameters alone or in combination reached statistical significance, neither by univariate analysis nor by multivariate logistic regression.

Operative Versus Conservative Treatment

No new data have been found, neither for observation versus cholecystectomy after conservative treatment nor for medical treatment versus cholecystostomy in critically ill patients. Sooner or later, a surgical intervention is indicated in patients with acute cholecystitis.

Choice of Surgical Approach and Procedure

Open Versus Laparoscopic Cholecystectomy

Two meta-analyses on timing, one randomized controlled trial (RCT) and two retrospective studies on cholecystostomy and one prospective study on the effect of conversion in gangrenous cholecystitis have recently been published, but no new data have been found on laparoscopic versus open cholecystectomy.

Early Versus Delayed Cholecystectomy

One of the meta-analyses [9] published is not a high-quality study since at least six of the criteria of the QUORUM checklist [5] for quality assessment of meta-analysis of RCT were not fulfilled. Some are of minor importance, but a selection bias by including a nonrandomized study and not other RCTs published at the time of the research and a lack of quality assessment of the studies included make the results uncertain and conclusions have to be drawn with caution. The other meta-analysis [14] was conducted following the criteria of the QUORUM checklist [5], but either laparoscopic or open cholecystectomies were analysed, including study from 1970 to 2003, a period of time during which peri- and postoperative care have changed. Only absolute risk by calculation of the risk difference was reported and data on laparoscopy may be extracted from a table but little information is available.

Cholecystostomy

A randomized clinical trial [1] compared two treatment regimens: cholecystostomy followed by early laparoscopic cholecystectomy (PCLC group) versus medical treatment followed by delayed laparoscopic cholecystectomy (DLC group) in high-risk patients. This was a medium-quality study, since six patients were excluded from the analysis in the PCLC group, thus violating the intention-to-treat principle. Patients were excluded because they failed to reach an APACHE II score of less than 12 within 120 h, which was required for surgery. Three patients were excluded from the DLC group, one patient died from multiple organ failure and the other two refused surgery. Definition of the risk is mainly based on the APACHE II score and therefore it is determined either by the comorbidity conditions or by the severity of the cholecystitis; however, associated diseases with an ASA score greater than 3 were reported in the majority of patients in both groups. Symptom relief time was significantly shorter in the PCLC group, being achieved within 24 h in all included patients compared with the 48–72 h in the DLC group ($P = 0.001$). Two patients in the DLC group experienced mild pancreatitis during the waiting period and this was taken into account in the mean hospital stay. The results of the laparoscopic cholecystectomies do not show differences in conversion rate (6.5% in the PCLC group versus 13.4% in the DLC group with P=0.42) and in postoperative hospital stay (1.58, standard deviation 0.72 in the PCLC group versus 1.66, standard deviation 0.72, in the DLC group, with $P = 1$). Two results favoured the PCLC group: total hospital stay, with 5.3 days versus 15.2 days ($P = 0.001$), and total cost, with US $ 2,612 versus 3735 ($P = 0.001$). Two retrospective uncontrolled studies were found on gallbladder aspiration [15] and the use of cholecystostomy [16] in high-risk patients, but no critical evaluation of these approaches was reported.

Conversion for Gangrenous Cholecystitis

In a prospective study on gangrenous cholecystitis [4], early conversion after initial visualization of the gallbladder, intermediate conversion after an initial attempt at dissection or late conversion after a protracted attempt at dissection do not influence significantly morbidity nor hospital stay, but just operative time from 1.8 to 2.1 and 2.7 h, respectively ($P < 0.01$).

Technical Aspects of Surgery

No new data are available other than those from a prospective study that reports aspiration of distended gallbladder with a Veress needle, but no critical evaluation of this technique was performed [11].

Peri- and Postoperative Care

No new data are available.

References

1. Akyürek N, Salman B, Yüksel O, Tezcaner T, Irkörücü O, Yücel C, Oktar S, Tatlicioglu E (2005) Management of acute calculous cholecystitis in high-risk patients: percutaneous cholecystotomy followed by early laparoscopic cholecystectomy. Surg Laparosc Endosc Percutan Tech 15(6):315–320
2. Beardsley SL, Shlansky-Goldberg RD, Patel A, Freiman DB, Soulen MC, Stavropoulos SW, Clark TW (2005) Predicting infected bile among patients undergoing percutaneous cholecystostomy. Cardiovasc Intervent Radiol 28(3):319–325
3. Bedirli A, Sakrak O, Sozuer EM, Kerek M, Guler I (2001) Factors effecting the complications in the natural history of acute cholecystitis. Hepatogastroenterology 48(41):1275–1278
4. Bingener J, Stefanidis D, Richards ML, Schwesinger WH, Sirinek KR (2005) Early conversion for gangrenous cholecystitis: impact on outcome. Surg Endosc 19(8):1139–1141
5. Clarke M (2000) The QUORUM statement. Lancet 355(9205):756–757
6. Eldar S, Sabo E, Nash E, Abrahamson J, Matter I (1997) Laparoscopic cholecystectomy for acute cholecystitis: prospective trial. World J Surg 21:540–545
7. Indar AA, Beckingham IJ (2002) Acute cholecystitis. BMJ 325:639–643
8. Kiviluoto T, Siren J, Luukkonen P, Kivilaakso E (1998) Randomised trial of laparoscopic versus open cholecystectomy for acute and gangrenous cholecystitis. Lancet 351(9099):321–325
9. Lau H, Lo CY, Patil NG, Yuen WK (2005) Early versus delayed-interval laparoscopic cholecystectomy for acute cholecystitis: a metaanalysis. Surg Endosc (in press). Epub 2005 Oct 24
10. Lee HK, Han HS, Min SK, Lee JH (2005) Sex-based analysis of the outcome of laparoscopic cholecystectomy for acute cholecystitis. Br J Surg 92(4):463–466
11. Lee KT, Shan YS, Wang ST, Lin PW (2005) Verres needle decompression of distended gallbladder to facilitate laparoscopic cholecystectomy in acute cholecystitis: a prospective study. Hepatogastroenterology 52(65):1388–1392
12. Merriam LT, Kanaan SA, Dawes LG, Angelos P, Prystowsky JB, Rege RV, Joehl RJ (1999) Gangrenous cholecystitis: analysis of risk factors and experience with laparoscopic cholecystectomy. Surgery 126:680–685

13. Shamiyeh A, Wayand W (2005) Current status of laparoscopic therapy of cholecysto-lithiasis and common bile duct stones. Dig Dis 23(2):119–126
14. Shikata S, Noguchi Y, Fukui T (2005) Early versus delayed cholecystectomy for acute cholecystitis: a meta-analysis of randomized controlled trials. Surg Today 35(7):553–560
15. Tazawa J, Sanada K, Sakai Y, Yamane M, Kusano F, Nagayama K, Ito K, Takiguchi N, Hiranuma S, Maeda M (2005) Gallbladder aspiration for acute cholecystitis in average-surgical-risk patients. Int J Clin Pract 59(1):21–24
16. Teoh WM, Cade RJ, Banting SW, Mackay S, Hassen AS (2005) Percutaneous cholecys-tostomy in the management of acute cholecystitis. ANZ J Surg 75(6):396–398
17. Urbach DR, Stukel TA (2005) Rate of elective cholecystectomy and the incidence of se-vere gallstone disease. CMAJ 172(8):1015–1019
18. Wilson RG, Macintyre IM, Nixon SJ, Saunders JH, Varma JS, King PM (1992) Laparo-scopic cholecystectomy as a safe and effective treatment for severe acute cholecystitis. BMJ 305(6850):394–396

Acute Pancreatitis – Update 2006

James Arbuckle, Alberto Isla

Definition, Epidemiology and Clinical Course

Acute pancreatitis is a common diagnosis requiring admission onto the surgical ward. Eighty percent of patients have mild acute pancreatitis, and will recover within a few days. Twenty percent have severe acute pancreatitis, and will require intensive management. This chapter aims to outline some fundamental principles of the disease, and to consider the specific management of mild gallstone pancreatitis.

Classification

The Atlanta classification is widely accepted as the standard system for describing acute pancreatitis [3]. A summary of terms and definitions from the Atlanta classification follows.

Acute pancreatitis is defined as an acute inflammatory process of the pancreas with variable involvement of other regional tissues or remote organ systems.

Severe acute pancreatitis is associated with organ failure and/or local complications, such as necrosis, abscess or pseudocyst. Scoring systems to characterise severe acute pancreatitis are discussed in the next section. The deterioration in physiological parameters is a reflection of the development of pancreatic necrosis.

Mild acute pancreatitis is associated with minimal organ dysfunction and an uneventful recovery. Approximately 75% of cases fall within this group.

Acute fluid collections occur early in the course of acute pancreatitis and are located in or near the pancreas. They always lack a wall of granulation or fibrous tissue. They occur in 30–50% of cases of severe pancreatitis, and more than half spontaneously regress.

Pancreatic necrosis is a diffuse or focal area of non-viable pancreatic parenchyma. Dynamic contrast-enhanced CT demonstrates a contrast density of less than 50 Hounsfield units in areas of necrosis (normal enhancement 50–150 Hounsfield units). The clinical distinction between sterile and infected necrosis is critical, the former being treated conservatively, and the latter surgically.

A *pseudocyst* is a collection of pancreatic juice enclosed by a wall of fibrous or granulation tissue arising as a result of acute or chronic pancreatitis, pancreatic trauma or surgery. The formation of a pseudocyst requires at least 4 weeks from the onset of acute pancreatitis.

Scoring Systems

The purpose of the various scoring systems available to the clinician is to identify the 20% of patients who present with acute pancreatitis with severe disease. No system has 100% sensitivity or specificity, but the prompt stratification of a patient on admission to a particular grade of severity is an essential step in the initial management of acute pancreatitis. Several scoring systems have been proposed to assess the severity of pancreatitis. Ranson, Glasgow and APACHE II all use physiological parameters to score the level of severity of the episode of pancreatitis.

In the classic paper of Ranson et al. [13] from 1976, 300 consecutive patients admitted with acute pancreatitis were assessed. Eleven factors (Table 20.1) were identified to be associated with increased morbidity and mortality in the first 100 patients. The 11 factors were then prospectively applied to the next 200 patients. The mortality rate in the first group of 100 patients was 15%. When the second group of 200 patients were assessed using the 11 factors identified in the first group, and treated according to the predicted severity of the episode of pancreatitis, the mortality rate was 3.5%. In the latter group of 200 patients, 38 patients had three or more positive factors, and 24 became seriously ill or died. Of the remaining 162 patients with fewer than three factors, only one patient died.

Imrie modified Ranson's criteria in 1978, and these factors were reviewed in 1984 in a series of 347 patients [2]. It was found that of the nine factors originally described by Imrie, omission of the aminotransferase values (to give an eight-factor score) increased the predictive value from 72 to 79% in attempting to classify mild or severe pancreatitis. This is the most widely used scoring system in daily UK clinical practice (Table 20.1).

Further scoring of severity by APACHE II (acute physiology and chronic health evaluation) to predict the severity of acute pancreatitis has been described [18]. The principal difference between the APACHE II and Ranson/Glasgow scoring systems is that physiological parameters (temperature, mean arterial pressure, heart rate, respiratory rate, Glasgow coma score) are combined with laboratory blood values in APACHE II. APACHE II scored as well as the established systems for gallstone pancreatitis, but less well for alcoholic pancreatitis.

A scoring system based on CT appearances (Table 20.2) has been developed by Balthazar et al. [1], taking into account the degree of inflammation

Table 20.1. Scoring systems for acute pancreatitis

Ranson		Glasgow
At admission	During initial 48 h	
Age above 55 years	Haematocrit value decrease over 10%	Age above 55 years
White blood count above 16×10^9/l	Blood urea nitrogen level rise over 5 mg%	White blood count above 15×10^9/l
Blood glucose levelabove 200 mg%	Serum calcium level below 8 mg%	Blood glucose above 10 mmol/l (no diabetic history)
Serum lactate dehydrogenase over 350 international units per litre	Arterial oxygen tensionbelow 60 mmHg	Serum urea above 16 mmol/l (no response to intravenous fluids)
Serum glutamic oxalacetic transaminase level over 250 Sigma Frankel units percent	Base deficit over 4 mEq/l	PaO$_2$ below 60 mmHg
	Estimated fluid sequestration over 6 l	Serum calcium below 2 mmol/l
		Serum albumin below 32 g/l
		Lactate dehydrogenase above 600 µl/l

PaO$_2$ partial pressure of oxygen in arterial blood

Table 20.2. Balthazar grading system based on CT appearances

Grade	Findings
A	Normal
B	Gland enlargement, small intrapancreatic fluid collection
C	Any of above, peripancreatic inflammation, less than 30% pancreatic necrosis
D	Any of above, single extrapancreatic fluid collection, 30–50% pancreatic necrosis
E	Any of above, extensive extrapancreatic fluid collection, pancreatic abscess, more than 50% pancreatic necrosis

of the pancreas, the presence of fluid collections, and the percentage of pancreatic necrosis. The severity of these changes has been shown to correlate with prognosis.

General Principles of Management of Acute Pancreatitis

Resuscitation of the patient with acute pancreatitis is the priority in the first 24 h of admission [11, 19]. Patients with fewer than two positive criteria may be carefully observed on a standard ward, but those with three or more should be managed in a high-dependency or intensive care unit.

Early, aggressive fluid resuscitation should be instituted because of the potential for sequestration of large volumes of fluid, specifically within the retroperitoneum. Intravenous cannulae to allow rapid infusion of fluids should be combined with a urinary catheter, together with central venous pressure monitoring and arterial pressure monitoring in severe cases. It may be necessary to infuse 5–10 l of fluid within the first 24 h in a case of severe acute pancreatitis. Meticulous observation of the patient to detect early signs of cardiac, respiratory or renal failure should be performed, with prompt treatment at the first sign of compromise.

Much has been written about feeding in severe acute pancreatitis. The principle of keeping patients nil by mouth to rest the pancreas has been discarded. There have also been several trials of parenteral versus enteral feeding. An international consensus conference in April 2004 [11] recommended that enteral nutrition should be used in preference to parenteral nutrition in severe acute pancreatitis. Nasojejunal feeding is preferable to nasogastric feeding, and it should be started after initial resuscitation. Parenteral nutrition can be used if enteral nutrition trials fail after 5 days, and the parenteral nutrition should be supplemented with glutamine to help maintain the gut mucosal barrier and prevent bacterial translocation. The importance of strict glycaemic control is emphasised. The most recent UK guidelines [17] are similar to the American recommendations and suggest use of the enteral route via a nasogastric tube.

The role of prophylactic antibiotics in severe acute pancreatitis remains a difficult subject. Many studies are underpowered, and use different regimes for varying durations. In light of these problems there is no consensus. The UK guidelines [17] do not recommend routine prophylaxis, but if it is used it should be given for a maximum of 14 days. The American group specifically recommend against the use of prophylactic antibiotics [11]. Both groups highlight the need for a high index of suspicion of fungal infection.

Acute Biliary Pancreatitis – Latest UK Guidelines (2005)

The most recent British guidelines for the management of acute pancreatitis were published in 2005 [17]. They recommend that urgent endoscopic retrograde cholangiopancreatography (ERCP) should be performed (ideally within the first 72 h of the onset of pain) in patients with severe pancreatitis of suspected or proven gallstone aetiology. Urgent ERCP should also be performed in cases associated with cholangitis, jaundice or a dilated common bile duct. They recommend that endoscopic sphincterotomy is performed in all cases, even if gallstones are not present in the common bile duct.

After an episode of gallstone pancreatitis, definitive treatment should be performed, usually laparoscopic cholecystectomy. In those patients who are unfit for surgery, endoscopic sphincterotomy is thought to be sufficient. However, a randomised trial by Targarona et al. [15] has shown that in elderly or high-risk patients surgical treatment was no more hazardous than endoscopic sphincterotomy in terms of morbidity and mortality, and was superior in terms of late complications of biliary origin. Ideally, cholecystectomy with intraoperative cholangiography should be performed on the same admission, after recovery from the acute inflammatory complications of pancreatitis. If the surgery is not performed at this time, it should be booked within 2 weeks of discharge, although this exposes the patient to the administrative risks associated with cancellation of surgery, and therefore a second, potentially fatal attack of acute pancreatitis.

Acute Biliary Pancreatitis – ERCP

One of the central questions in the management of acute biliary pancreatitis is the role of preoperative ERCP and sphincterotomy. If the surgical expertise exists to perform laparoscopic common bile duct exploration and clearance at the same time as laparoscopic cholecystectomy, is preoperative ERCP and sphincterotomy necessary?

There have been three published trials examining the role of preoperative ERCP. Neoptolemos et al. [12] published a trial in the Lancet in 1999 of 121 patients with acute pancreatitis thought due to gallstones. Fifty-nine had an ERCP within 72 h of admission, 62 did not. There was no difference in overall mortality between the groups, but the overall complication rate was 12% in the group who had ERCP within 72 h, and 24% in those who did not have ERCP. The major complications in the non-ERCP group were more frequent pseudocyst formation, and organ failure (respiratory, cardiac, renal – in decreasing order of frequency). They also observed that when the episode of acute pancreatitis was mild, the complication rate was similar in both groups; however, in severe pancreatitis, the difference in complications between the ERCP and non-ERCP groups was highly significant, being much higher in the non-ERCP group.

The study of Fan et al. [6] from Hong Kong involved random assignment of 195 patients with acute pancreatitis to ERCP within 24 h (97 patients), or conservative management (98 patients). No symptoms of biliary sepsis developed in the ERCP group, but 12 patients in the non-ERCP group developed biliary sepsis. Interestingly, there was no significant difference in complication rates between the two groups, in contrast to the case for the study of Neoptolemos et al.

The third trial, by Fölsch et al. [7], was multicentre, and randomised 126 patients to ERCP within 72 h of symptom onset, and 112 to conservative management. Patients with obvious biliary obstruction were excluded (more than 5mg/dl bilirubin). They found that there was no significant difference in mortality or complication rate between the two groups.

Therefore, although ERCP appears to be appropriate if biliary obstruction or sepsis is present, the role is not so clear if these conditions are absent.

Single-Stage and Two-Stage Management: the Debate

The traditional view of two-stage management of acute biliary pancreatitis (preoperative ERCP followed by laparoscopic cholecystectomy) has been challenged by single-stage management (laparoscopic cholecystectomy with intraoperative cholangiogram, and laparoscopic exploration of the common bile duct if the cholangiogram shows filling defects suggestive of stones). A European multicentre trial has shown equivalent success rates, but much shorter hospital stays with the single-stage treatment [4].

The rationale behind this change in management is based on observations that most gallstones spontaneously pass through the common bile duct within 7 days of the onset of pancreatitis.

Uhl et al. [16] noted that, in patients diagnosed with acute biliary pancreatitis, when ERCP was performed within a median time of 14 h from admission to hospital, 74% of patients had stones in the common bile duct. The study of Fan et al. [6] showed that the incidence of common bile duct stones in those undergoing emergency ERCP for acute biliary pancreatitis within 24 h of admission was 38%. The study of Fölsch et al. [7] shows that this figure drops to 46% if ERCP is performed within 72 h of symptom onset.

The study of Neoptolemos et al. [12] was based on ERCP performed within 72 h of admission, rather than symptom onset, and shows common bile duct stones to be present in 25% of those patients with mild pancreatitis and 63% of those with severe pancreatitis. In the other arm of the study which had ERCP between 6 and 30 days, common bile duct stones were detected in 21% of cases. The incidence of common bile duct stones has been shown to be between 5 and 10% at 10 week after admission [14].

In a study performed in our unit [8], 45 patients with mild acute biliary pancreatitis underwent management with the single-stage approach. Thirty-nine patients required laparoscopic cholecystectomy only. The remaining six patients underwent laparoscopic common bile duct exploration in addition to laparoscopic cholecystectomy. In one of the six patients, the intraoperative cholangiogram revealed a false positive result (probable air bubbles in the common bile duct) and the common bile duct exploration was therefore negative (transcystic approach). In the remaining five of the six patients, the common bile duct was explored through a choledochotomy in four patients, and transcystically in one. All cases were completed laparoscopically, and there were two complications (umbilical port bleed-discharged on the second postoperative day, and T-tube dislodgement requiring a second operation for replacement). As a result of problems associated with T-tubes, they are not routinely used in our practice (our current approach is described later in this chapter). No cases of recurrent pancreatitis occurred in the median follow-up period of 25 months (interquartile range 14–42 months).

If only one patient in ten has common bile duct stones 1 week after admission with acute biliary pancreatitis, then ERCP performed within 24–72 h is not necessary in nine cases. ERCP and endoscopic sphincterotomy is not without risk (morbidity includes 1% pancreatitis, 0.8% ascending cholangitis, 0.4% bleeding requiring transfusion, and 0.2% mortality [5]).

Therefore we feel that, apart from the absolute indications for ERCP in acute pancreatitis (obstructive jaundice and cholangitis), patients with mild acute biliary pancreatitis should not undergo routine ERCP. Rather, they should have the single-stage approach with laparoscopic cholecystectomy, intraoperative cholangiogram and laparoscopic common bile duct exploration, dependent on the results of the cholangiogram. Only in patients who are unfit for surgery should ERCP with endoscopic sphincterotomy be routinely performed. The rationale for this approach is that 90% of common bile duct stones spontaneously pass within approximately 7 days [15].

It is accepted that laparoscopic common bile duct exploration may not be successful in all patients, and therefore postoperative ERCP may be necessary in a limited number of cases.

Single-Stage Management: Technique for Laparoscopic Cholecystectomy, Intraoperative Cholangiogram and Common Bile Duct Exploration.

In view of the evidence presented here, we feel that the single-stage approach should be the standard treatment for patients who present with mild acute biliary pancreatitis.

Intraoperative cholangiography is performed through a catheter advanced via the cystic duct into the common bile duct. Common bile duct exploration may be performed transcystically or through a choledochotomy. Laparoscopic choledochotomy is indicated if the common bile duct is dilated to 8 mm or more, if calculi are 1 cm or more, or are multiple, impacted or intrahepatic. Laparoscopic choledochotomy has been associated with higher morbidity rates, mainly related to T-tube insertion [10].

If the intraoperative cholangiogram is suggestive of stones within the common bile duct, a 10-mm longitudinal choledochotomy is performed. The choledochotomy is performed at the level of the cystic duct and common bile duct junction, away from the upper border of the duodenum. As previously described [9], after stone extraction, a 10 French biliary stent is placed into the common bile duct with the distal end protruding into the duodenum, and the proximal end distal to the lower edge of the choledochotomy. We have found this technique to have fewer complications than traditional T-

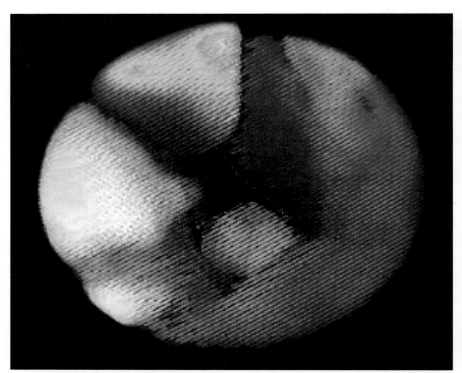

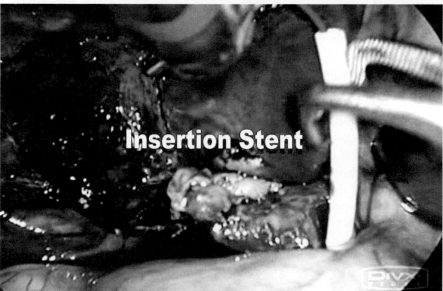

Fig. 20.1. View of stone in common bile duct being retrieved with Dormia basket, and insertion of stent

tube insertion, and it is probably safer than primary closure. The common bile duct is closed with interrupted 4/0 absorbable sutures (Vicryl), and a drain is placed in the gallbladder fossa. The stent may be removed 4 weeks later at upper gastrointestinal endoscopy.

The technique outlined previously and illustrated in Fig. 20.1 is appropriate for most cases of mild pancreatitis. It is not intended to be performed in cases of severe acute pancreatitis with signs of biliary sepsis or obstruction, where an urgent ERCP is clearly indicated.

Summary

Acute pancreatitis is a common surgical problem, with approximately 50% of cases attributable to gallstones. The definitive management involves eradication of the gallstones from the gallbladder and bile duct. Laparoscopic cholecystectomy should be performed as soon as the general condition of the patient allows. Because most common bile duct stones have passed within 10 week of the episode of mild acute biliary pancreatitis, if expertise is available, we recommend the single-stage approach with laparoscopic cholecystectomy, and intraoperative cholangiogram, proceeding to laparoscopic common bile duct exploration if necessary. If the expertise is not available, we recommend non-invasive imaging of the common bile duct before preoperative ERCP, MRI cholangiogram or endoscopic ultrasound.

References

1. Balthazar EJ, Robinson DL, Megibow AJ, Ranson JH (1990) Acute pancreatitis: value of CT in establishing prognosis. Radiology 174:331–336
2. Blamey SL, Imrie CW, O'Neill J, Gilmour WH, Carter DC (1984) Prognostic factors in acute pancreatitis. Gut 25:1340–1346
3. Bradley EL 3rd (1993) A clinically based classification system for acute pancreatitis. Arch Surg 128:586–590
4. Cuschieri A, Lezoche E, Morino M, Croce E, Lacy A, Toouli J, Faggioni A, Ribeiro VM, Jakimowicz J, Visa J, Hanna GB (1999) E.A.E.S. multicenter prospective randomized trial comparing two-stage vs single-stage management of patients with gallstone disease and ductal calculi. Surg Endosc 13:952–957
5. Deans GT, Sedman P, Martin DF, Royston CMS, Leow CK, Thomas WEG, Brough WA (1997) Are complications of endoscopic sphincterotomy age related? Gut 41:545–548
6. Fan ST, Lai ECS, Mok FPT, Lo CML, Zheng SS, Wong J (1993) Early treatment of acute biliary pancreatitis by endoscopic papillotomy. N Engl J Med 328:228–232
7. Fölsch UR, Nitsche R, Ludtke R, Hilgers RA, Creutzfeldt W, the German Study Group on Acute Biliary Pancreatitis (1997) Early ERCP and papillotomy compared with conservative treatment for acute biliary pancreatitis. N Engl J Med 336:237–242
8. Isla A, Griniatsos J, Rodway A (2003) Single-stage definitive laparoscopic management in mild acute biliary pancreatitis. J Laparoendosc Adv Surg Tech A 13:77–81
9. Isla AM, Griniatsos J, Wan A (2002) A technique for safe placement of a biliary endoprosthesis after laparoscopic choledochotomy. J Laparoendosc Adv Surg Tech A 12:207–211

10. Isla AM, Griniatsos J, Karvounis E, Arbuckle JD (2004) Advantages of laparoscopic stented choledochorrhaphy over T-tube placement. Br J Surg 91:862–866
11. Nathens AB, Curtis JR, Beale RJ, Cook DJ, Moreno RP, Romand JA, Skerrett SJ, Stapleton RD, Ware LB, Waldmann CS (2004) Management of the critically ill patient with severe acute pancreatitis. Crit Care Med 32:2524–2536
12. Neoptolemos JP, Carr-Locke DL, London NJ, Bailey IA, James D, Fossard DP (1988) Controlled trial of urgent endoscopic retrograde cholangiopancreatography and endoscopic sphincterotomy versus conservative treatment for acute pancreatitis due to gallstones. Lancet 2:979–983
13. Ranson JH, Rifkind KM, Turner JW (1976) Prognostic signs and nonoperative peritoneal lavage in acute pancreatitis. Surg Gynecol Obstet 143:209–219
14. Schachter P, Peleg T, Cohen O (2000) Interval laparoscopic cholecystectomy in the management of acute biliary pancreatitis. HPB Surg 11:319–323
15. Targarona EM, Perez Ayuso RM, Bordas JM, Ros E, Pros I, Martínez J, Terés J, Trías M (1996) Randomised trial of endoscopic sphincterotomy with gallbladder left in situ versus open surgery for common bileduct calculi in high-risk patients. Lancet 347:926–929
16. Uhl W, Müller CA, Krähenbühl L, Schmid SW, Scholzel S, Büchler MW (1999) Acute gallstone pancreatitis: timing of laparoscopic cholecystectomy in mild and severe disease. Surg Endosc 13:1070–1076
17. UK Working Party on Acute Pancreatitis (2005) UK guidelines for the management of acute pancreatitis. Gut 54(Suppl III):iii1–iii9
18. Wilson C, Heath DI, Imrie CW (1990) Prediction of outcome in acute pancreatitis: a comparative study of APACHE II, clinical assessment and multiple factor scoring systems. Br J Surg 77:1260–1264
19. Yousaf M, McCallion K, Diamond T (2003) Management of severe acute pancreatitis. Br J Surg 90:407–420

Acute Appendicitis – Update 2006

Stefan Sauerland

Definition, Epidemiology and Clinical Course

Acute appendicitis, defined as an acute inflammation of the vermiform appendix, is the most frequent condition leading to emergent abdominal surgery in children and young adults. The clinical course of the disease is characterized by loss of appetite, nausea, mild fever, and pain in the lower-right abdominal quadrant. Although signs and symptoms are typical in many patients, there are about 20% of atypical presentations.

Noninvasive Diagnostics

Laboratory investigations are considered to be a standard in any patient with abdominal pain. Other diagnostic tests may be used additionally depending on symptoms. Ultrasonography has been studied extensively, but as yet no definitive conclusions can be drawn, most probably owing to the large interobserver variability of the technique. Computed tomography is being used at increasing rates. The diagnostic accuracy in terms of sensitivity and specificity is about 95%, but there is no comparison yet with diagnostic laparoscopy.

Invasive Diagnostics

There are no new data available on the value of diagnostic laparoscopy; therefore, the consensus statement is correct in recommending diagnostic laparoscopy in patients with symptoms and diagnostic findings suggestive of acute appendicitis. Of course, the potential benefit of diagnostic laparoscopy is greater the larger the uncertainty of the diagnosis is.

Operative Versus Conservative Treatment

Acute appendicitis generally requires appendectomy, although some cases may resolve without therapy or under conservative treatment [14]. Controversy surrounds those situations, where the surgeon finds a normal-appearing appendix. If no other cause for the patient's problem can be detected, removal of the appendix is considered to be the safest option. However, if the patient's symptoms can be ascribed to an abdominal pathology other than appendicitis, it is better to leave a normal-appearing appendix, as stated in the EAES recommendations.

Choice of Surgical Approach and Procedure

The relative advantage of laparoscopic over conventional appendectomy has been under debate for more than a decade. According to the most recent Cochrane review [12], laparoscopic appendectomy offers certain advantages, although the difference from open appendectomy is not large. Accordingly, the EAES recommends laparoscopic over open appendectomy. This statement holds true, although some new data have been published recently. In 2006, paediatric trials comparing laparoscopic and open appendectomy were summarized in a meta-analysis [2], which mainly confirmed the findings of the Cochrane review. However, some advantages of laparoscopic appendectomy reached statistical significance, because nonrandomised trials were also included in the meta-analysis.

One randomized controlled trial (RCT) published on appendectomy in adults by Katkhouda et al. [8] only concluded that "choice of the procedure should be based on surgeon or patient preference", because postoperative pain was similar in both therapy groups of this blinded trial. Other results were in line with previous studies. A trial from Israel compared inflammatory markers after open and laparoscopic appendectomy [1], but no clinical data were collected (M. Almagor, personal communication). A third new trial, by Olmi et al. [11], failed to have a formal randomization, as the admission code numbers were used to assign patients to treatment groups. The results of this pseudo-randomized trial, however, clearly favoured laparoscopic appendectomy.

In summary, the relative advantages of laparoscopic over open appendectomy are small but well-proven; therefore, the EAES recommendation holds true, although in everyday practice surgical expertise, patient expectations and cost considerations also need to be considered [6]. Hospital costs of laparoscopic appendectomy are still slightly higher than those for open appendectomy [4, 5].

Technical Aspects of Surgery

Needlescopic instruments were used in a recent RCT from Hong Kong [10]. Pain levels were similar in needlescopic and conventional laparoscopic appendectomy, but operating time was longer. This is not in full agreement with the first RCT on this topic [7], but in general needlescopic appendectomy seems to offer few additional advantages compared with standard laparoscopic appendectomy.

Appendix stump closure is another important aspect of the laparoscopic technique. An inspection of more recent data suggests that wound infection is less likely to occur if the appendiceal base is secured with staples [3, 9, 13]. Again, cost considerations will have a strong impact on the acceptability of the ENDO GIA.

Peri- and Postoperative Care

No new data are available.

References

1. Almagor M, Mintz A, Sibirsky O, Durst A (2005) Preoperative and postoperative levels of interleukin-6 in patients with acute appendicitis: comparison between open and laparoscopic appendectomy. Surg Endosc 19:331–333
2. Aziz O, Athanasiou T, Tekkis PP, Purkayastha S, Haddow J, Malinovski V, Paraskeva P, Darzi A (2006) Laparoscopic versus open appendectomy in children: a meta-analysis. Ann Surg 243:17–27
3. Beese-Hoffmann E (2005) Röderschlinge versus Endo-GIA: eine prospektiv randomisierte Studie zur Technik der Stumpfversorgung bei der laparoskopischen Appendektomie. Thesis. Humboldt University, Berlin, pp 1–80
4. Bresciani C, Perez RO, Habr-Gama A, Jacob CE, Ozaki A, Batagello C, Proscurshim I, Gama-Rodrigues J (2005) Laparoscopic versus standard appendectomy outcomes and cost comparisons in the private sector. J Gastrointest Surg 9:1174–1181
5. Cothren CC, Moore EE, Johnson JL, Moore JB, Ciesla DJ, Burch JM (2005) Can we afford to do laparoscopic appendectomy in an academic hospital? Am J Surg 190:950–954
6. Guller U, Jain N, Curtis LH, Oertli D, Heberer M, Pietrobon R (2004) Insurance status and race represent independent predictors of undergoing laparoscopic surgery for appendicitis: secondary data analysis of 145,546 patients. J Am Coll Surg 199:567–577
7. Huang MT, Wei PL, Wu CC, Lai IR, Chen RJ, Lee WJ (2001) Needlescopic, laparoscopic, and open appendectomy: a comparative study. Surg Laparosc Endosc Percutan Tech 11:306–312
8. Katkhouda N, Mason RJ, Towfigh S, Gevorgyan A, Essani R (2005) Laparoscopic versus open appendectomy: a prospective randomized double-blind study. Ann Surg 242:439–450
9. Kouwenhoven EA, Repelaer van Driel OJ, van Erp WF (2005) Fear for the intraabdominal abscess after laparoscopic appendectomy: not realistic. Surg Endosc 19:923–926
10. Lau DHW, Yau KKK, Chung CC, Leung FCS, Tai YP, Li MKW (2005) Comparison of needlescopic appendectomy versus conventional laparoscopic appendectomy: a randomized controlled trial. Surg Laparosc Endosc Percutan Tech 15:75–79
11. Olmi S, Magnone S, Bertolini A, Croce E (2005) Laparoscopic versus open appendectomy in acute appendicitis: a randomized prospective study. Surg Endosc 19:1193–1195
12. Sauerland S, Lefering R, Neugebauer E (2004) Laparoscopic versus open surgery for suspected appendicitis [Cochrane review]. In: The Cochrane Collaboration (ed) The Cochrane database of systematic reviews, vol IV/2004 CD-ROM. Update Software, Oxford
13. Strickland AK, Martindale RG (2005) The increased incidence of intraabdominal infections in laparoscopic procedures: potential causes, postoperative management, and prospective innovations. Surg Endosc 19:874–881
14. Styrud J, Eriksson S, Nilsson I, Ahlberg G, Haapaniemi S, Neovius G, Rex L, Badume I, Granström L (2006) Appendectomy versus antibiotic treatment in acute appendicitis. A prospective multicenter randomized controlled trial. World J Surg 30:1033–1037

Acute Nonspecific Abdominal Pain – Update 2006

Ferdinando Agresta

Definition and Epidemiology

Nonspecific acute abdominal pain (NSAP) is a significant problem in general surgery and accounts for up to an estimated 40% of all emergency surgical admissions [14]. It is defined as a condition of acute abdominal pain of less than 7 days' duration in which, after examination and (radiological and laboratory) investigations, the diagnosis still remains uncertain [6, 7, 19]. The diagnosis is important in order to avoid an unnecessary laparotomy (as high as 29%) and/or in order to plan the right abdominal incision [1, 6, 7, 17, 19]. With the traditional "wait-and-see management" the mean hospital stay for patients admitted with a NSAP ranges between 4 and 6 days, which it is costly owing to the repeated clinical, radiological and laboratory investigations [1, 10, 12, 14].

Diagnosis

The accuracy of conventional radiography in NSAP, although considered an essential part of the patient's workup, reaches only 50%, whereas that of abdominal ultrasound is 60–89%. The CT scan is more accurate (84–98%) but is expensive and is not always possible to perform in all hospital situations, 24 h a day [2, 10, 13, 14, 18, 19]. A delay in surgical intervention while further investigations are performed may increase morbidity and prolong hospital stay (average delay period of 6.12 days), especially if it is taken into account that patients admitted with NSAP might be old, obese, critically ill and with comorbidity situations (such as diabetic and immunosuppressive therapy) [6, 10, 11].

Operative Versus Conservative Treatment

When patients are admitted to hospital with acute abdominal pain, clinicians, irrespective of a specific diagnosis, select three diagnostic classes: operation definitely required; operation definitely not required, need for operation uncertain [12, 17].

Choice of Surgical Approach and Procedure

If a surgical exploration is required, and if there are no absolute contraindications to the approach, a laparoscopic exploration should be preferred [1, 4, 7]. This is due not only to its diagnostic value/accuracy (89–100%) but also to the potential—which is mainly related to the human factor (surgeons' skills)—for therapeutic manipulation during the same setting (up to 88.2%) (or to plan the right abdominal approach) [1, 6–8, 10, 14, 19, 21]. It is reported in the literature that with an open approach such as in suspected appendicitis, the accurate on-table diagnosis is missed in up to 14.3% of cases and that the sensitivity for diagnosing normal appendices is low at 51.3%, thus suggesting that almost half of normal appendicitis cases might be misdiagnosed as pathological, with the risk of no further exploration for other pathologies [17, 20, 22]. As already described, laparoscopic surgery is advantageous for many abdominal diseases, which may also turn out to be the underlying cause of the hospital admission. Thus, especially in lower abdominal and pelvic pain among female patients during their reproductive years, a laparoscopic approach might lead to correction of an erroneous preoperative diagnosis in up to 40% of cases and/or exclude other pathologies (which may be present in approximately 20% of cases) [3, 6, 16, 22].

To undertake emergency laparoscopic operations, the surgeon must be experienced [1, 6]. A possible small operating theatre together with the wide variety of therapeutic findings require a well-trained and experienced surgeon as well as a well-trained surgical team. Mastery of two-handed dissection is suggested, as laparoscopic suturing technique has to be considered as an absolute requirement. Good judgment is needed for a timely decision to convert the procedure (and plan a "target" incision) in order not to jeopardize and prolong the attempts to complete the operation laparoscopically [1]. The morbidity (0.6–24%) and mortality (less than 1%) of a laparoscopic approach in an emergency situation are comparable if not lower than those reported with laparotomy, and converted cases (up to 16%) have a similar outcome compared with primarily open cases [1, 6, 8, 9].

As stated by the controlled trials in which an early laparoscopy is compared with observation for NSAP, diagnostic laparoscopy benefits patients by avoiding unnecessary surgery, avoiding a possibly deleterious delay in diagnosis and treatment, shortening the operative and hospitalized period and reducing the readmission rate and helps in containing health-care costs [5, 7, 9, 15] (EL 1b). On the basis of these data, it seems justified to lower the threshold for surgical exploration when using laparoscopy rather than laparotomy [1, 4]. However, it has to be kept in mind that laparoscopy provides only an alternative not a substitute for traditional diagnostic and clinical procedures and will never lessen the importance of a needed conventional laparotomy.

References

1. Agresta F, Michelet I, Colucci G, Bedin N (2000) Emergency laparoscopy. Surg Endosc 14:484–487
2. Ahn HS, Mayo-Smith WW, Murphy BL, Reinert SE, Cronan JJ (2002) Acute nontraumatic abdominal pain in adult patients: abdominal radiography compared with CT evaluation. Radiology 225:159–164
3. Aulestia SN, Cantele H, Leyba JL, Navarrete M, Llopla SN (2003) Laparoscopic diagnosis and treatment in gynecologic emergencies. JSLS 7(3):239–242
4. Branicki FJ (2002) Abdominal emergencies: diagnostic and therapeutic laparoscopy. Surg Infect 3(3):269–282
5. Champault G, Rizk N, Lauroy J, Olivares P, Belhassen A, Boutelier P (1993). Douleurs ilaques droites de la femme. Approche diagnostique conventionelle versus laparoscopie première. Etude controlée (64 cas). Ann Chir 47:316–319
6. Cuesta MA, Eijsbouts QAJ, Gordijn RV, Borgstein PF, de Jong D (1998) Diagnostic laparoscopy in patients with an acute abdomen of uncertain etiology. Surg Endosc 12 915–917
7. Decadt B, Sussman L, Lewis MPN, Secker A, Cohen L, Rogers C, Patel A, Rhodes M (1999) Randomized clinical trial of early laparoscopy in the management of acute nonspecific abdominal pain. Br J Surg 86(11):1383–1386
8. Fahel E, Amaral PC, Filho EM, Ettinger JE, Souza EL, Fortes MF, Alcantara RS, Regis AB, Neto MP, Sousa MM, Fogagnoli WG, Cunha AG, Castro MM, Santana PA (1999) Non-traumatic acute abdomen: videolaparoscopic approach. JSLS 3(3):187–192
9. Gaitan H, Angel E, Sanchez J, Gomez I, Sanchez L, Aguledo C (2002). Laparoscopic diagnosis of acute lower abdominal pain in women of reproductive age. Int J Gynaecol Obstet 76(2):149–158
10. Golash V, Willson PD (2005) Early laparoscopy as a routine procedure in the management of acute abdominal pain. Surg Endosc 19:882–885
11. Hackert T, Kienle P, Weitz J, Werner J, Szabo G, Hagl S, Buchler MW, Schimdt J (2003) Accuracy of diagnostic laparoscopy of early diagnosis of abdominal complications after cardiac surgery. Surg Endosc 17:1671–1674
12. Kirshtein B, Roy-Shapira A, Lantsberg L, Mandel S, Avinoach E, Mizrahi S (2003) The use of laparoscopy in abdominal emergencies. Surg Endosc 17:1118–1124
13. MacKersie AB, Lane MJ, Gerhardt RT, Claypool HA, Keenan S, Katz DS, Tucher JE (2005) Nontraumatic acute abdominal pain: unenhanced helical CT compared with three-view acute abdominal series. Radiology 237(1):114–122
14. Majeski W (2000) Diagnostic laparoscopy for the acute abdomen and trauma. Surg Endosc 14:930–937
15. Morino M, Castagna E, Roisso E, Mao P (2004) Non-specific acute abdominal pain: a randomized controlled trial comparing early laparoscopy vs Observation [abstract]. Surg Endosc 18(Suppl):S2
16. Ou CS, Rowbotham R (2000) Laparoscopic diagnosis and treatment on non-traumatic acute abdominal pain in woman. J Laparoendosc Adv Surg Tech 10(1):41–45
17. Paterson-Brown S, Eckersley JR, Sim AJ, Dudley HA (1986) Laparoscopy as an adjunct to decision making in the "acute abdomen". Br J Surg 73(12):1022–1024
18. Salem TA, Molly RG, O'Dwyer PJ (2005) Prospective study on the role of the CT scan in patients with an acute abdomen. Colorectal Dis 7(5):460–466
19. Salky BA, Edye MB (1998) The role of laparoscopy in the diagnosis and treatment of abdominal pain syndromes. Surg Endosc 12:911–914
20. Shum CF, Lim JF, Soo KC, Wong WK (2005) On-table diagnostic accuracy and the clinical significance of routine exploration in open appendectomies. Asian J Surg 28(4):257–261
21. Udwadia TE (2004) Diagnostic laparoscopy. Surg Endosc 18:6–10
22. Van Dalem R, Bagshaw PF, Dobbs BR, Robertson GM, Lynch AC, Frizelle FA (2003) The utility of laparoscopy in the diagnosis of acute appendicitis in women of reproductive age. Surg Endosc 17:1311–1313

Adhesions and Small Bowel Obstructions – Update 2006

Benoit Navez

Introduction

Acute small bowel obstruction (ASBO) remains a significant surgical problem and is commonly caused by postoperative adhesions.

Definition

Adhesions consist of obstructive bands and/or matted adhesions. The mechanism of ASBO can be either strangulation or volvulus of one or several bowel loops.

Epidemiology and Clinical Course

Colorectal surgery (odds 2.7) and vertical incisions (odds 2.5) more frequently produce intestinal obstruction (reported rate of ASBO of 3.6% at 3 years' time interval) and predispose to multiple matted adhesions than an obstructive band [6, 8].

In a retrospective study, it seems that ASBO requiring hospitalization with conservative management occurs less frequently after laparoscopic bowel resection than after open surgery; however, the need for surgical release of ASBO is similar [2].

The risk of ASBO recurrence increases with the number of ASBO episodes. Surgical treatment decreases the risk of future admissions for ASBO but not the risk of new surgically treated ASBO [4].

Diagnostics

Computed tomography (CT) has proven useful in the diagnosis of mechanical ASBO. Its specificity is superior to that of plain abdominal film. Although CT can seldom identify the obstructive adhesion, it has the advantage of eliminating another cause of obstruction (e.g. tumour) [3]. The highly specific CT criteria used for differentiating simple from strangulated ASBO include the poor or no enhancement of the bowel wall, a serrated beak, a large amount of ascites, diffuse mesenteric changes and an abnormal mesenteric vascular course. However, to improve the diagnostic accuracy of CT and to avoid unnecessary surgical exploration, CT findings must be correlated with clinical and biochemical criteria [5].

Operative Versus Conserative Treatment

Use of an oral water-soluble contrast medium is a useful predictive test for non-operative resolution of adhesive ASBO. The appearance of contrast medium in the caecum on an abdominal radiograph within 24 h of its administration predicts the resolution of an obstruction with a sensitivity and specificity of 96%. However Gastrografin is only a predictive test and does not cause resolution of ASBO [1]. In the absence of clinical and CT signs of acute intestinal ischemia requiring an urgent operation, it seems to be safe to attempt a non-operative management of ASBO. The use of a short versus a long tube for gastrointestinal decompression remains under debate as well as the duration of conservative treatment (from 1 day to several days). When non-operative treatment is unsuccessful, emergency surgery is required.

Choice of Surgical Approach and Procedure

There are no prospective randomized trials comparing open and laparoscopic adhesiolysis for ASBO. The benefits of laparoscopic approach in ASBO that have been reported in case series and in one retrospective matched-pair analysis are the same as in laparoscopy for other conditions: quicker return of intestinal function, lower morbidity, shorter hospital stay [9]. However, laparoscopic adhesiolysis in an emergency has not gained wide acceptance because of the limited visualization of the abdominal cavity secondary to the distended bowel and because of the risk of iatrogenic intestinal injury. The high conversion rate is also an issue, ranging from 15 to 43%. The best cases for laparoscopic approach are patients with moderate abdominal distension (proximal obstruction), a bowel diameter not exceeding 4 cm, a few adhesions and a limited number of previous scars [7].

Technical Aspects of Surgery

In order to limit the risk of injury to the underlying adherent bowel, open Hasson technique is required to enter the abdominal cavity. Instrumental manipulation of fragile dilated bowel loops should be avoided. It is recommended to run the flat small bowel with atraumatic graspers from the ileocaecal valve until the site of obstruction is found. Only pathologic adhesions should be cut. In case of any doubt about the viability of the bowel, a minilaparotomy can be performed to check the intestinal blood supply and if necessary bowel resection [7].

Peri- and Postoperative Care

No new data are available.

References

1. Abbas S, Bisset IP, Parry BR (2005) Oral water soluble contrast for the management of adhesive small bowel obstruction. Cochrane Database Syst Rev 25(1):CD004651
2. Duepree HJ, Senagore AJ, Delaney CP, Fazio VW (2003) Does means of access affect the incidence of small bowel obstruction and ventral hernia after bowel resection? Laparoscopy versus laparotomy. J Am Coll Surg 197(2):177–181
3. Duron JJ (2003) Pathologie occlusive postopératoire. Occlusions mécaniques postopératoires du grêle par brides ou adhérences. J Chir 140:325–334
4. Fevang BS, Fevang J, Lie SA, Soreide O, Svanes K, Viste A (2004) Long-term prognosis after operation for adhesive small bowel obstruction. Ann Surg 240:193–201
5. Kim JH, Ha HK, Kim JK, Eun HW, Park KB, Kim BS, Kim TK, Kim JC, Auh YH (2004) Usefulness of known computed tomography and clinical criteria for diagnosing strangulation in small bowel obstruction: analysis of true and false interpretation groups in computed tomography. World J Surg 28:63–68
6. Miller G, Boman J, Shrier I, Gordon PH (2000) Natural history of patients with adhesive small bowel obstruction. Br J Surg 87:1240–1247
7. Nagle A, Ujiki M, Denham W, Murayama K (2004) Laparoscopic adhesiolysis for small bowel obstruction. Am J Surg 187:464–470
8. Ryan MD, Wattchow D, Walker M, Hakendorf P (2004) Adhesional small bowel obstruction after colorectal surgery. ANZ J Surg 74(11):1010–1012
9. Wullstein C, Gross E (2003) Laparoscopic compared with conventional treatment of acute adhesive small bowel obstruction. Br J Surg 90:1147–1151

Abdominal Trauma – Update 2006

Abe Fingerhut, Selman Uranues

To the best of our knowledge, there have been no new randomized controlled trials concerning laparoscopy in the trauma setting since the consensus report published by Sauerland et al. [1] in 2005.

One recent prospective evaluation study from Japan [2] involving 399 hemodynamically stable patients suspected of having blunt bowel injury (BBI) showed that a physical examination and contrast CT scanning at admission and once again approximately 12 h (range, 6–24 h) after admission was safe and could prevent nontherapeutic laparotomy and delayed diagnosis in patients with suspected BBI.

A new role for laparoscopic surgery was heralded when in a two-center study of post-non-operative management of severe (grades 3–5) hepatic injuries, laparoscopy was used to diagnose and treat biliary complications [3].

Laparoscopy may also have a potential role in setting up direct intraabdominal pressure measurement using a continuous indwelling compartment pressure monitor [4], and therefore may facilitate the early detection of the abdominal compartment syndrome. Caution must be exercised, however, not to use high insufflation pressures for the exploration in order not to unduly increase the abdominal compartment syndrome.

References

1. Sauerland S, Agresta F, Bergamaschi R, Borzellino G, Budzynski A, Champault G, Fingerhut A, Isla A, Johansson M, Lundorff P, Navez B, Saad S, Neugebauer EA (2005) Laparoscopy for abdominal emergencies. Evidence-based guidelines of the European Association for Endoscopic Surgery. Surg Endosc 20:14–29
2. Kitano M, Sasaki J, Nagashima A, Doi M, Hayashi S, Egawa T, Yoshii H (2005) Computed tomographic scanning and selective laparoscopy in the diagnosis of blunt bowel injury: a prospective study. J Trauma 58:696–703
3. Kozar RA, Moore JB, Niles SE, Holcomb JB, Moore EE, Cothren CC, Hartwell E, Moore FA (2005) Complications of nonoperative management of high-grade blunt hepatic injuries. J Trauma 59:1066–1071
4. Brooks AJ, Simpson A, Delbridge M, Beckingham IJ, Girling KJ (2005) Validation of direct intraabdominal pressure measurement using a continuous indwelling compartment pressure monitor. J Trauma 58:830–832

Laparoscopic Surgery: Strategies for Future Outcome Studies

Henrik Kehlet

The concept of minimally invasive surgery, including laparoscopic procedures, represents a major breakthrough as one of the important components of multimodal rehabilitation (fast-track surgery) to improve postoperative outcome. It is well documented that minimally invasive surgery reduces wound size, surgical stress responses and organ dysfunctions, mostly as a result of decreased pain and inflammatory responses. These effects have during the last 10 years translated into major improvements in clinical outcome in certain operations where the alternative was a large incision i.e. surgery for gastro-oesophageal reflux, hiatal hernias, adrenalectomy, bariatric surgery, splenectomy, nephrectomy, etc., most of which can be performed as day cases or with the need of 1–2 days' hospitalisation. So what is the problem? Do we need more scientific, randomised studies before we have a more widespread implementation of laparoscopy? Do we need more research and improvement? The answer is complex and has not been solved, except in the aforementioned procedures where there is no need for randomised studies to show improvements in *early* postoperative outcome compared with conventional open surgery. However, in many other, more common procedures, the role of laparoscopy is still debatable despite initial positive results reported in several randomised trial and meta-analyses in hernia surgery, cholecystectomy, colonic surgery, hysterectomy, etc. On the positive side, these studies have repeatedly demonstrated some improvements with laparoscopy because of less pain, need for hospitalisation, and convalescence. On the other hand, it is also well established that a significant learning curve is required for optimal results of laparoscopy, amounting to about 60 patients in colonic procedures and up to 100–200 patients with groin hernia repair. In addition, there may be increased direct costs from laparoscopy, which to some extent have been outweighed by the demonstrated postoperative benefits.

However, the main reason for a required new debate on the advantages of laparoscopy and the future strategies for further improvement is the concomitant developments within multimodal perioperative rehabilitation (i.e. fast-track surgery) [10, 12]. This concept, which ideally includes minimally invasive surgery (laparoscopy), combines improved preoperative patient information with optimal, dynamic pain relief, reduction of surgical stress responses, revision of perioperative care principles adjusted to evidence (tubes, drains, restrictions, etc.) and revision of nurse care principles to utilise the benefits of stress reduction and pain relief into early oral nutrition and mobilisation [2, 10]. The concept has repeatedly been demonstrated to lead to major improvements in recovery of organ functions, reduction of medical morbidity, need for hospitalisation, and convalescence in a variety of procedures [8, 10]. In many areas, the results have been more impressive by this approach compared with the effects reported by laparoscopy and where revision of perioperative care principles were not reported or instituted. Thus, several fast-track colonic resection series have documented hospital stays between 2 and 4 days where randomised studies comparing a laparoscopic vs. an open approach have shown hospital stays of 5–7 and 7–9 days, respectively [8, 11].

One of the outcome parameters often quoted in randomised studies comparing open vs. laparoscopic surgery is postoperative convalescence. Although convalescence is an important outcome parameter, unfortunately most studies have insufficient or no information on postdischarge pain intensity, analgesic treatment or advice given for duration of convalescence. Thus, it is well established that the duration of convalescence is highly dependent on traditions and recommendations and several studies have documented a shorter duration of convalescence, for example after cholecystectomy or inguinal herniorrhaphy, when short recommendations have been given [5] compared with longer convalescence times reported in randomised studies. Most existing data from previous randomised studies are therefore difficult to interpret since the reported duration of convalescence may also depend on bias induced by surgeons or patients expecting shorter convalescence after a laparoscopic approach, but where the patients operated on with an open technique were often treated with traditional, unadjusted convalescence recommendations [5].

A logical approach to document the exact role of minimally invasive surgery is therefore a combined approach where laparoscopy is integrated with the principles of fast-track surgery [5, 10], thereby minimising the effects of traditional and restrictive care principles on functional recovery. Unfortunately, only two such randomised studies have been performed, where the surgical approach was blinded by an opaque abdominal dressing, thereby eliminating the bias from previous studies where surgeon and patient expectances may have influenced the outcome results. One study in elderly high-risk colonic resection patients showed no differences in a detailed assessment of functional recovery, and with a median hospital stay of 2 days in both groups [1], significantly shorter than reported in previous unblinded, randomised studies [11]. The other study in appendectomy [4] did not show relevant clinical differences in outcome. A third randomised study [14] with blinding of the surgical approach in cholecystectomy did not include the principles of multimodal rehabilitation and therefore showed no differences in outcome between a laparoscopic vs. an open technique, since hospital stay was 3 days in both groups and with 3–4 weeks' convalescence reflecting traditions of care, rather than the influence of the surgical approach per se [5].

So, what are the future strategies for further development and improvement of the effects of laparoscopy on outcome. First of all, laparoscopy should be combined with evidence-based principles of perioperative care (i.e. fast-track surgery) [2, 10, 11, 13]. Secondly, perioperative pain management should be further developed to be opioid-free, multimodal analgesia [6] in order to avoid opioid-related side effects and thereby improve functional recovery. In addition, such pain therapy should be procedure-specific, adjusted to available evidence [7]. Thirdly, future studies should combine laparoscopy and the principles of fast-track surgery with additional pharmacological modification of stress responses [9]. Thus, several techniques are available (i.e. glucocorticoids, beta-blockers, anabolic steroids, insulin, statins, etc.), all of which may further reduce hormonal as well as inflammatory responses, thereby aiming at a "stress and pain free" patient [9], with subsequent improvement in recovery and reduction in morbidity, hospital stay, and convalescence. Finally, evidence-based principles of perioperative fluid management should be integrated in such strategies [3], with a focus on early, goal-directed haemodynamic optimisation and balancing volume administration to avoid fluid excess and hypovolaemia [3].

In future outcome studies it is crucial to include a detailed description/revision of perioperative patient information (convalescence recommendations, etc.), techniques of perioperative analgesia, resource utilisation (nurse workload, direct and indirect costs, including additional postdischarge costs on readmission, use of home nurses, visits to general practitioners, etc.). Also potential benefits of laparoscopy on late sequelae such as bowel obstruction due to adhesions, chronic pain and ventral hernias must be assessed [11].

In summary, the future is open for further fascinating improvements in surgical outcome and where laparoscopy is a rational, but not the only component since the pathogenesis of perioperative morbidity includes multifactorial components [10]. Hopefully, minimally invasive surgeons will adopt the principles of multimodal rehabilitation in their daily clinical practice as well as in future research.

References

1. Basse L, Jacobsen DH, Bardram L et al (2005) Functional recovery after open vs laparoscopic colonic surgery. A randomised blinded study. Ann Surg 241:416–423
2. Fearon K, Ljungqvist O, Meyenfeldt MV et al (2005) Enhanced recovery after surgery: a consensus review of clinical care for patients undergoing colonic resection. Clin Nutr 24:466–477
3. Holte K, Kehlet H (2006) Fluid therapy and surgical outcome in elective surgery – a need for reassessment in fast-track surgery. A systematic review. J Am Coll Surg (in press)
4. Katkhouda N, Mason RJ, Towfigh S et al (2005) Laparoscopic versus open appendectomy. A prospective randomised double-blind study. Ann Surg 242:439–450
5. Kehlet H (2002) Clinical trials and laparoscopic surgery. The second round will require a change of tactics. Surg Laparosc Endosc Percutan Tech 12:137–138
6. Kehlet H (2005) Postoperative opioid-sparing to improve outcome – what are the issues? Anesthesiology 102:1083–1085
7. Kehlet H (2005) Procedure specific postoperative pain management. Anesthesiol Clin N Am 23:203–210
8. Kehlet H (2005) Fast-track colonic surgery – status and perspectives. Recent Results Cancer Res 165:8–13
9. Kehlet H (2006) Surgical stress and outcome – from here to where? Reg Anesth Pain Med 31:47–52
10. Kehlet H, Dahl JB (2003) Anaesthesia, surgery and challenges in postoperative recovery. Lancet 362:1921–1928
11. Kehlet H, Kennedy R (2006) Laparoscopic colonic surgery–mission accomplished or work in progress? Colorectal Dis (in press)
12. Kehlet H, Wilmore DW (2005) Fast-track surgery. Br J Surg 92:3–4
13. Kehlet H, Büchler MW, Beart RW et al (2006) Care after colonic surgery – is it evidence-based? Results from an multinational survey in Europe and the USA. J Am Coll Surg 202:45–54
14. McMahon AJ, Russell IT, Baxter JN et al (1994) Laparoscopic vs mini laparotomy cholecystectomy: a randomised trial. Lancet 343:135–138

Subject Index

D

H

I

Printing: Krips bv, Meppel
Binding: Stürtz, Würzburg